Special P.
RecoveryMind Training

"In his book, *RecoveryMind Training*, Dr. Paul Earley has created an immensely powerful, integrative, holistic, and coherent approach to addiction treatment and ongoing recovery. This creative and comprehensive book has been much needed in our field and will be of great benefit to addicted patients and the staff who treat them."

Daniel H. Angres, MD
Medical Director, Positive Sobriety Institute
Chief Medical Officer, Addiction Services, RiverMend Health
Adjunct Associate Professor of Psychiatry
Northwestern Feinberg School of Medicine

"In the early twenty-first century's opioid epidemic, this new book synthesizes a modern, integrated solution. With clear, articulate prose, the doctor's doctor, Paul Earley, MD, teaches healthcare professionals a refined, comprehensive approach, eschewing the formulaic and ideological. He convincingly posits addiction as an alien drive system, not the individual's essence, thereby helping to ameliorate shame and facilitate a new, self-protective identity narrative. With concrete assignments and skills practice, Earley helps providers help patients repair their AddictBrain, and replenish the human organism, including its soul, with self-acceptance, self-efficacy, love, and spiritual contentment—all through RecoveryMind Training."

David R. Gastfriend, MD, DFASAM
Scientific Advisor, Treatment Research Institute
Cofounder, DynamiCare Health

"RecoveryMind Training (RMT) is based upon the principles of neuroscience and neurology, but implements practical techniques to modify and even change brain behavior pathways. This evidence-based textbook can also be used as a clinical manual helping clinicians understand the complexities of addiction treatment and recovery.

"Paul has done an outstanding job in refining RMT, making it more treatment-friendly and focused on long-term outcomes. When so many addiction specialists concentrate on detoxification and short-term results, Dr. Earley reminds everyone that treatment and recovery both require hard work and commitment to remedy AddictBrain and the disease of addiction."

Mark S. Gold, MD, DFASAM, DLFAPA
Chairman, Scientific Advisory Boards, RiverMend Health
Adjunct Professor, Washington University School
of Medicine, Department of Psychiatry

"Addictive disease has long been misunderstood and stigmatized. With recent findings demonstrating significant value from pharmacotherapy in some cases, other forms of therapy with great efficacy have been ignored by many. Dr. Earley brings decades of experience with thousands of patients suffering from addictive disease to his text, weaving a science-based underpinning into the need for a complete biopsychosocial and spiritual model of treatment. The resulting book will serve patients and clinicians equally well."

Stuart Gitlow, MD, MPH, MBA, DFAPA, DFASAM
Executive Director, Annenberg Physician Training Program in
Addictive Disease
Associate Professor, University of Florida
Immediate Past President, American Society of Addiction Medicine

"With his presentation of *RecoveryMind Training*, Paul Earley draws on his vast knowledge and experience with addiction and the neurosciences to present a tour de force in addiction treatment. This book manages to accomplish the delicate task of being elegant, simple, comprehensive, and practical without being formulaic or mechanical. In this book, he provides the reader with a straightforward explanation, free of jargon, on how addiction changes the brain neurobiologically and how his model of treatment, RecoveryMind Training, reverses this process. A must-read for anyone who works with this population."

Philip J. Flores, PhD, ABPP, CGP, FAGPA
Author of *Addiction as an Attachment Disorder*

"RecoveryMind Training is an impressive undertaking. Dr. Earley has beautifully described what happens in the brain and in the mind during the downhill spiral of addiction and the uplifting journey of recovery. This book will jar many readers' mental models and, hopefully, it will guide professional healers to adopt new approaches and establish more realistic goals for treatment so that the investments in time, energy, and money that are devoted to the addiction treatment process can bear the most fruit for individuals, for their families, for their employers, and for their communities."

Michael M. Miller, MD
Medical Director, Herrington Recovery Center
Past President, American Society of Addiction Medicine
Director, American Board of Addiction Medicine
and the Addiction Medicine Foundation

RecoveryMind Training

RecoveryMind Training

A Neuroscientific Approach to Treating Addiction

Paul H. Earley

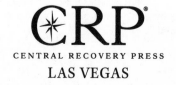

CENTRAL RECOVERY PRESS

LAS VEGAS

Central Recovery Press (CRP) is committed to publishing exceptional materials addressing addiction treatment, recovery, and behavioral healthcare topics.

For more information, visit www.centralrecoverypress.com.

© 2017 by Earley Consultancy, LLC
All rights reserved. Published 2017. Printed in the United States of America.

No part of this publication may be reproduced, stored in a retrieval system, or transmitted in any form or by any means, electronic, mechanical, photocopying, recording, or otherwise, without the written permission of the publisher.

Publisher: Central Recovery Press
　　　　　3321 N. Buffalo Drive
　　　　　Las Vegas, NV 89129

22 21 20 19 18 17　　1 2 3 4 5

Library of Congress Cataloging-in-Publication Data
Names: Earley, Paul H.
Title:Recoverymindtraining:aneuroscientificapproachtotreatingaddiction/PaulH.Earley.
Description: Las Vegas: Central Recovery Press, 2017.
Identifiers: LCCN 2016032444 (print) | LCCN 2016037904 (ebook) | ISBN 9781942094326 (paperback) | ISBN 9781942094333
Subjects: LCSH: Substance abuse--Treatment. | Addicts--Rehabilitation. | Psychology. | Neurosciences. | BISAC: SELF-HELP / Substance Abuse & Addictions / General. |
MEDICAL / Neuroscience. | PSYCHOLOGY / Psychopathology / Addiction.
Classification: LCC RC563 .E27 2017 (print) | LCC RC563 (ebook) | DDC 362.29--dc23
LC record available at https://lccn.loc.gov/2016032444

Photo of Paul Earley by Eric Bern of Eric Bern Studio. Used with permission.

Every attempt has been made to contact copyright holders. If copyright holders have not been properly acknowledged please contact us. Central Recovery Press will be happy to rectify the omission in future printings of this book.

THE ACCIDENTAL MIND: HOW BRAIN EVOLUTION HAS GIVEN US LOVE, MEMORY, DREAMS, AND GOD by David J. Linden, Cambridge, Mass.: The Belknap Press of Harvard University Press, Copyright © 2007 by the President and Fellows of Harvard College.

Publisher's Note: This book is not an alternative to medical advice from your doctor or other professional healthcare provider. CRP books represent the experiences and opinions of their authors only. Every effort has been made to ensure that events, institutions, and statistics presented in our books as facts are accurate and up-to-date. To protect their privacy, the names of some of the people, places, and institutions in this book may have been changed.

Cover design by David Hardy
Interior design by Deb Tremper, Six Penny Graphics

This book is dedicated to my wife, Wanda C. Faurie, PhD. Although our partnership supports me in innumerable ways, her unflappable belief in me has repeatedly pulled me out of the downward spiral of writer's self-doubt. Her abiding encouragement sustained me during many long years battling this manuscript. Without her discriminating ear and veracious feedback, this book would have never been written.

I want to thank the hundreds of patients who taught me how to walk alongside as each found their own path out of the quagmire of addiction.

TABLE OF CONTENTS

Foreword

Addiction is a devastating brain disease affecting over twenty-three million individuals, including their loved ones, in the US alone. Addiction does not discriminate and often negatively affects a person physically, mentally, emotionally, and spiritually. As Dr. Paul Earley eloquently states in the Introduction of this book: "Addiction is the most complex illness of humankind. It can impact nearly every organ of the body. Dangerous by itself, it exacerbates other physical and mental disorders, generating a maelstrom of confusing symptoms and conditions." Add to that the current epidemic of overdoses from opioid painkillers, legalized marijuana, and persistently high rates of alcohol and stimulant use disorders, and you have a recipe for a disastrous meltdown challenging our entire public health system. The need for effective and compassionate addiction treatment has never been greater.

Dr. Earley is a superb clinician and in *RecoveryMind Training* (RMT) presents a comprehensive treatment model based upon the concept that addiction recovery is a learned skill. To be successful, the learning involved in recovery has to overcome the complex and hardwired entrainment produced by the use of highly reinforcing drugs—including alcohol. RMT describes the dynamics of active addiction with regard to its effects on the brain—motivations, drives, memories, and cognitive distortions—with the term "AddictBrain." Recovery is facilitated through the learning of a structured set of skills that promote changes in a person's thoughts, beliefs, and actions, and bring about "RecoveryMind."

RecoveryMind Training fits well with both the American Society of Addiction Medicine's (ASAM) assessment dimensions and levels of care structures. It reviews and expands on the ASAM definition of addiction, clarifying the parts of the brain involved and the interplay with neurophysiology and behavior. Dr. Earley takes a head-on approach to those who would explain addiction as a weakness or moral failing. The guilt and shame associated with these misconceptions are some of the most common obstacles for people new to recovery; however, with information and clinical suggestions and exercises, Dr. Earley guides us toward a clear and useful approach to this complicated disease. I am particularly pleased that rather than abandoning tried-and-true evidence-based methods, this book enhances and builds on what we already know to be effective. RMT incorporates and unifies multiple treatment modalities into a cohesive patient-centric system. Moreover, it complements twelve-step recovery and in fact, *RecoveryMind Training* (the book) points out the efficacy of twelve-step programs and actively encourages twelve-step program participation.

The book is divided into two sections. Section One focuses on active addiction and the AddictBrain concept and Section Two details the recovery process and the RecoveryMind Training model. Dr. Earley's approach uses a combination of techniques, including disease containment, twelve-step work, cognitive-behavioral therapy, mindfulness training, emotional regulation, eliminating negative self-talk, healthy attachment to others, a personal spiritual process, and relapse prevention therapy. RMT articulates complex concepts in detailed yet user-friendly language.

Dr. Earley understands the distinctions between treatment and recovery, and views RecoveryMind Training as an effective means to clarify the focus of treatment for patients and help jumpstart the change processes that facilitate recovery. In RMT, Dr. Earley supports the view that addiction is one disease with many manifestations, and it is a disorder that extends well beyond the use of substances and/or addictive behaviors. RMT is well researched, instructive, and seeks to clarify (and unify) some of the confusion relating to addiction treatment and the terms used within the treatment industry.

As the Chief Medical Officer of an inpatient program and with over thirty-five years of experience treating addiction and chronic pain, I found this book to be extremely helpful in approaching treatment for people with addiction. RMT organizes and outlines the neuroscience and neurology of the human brain in a compelling and digestible way. When I work with patients today, I have the structure and support of a sophisticated treatment team to educate patients and their families. I look forward to utilizing Dr. Earley's RMT to solidify gains and enhance treatment with better results and outcomes.

Mel Pohl, MD, DFASAM
Chief Medical Officer
Las Vegas Recovery Center

Introduction

Addiction is a serious illness. Dangerous by itself, it exacerbates other physical and mental disorders, generating a maelstrom of confusing symptoms and conditions. Addiction is baffling and subversive by nature. Many of its victims never get a clear view of the monster that steals their health, self-esteem, and joy. Some die a slow painful death because they cannot extricate themselves from its clutches.

Addiction is the most complex illness of humankind. It can impact nearly every organ of the body. It creates wholesale and nearly unfathomable changes to the most intricately organized structure in the known universe—the human mind—including, but not limited to, altering the brain's primitive drives, our perception of reality, and how "the self" is conceptualized. It actively thwarts attempts to intervene, often to the point of death. Addiction has resulted in a spate of laws throughout our society; it creates its own social strata and has brought entire countries to their knees. Working in therapy and treatment with persons with addiction is extremely complex. This complexity has led to frustration, compassion fatigue, professional burnout, and a sense of hopelessness in caregivers—both professionals and laypersons. No wonder we have not yet found universally effective treatment.

In many ways, we have not won the war because we do not understand our enemy. RecoveryMind Training (RMT) brings a clearer understanding to this muddle, and this book is, at best, an attempt to move the needle forward in that direction.

RecoveryMind Training (the book) is addressed to therapists, physicians, educators, and other professional caregivers who diagnose and treat addiction. It will prove helpful to the social worker, psychologist, or anyone who works with individuals with alcohol and other drug use disorders and/or those suffering from a behavioral addiction. Although it is not designed for patients or clients, affected family members, or friends of persons with addiction, it may prove helpful to such individuals if they are sufficiently inquisitive. And while not a self-help book per se, the principles herein detail a series of changes in thoughts, actions, and beliefs that promote a durable recovery.

This text assumes a general knowledge of addiction and its treatment. It will not presume the reader has a complete understanding of addiction. RecoveryMind Training rethinks much of addiction treatment and may seem odd or prove jarring to those with extensive addiction treatment experience. Therefore, the seasoned veteran may struggle more with this book than the interested novice.

RecoveryMind Training is best implemented in an organized treatment setting, but most of the skills embodied in RMT can be taught by an individual therapist or recovery coach and practiced in that same setting. This book will stimulate you to reconsider addiction, to look at it from a different point of view. As you read, keep an open mind as some of the concepts may seem unconventional, radical, or even disturbing.

I had my own serious doubts when my mentor, Tom Butcher, PhD, tried to push the antecedents of RMT into my brain twenty-five years ago. My mind revolted; it seemed "not of this world" to describe those afflicted with addiction as hapless victims, suffering at the hand of renegade neural circuitry inside their own brain. Nevertheless, I tested his seminal ideas and found, to my surprise, they held together in a coherent whole. My patients grabbed onto his concepts like shipwreck victims endlessly adrift in the vast Pacific. Over the years, I have expanded Dr. Butcher's teachings, creating an entire system from what twenty-five years ago appeared to be a quirky way of looking at the illness.

I have also been influenced by interacting with colleagues in the American Society of Addiction Medicine (ASAM), a 4,000-member professional society of addiction specialist physicians and others, as we developed a document that was adopted by ASAM in 2011: the oft-cited ASAM Definition of Addiction. Michael Miller, MD, a past president of ASAM and Raju Hajela, MD, a past president of the Canadian Society of Addiction Medicine, were both friends and mentors as we formulated this description of a bio-psycho-social-spiritual disease of the brain, the mind, and the spirit.

But why should *you* read this book? First, the text creates a cohesive framework for addiction care. In many ways, it is a training manual that teaches its reader a systematic way of observing and understanding addiction. The training pulls together the most useful knowledge from neuroscience with the best therapy and behavioral techniques. The RecoveryMind framework will help systematize your approach to addiction and prioritize interventions—putting order to the chaos. Second, RMT helps you see addiction from a different vantage point, one that is often accompanied by startling insights. My hope is that new doors will open with your clients or patients through the use of RecoveryMind Training.

People do not develop addiction overnight, despite all the sensationalistic stories we read in novels and the press. Addiction develops over a period of time, which varies from person to person, and it develops in a certain subset of individuals who expose themselves to powerful rewards, including alcohol, nicotine, and rewarding behaviors such as gambling. This book is an exploration of how that change occurs and, more importantly, how to unwind the vast array of effects addiction has on the brain and on the mind. Addiction is an unrelenting, progressive malady that eats away at what it means to be a freethinking, choice-making, vibrant human being. As stated in the Narcotics Anonymous Basic Text, addiction leads to "jails, institutions, and death."[1] Not fun. Not happy. Not healthy.

Many books have been written about addiction treatment. So how is this book different? The most important difference is its approach to addiction, combining recent scientific findings and theories derived from neuroscience and my thirty years of trying myriad techniques—with decidedly mixed success. Listening closely to my patients, as well, helped hone the AddictBrain concept. I have collected all this into a cohesive framework, naming it RecoveryMind Training. RMT is understandable and practical. It approaches addiction recovery as a set of multifaceted but learnable skills that increase the afflicted to rethink, react, and reengineer their lives, putting the illness in remission and building a new life in recovery. This book provides in-depth knowledge of how addiction rewires the brain, followed by a road map for the way out. It is based upon current addiction research that establishes this illness as a complex brain disease with biological, psychological, spiritual, and social elements.

I believe the most hopeful approach to the treatment of addiction is to see it is as something best solved through retraining. It might seem strange that RMT sees addiction as a biological disease that is treated by learning and reeducation; however, addiction trains the brain to act one way, so it only makes sense that we have to train the brain to act another. Part of this training involves visualizing the problem. RecoveryMind Training provides a clear view of what addiction is, and seeing it with clarity helps move the patient from contemplation to action. Neurophysiologist Richard Davidson, PhD, has proposed that "qualities such as patience, calmness, cooperation, and compassion are best regarded as skills that can be trained."[2] In a similar manner, I assert that RecoveryMind Training is an intricate set of skills that once learned and faithfully practiced result in abstinence and recovery. As I discuss later in the book, the retraining must extend over many areas, including learning about how the brain is altered by addiction, learning to trust others, and practicing behavioral skills that reduce the risk of relapse.

A patient of mine, who was successful at most things she put her mind to, stated that she "just needed a deep-seated conviction that drinking was bad for me." Unfortunately, one never recovers from this devastating illness by simply changing one's mind, no matter how heartfelt. It requires learning, feeling, and practicing the new skill sets of RecoveryMind Training.

The book is divided into two sections. The first section focuses on AddictBrain and the second section on RecoveryMind Training. These two concepts are inextricably interlinked and form the foundation of RMT. Section One explains the problem. Section Two outlines the solution. In this text, I use the levels of care described in the ASAM Criteria,[3] the most widely accepted and used guide to assigning patients to various intensities and durations of addiction treatment based on an assessment of various aspects of their clinical condition.

The RMT treatment system has been developed with the knowledge that many treatment providers have to build a care plan limited by too little time in treatment and funded by insufficient treatment dollars. For example, some patients with a longstanding addiction disorder may wind up in an evening intensive outpatient program (abbreviated IOP and designated as an ASAM Criteria Level 2.1 program). Such individuals may only have four weeks in this care level to contain their illness using the techniques in Domain A and learn and practice Recovery Basics (Domain B). Such a program would focus on these first two RMT domains for the majority of their care. If time permits or it is therapeutically appropriate, a patient may begin work in one or more additional domains in such a setting. The hope is that such patients will continue to work in the subsequent domains once they have stepped down to ASAM Level 1 (outpatient services). A patient in a day hospital (ASAM Criteria Level 2.5) may proceed further in his or her domain work at a subsequent, less intense level of care. If in a residential program, a patient would have the opportunity to embrace an even more comprehensive treatment process that encompasses all six domains.

Similarly, patients who relapse after a period of substantive abstinence and/or recovery begin their treatment with a brief revisit of Domain A (Containment). This will help them recapture their previous abstinence. A review of the remainder of the domains is then indicated. Did they have problems with a harsh or self-sabotaging Internal Narrative (Domain D)? Were they plagued with problems in recognizing and managing strong emotions (Domain C)? Did they simply lack sufficient relapse preventions skills (Domain F)? Or, were there problems in several RecoveryMind domains that require attention in their second treatment? The in-depth, multifaceted qualities of RecoveryMind Training build a comprehensive treatment model and avoid becoming formulaic.

Definitions

Before moving on, I want to explain some of the language used in this book. Clear definitions make clear understanding. If you are a seasoned physician, counselor, or therapist familiar with most of the terms within this text, you may want to skip to the next chapter. Others should plow ahead. Addiction treatment, like any other field, has its assumed definitions and meanings. Addiction itself can be defined and described in various ways. I encourage the reader to become familiar with the Definition of Addiction as developed and approved by the American Society of Addiction Medicine.

Before we get into all the details, let me share a story. I met a group of friends for dinner at a local restaurant several months ago. One member of our party was a recent acquaintance. When the end of the meal came, he stated, "No dessert for me, I am a diabetic." He stated this without embarrassment or self-deprecation. Using identifiers such as diabetic (or alcoholic) promotes clarity—I implicitly grasped my dinner companion's situation. The problem is not the word "addict" or "alcoholic," it is society's deeper prejudice about the illness itself. Changing terms will do little to move the needle on discrimination. Only a deeper appreciation, understanding, and acceptance of addiction as a disease will begin to sway the tide of negative sentiment against those who have it.

The first term to get clear about is what we call the individual who is under our care. I will most often use the word "patient" because I was trained as a physician and that is the word I learned to use for those who seek medical services. This text is clearly not for physicians alone. Our patients and clients consult an array of providers from multiple areas of healthcare to help them recover. Therefore, I will use the word "client" from time to time to honor the many providers who use this term.

But more fundamentally, I use the term "person with addiction" rather than that familiar, briefer term: addict. For too long—for most of human history—persons with addiction involving alcohol, opium, or other drugs, have been considered less than full persons or even as non-persons. The inability of a person with active addiction to function fully in his family, at his job, or in his community, commonly leads to approbation and scorn. Persons with addiction face discrimination in society as they are deemed not deserving or worthy of the same status and rights accorded the rest of us. Segregating persons with addiction from others, in our minds, in our attitudes, or through our actions, depends on considering them "non-people." First in my orientation is to consider persons with this disease as people. Dr. Ed Salsitz, a New York City internal medicine physician who subspecializes in addiction, has spoken eloquently about this.

Recently, the *Journal of Addiction Medicine*, through its editor, Richard Saitz, MD, MPH, has called for a revision of our language in addiction care.[4] Dr. Saitz called for "person first" language (e.g., referring to an "alcoholic" as a "person with an alcohol use disorder"). I have adopted such language wherever possible in this text despite the fact that it generates awkward syntax at times. However, I want to make it clear that many experienced providers continue to use the term addict or alcoholic. I disagree that this term is invariably pejorative. It offers clarity of communication that appeals to me. Those who are outside the field may hear the words "addict" or "alcoholic" as negative, most often because they harbor negative feelings about addiction. For those of us with many years in the field of addiction, the word "addict" is used with kindness and affection. Nonetheless, I understand the need to eliminate potential prejudice. Therefore, I will not use the term addict or alcoholic in this book, except in unavoidable circumstances.

Decisions about the use of specific terms come down to timing. When a patient is fighting the truth about being ill with addiction, it is best to use terms she can agree with while leaving the door open to more accurate self-determination. As acceptance grows, the therapist nudges the patient toward more definitive terms. "I drink too much" becomes "my alcohol use was out of control." Many individuals are more comfortable saying, "I have a problem with alcohol" or "I have a problem with pills" or "I have a problem with gambling" than they are saying they have a disease that has changed their brain. In time the person in treatment or in recovery may say, "I was addicted to alcohol." In the end, if a patient or client chooses to self-identify as an alcoholic or addict, she has acquired precious insight. Some would argue that we should not take away simple words like "alcoholic" and replace them with phraseology that may be politically correct but dangerously ambiguous.

Another point worth addressing is that as addiction takes hold, the brain cares little as to whether the chemical involved is legal or not. Some drugs are legal (e.g., alcohol,[5] nicotine and, increasingly, in the United States, cannabis) others are illegal (e.g., methamphetamine, cocaine, and heroin). Your brain is not wired by legal definitions. Most of us who work in the addiction field accept the concept that addiction to one substance dramatically increases the probability that other addicting substances, tried or not, will generate the same addictive demise. The compulsion for abusing one substance renders one vulnerable for compulsion with other addictive substances or behaviors. For example, a person with an alcohol use disorder may stop drinking ethanol and try benzodiazepine drugs,[6] such as alprazolam (Xanax).[7] Alternatively, the person with addiction to cocaine may stop using cocaine, and his compulsive sexual behaviors may then accelerate into a downhill spiral of sex addiction. Addiction is an illness with many changing facets; over time, it takes on different preferred chemical rewards and rewarding behaviors for its own end. I will explore these facets in depth, as well, in a subsequent chapter.

Addiction treatment is a confusing beast of a term as well. For the purposes of this text, treatment is any organized endeavor by trained professionals used to help the patient or client with the process of recovery (this is described in some detail in a Public Policy Statement on Treatment of Addiction adopted by ASAM). Treatment can begin with a verbal contract between the client and his or her individual therapist. Treatment can be following a set of spiritual rules in a faith-based approach to healing. Treatment may be attending twelve-step support group meetings such as Alcoholics Anonymous, Narcotics Anonymous or Gamblers Anonymous. Treatment may involve a prolonged stay in a residential program or living in a supportive living environment. It is difficult to build an all-encompassing view because there is no single approach that works for everyone. (See the *Principles of Drug Addiction Treatment* first published by the National Institute on Drug Abuse in 1999. The First Principle states, "Addiction is a complex but treatable disease that affects brain function and behavior." The second of the fourteen principles states explicitly, "No single treatment is appropriate for everyone.")

In contrast, if you tell a friend that your physician has diagnosed you with high blood pressure, she may ask, "Have you started treatment?" In your friend's mind, she visualizes you being prescribed and taking one or more high blood pressure medications and checking your blood pressure to track results. The treatment is clear and universally understood.

If, however, you tell your friend you started treatment for addiction, she would not intuitively understand what you are doing, and generally the first thing that would come to mind would not be "going to my doctor and getting a prescription for a drug to *treat* addiction." Why is this? One answer comes from our limited research in understanding treatment effectiveness. Billions of research dollars have gone into understanding high blood pressure, cardiovascular disease, and stroke, and their effective management. Despite the fact that addiction will strike one in ten people during his or her lifetime, a paltry sum of money has gone into the social, psychological, and biological causes of addiction, and an infinitesimal amount of money has gone to determine what constitutes proper treatment for this condition. While significant research has been conducted on the neurobiology of addiction, virtually none has been devoted to understanding the neurobiology of recovery. Even so, addiction treatment is surprisingly successful, as successful as treatment for other common chronic diseases.[8, 9] Limited research into effectiveness results in a confusing hodgepodge of treatment approaches and promises of magical cures. Your friend, with whom you discussed your upcoming treatment, might visualize any number of potential interventions, ranging from "going off to treatment" in a center across the country to signing up for three sessions of acupuncture. Treatment is plagued by a dizzying array of methodologies with few standards. In many ways, addiction care in the twenty-first century is where cancer treatment was in the 1960s.

Just to make the treatment conundrum more complicated, it is hard to define how long treatment should last. We do know, however, that the best prognosis comes from a prolonged relationship with a treatment provider, program, or process. The longer a patient has some type of therapeutic relationship, the better the outcome. In fact, the length of time in treatment for this chronic relapsing and remitting disease is much more important than its intensity. More intense treatment has a tendency to produce a more rapid initial change, but longer care produces the best outcome.

Our society is attached to the quick fix. With addiction, any quick fix is a formula for failure. In medicine, the word for the surgical removal of a diseased part of the body comes from the name of the body part followed by the suffix: "-ectomy." If your appendix is inflamed, the surgeon performs an appendectomy. In addiction medicine, there is no "addictionectomy." Despite this truth, most of the well-known and highly respected addiction treatment programs use an acute care model for a chronic disease. In doing so, treatment is structured in a fundamentally flawed way and almost assures recurrences of symptoms (relapse). No one would think of offering treatment for diabetes for just twenty-eight days or three months, then withdrawing professional help and "seeing what the patient looks like" at some point down the line. When you only offer acute interventions for a chronic problem—well, that's a problem, too. People still go to three or four weeks of addiction treatment and expect to be "all better." It is no surprise that such treatment does not generate lasting beneficial effects.[10]

Can we say how long it takes to heal? Once the neuroadaptations of addiction have taken hold, leading to changes in how the brain thinks and guides motivation and behavior and the individual's interpersonal interactions, the damage to the body and one's family and social situation, and, very importantly, damage to the spirit cannot be resolved with a quick fix. For people with severe addiction, healing time is measured in years. Removing the behavior of unhealthy use of chemicals (e.g., alcohol) or eliminating the unhealthy the behavior (e.g., compulsive gambling) is the first step in the healing process. As afflicted individuals begin their journey out of addiction, the path is long and arduous. They may see it as dull, lifeless, and plodding. This is not the way recovery unfolds for most people. The journey out of addiction is filled with strange new experiences. Like a long hike, there may be parts that are flat and uninteresting. At other times, the journey is challenging. Along the way, there will be excitement and beauty. The beauty will come for most people if they consider recovery as a journey of self-discovery. We should encourage them to open their eyes and their hearts along the way. Regardless, everyone on the recovery path should plan on measuring the hike in terms of months or years, not days.

Introduction Notes

1. Narcotics Anonymous, *Narcotics Anonymous*, Sixth ed. (Van Nuys: Narcotics Anonymous World Services, Inc., 2008).

2. R. J. Davidson, "The Heart-Brain Connection: The Neuroscience of Social, Emotional, and Academic Learning," by Edutopia, *CASEL Forum* (2007).

3. ASAM, *The ASAM Criteria: Treatment Criteria for Addictive, Substance-Related and Co-Occuring Disorders*, Third ed., ed. David Mee-Lee (Carson City: The Change Companies, 2013).

4. R. Saitz, "Things That Work, Things That Don't Work, and Things That Matter— Including Words," *J Addict Med* 9, no. 6 (2015): 429–30.

5. Alcohol is one of the drugs that have the capacity to produce addiction. Despite being one of the oldest drugs of humankind and its pervasive consumption in many cultures, it is a drug, nothing more.

6. In the 1980s, addiction medicine physicians used to joke that some of our less informed physician colleagues believed alcoholism was a syndrome that resulted from a deficiency of Valium.

7. In the United States, the trade name for alprazolam is Xanax. To avoid confusion throughout this book, I will use generic names for medications and only occasionally mention trade names.

8. A. T. McLellan, J. R. McKay, R. Forman, J. Cacciola, and J. Kemp, "Reconsidering the Evaluation of Addiction Treatment: From Retrospective Follow-up to Concurrent Recovery Monitoring," *Addiction* 100, no. 4 (2005): 447–58.

9. A. T. McLellan, L. Luborsky, C. P. O'Brien, G. E. Woody, and D. K. A., "Is Treatment for Substance Abuse Effective?" *JAMA* 247, no. 10 (1982): 1423–28.

10. A. T. McLellan, D. C. Lewis, C. P. O'Brien, and H. D. Kleber, "Drug Dependence, a Chronic Medical Illness: Implications for Treatment, Insurance, and Outcomes Evaluation," *JAMA* 284, no. 13 (2000): 1689–95.

SECTION ONE

CHAPTER ONE

RecoveryMind Training: A Path of Change

The Seven Elements of RecoveryMind Training

Although it is well meaning, addiction treatment has evolved into a hodgepodge of treatment techniques. One treatment center uses techniques that are vastly different from another. Patients or clients in treatment are confused by nebulous goals. Meaningful outcome studies that compare the effectiveness of one center to another are uninterpretable because such studies wind up comparing apples to oranges. RecoveryMind Training is an evolving attempt to correct all that. It strives for clarity of language, clarity of metaphor, and clarity of treatment goals.

Over the years, I have been asked, "What is RecoveryMind?" This question always makes my mind race in an effort to produce a succinct description of RecoveryMind Training, but such summaries tend to leave out much of the meaningful and robust qualities of this addiction treatment system. With some reservation, let me posit a short list that summarizes RecoveryMind Training, which asserts that

1. When one develops an addiction disorder, addiction overrides many of the brain's control mechanisms, including the reward, motivation, attentional systems and the memory and

consciousness networks. Addiction hijacks all these brain systems to its own ends, setting up a second tightly organized and efficient command-and-control center in the brain;

2. This second brain system is called **AddictBrain**. AddictBrain is produced by a complex set of brain systems that collude together, establishing a *biological imperative* to continue alcohol or other drug use. Recognizing and accepting that AddictBrain is trying to destroy its host helps rally its victims, helping patients engage in treatment;

3. The process of addiction recovery is, at its core, a learning process. The learning required is procedural (learning "how") and not declarative (learning "what"). All useful recovery skills must be acquired and practiced in treatment. Listening to lectures has little value;

4. These skills (called Recovery Skills) are divided into six domains:
   • Domain A: Addiction Containment
   • Domain B: Basic Recovery Skills
   • Domain C: Emotional Awareness and Resilience
   • Domain D: Internal Narrative
   • Domain E: Connectedness and Spirituality
   • Domain F: Relapse Prevention;

5. The aggregate of definitions, domains, and skills create a treatment system called **RecoveryMind Training**. When recovery skills are acquired and practiced, the individual with addiction develops RecoveryMind, out of which recovery emerges. **Recovery** is a state of significant change and often a substantive transformation for the afflicted individual. As this recovery builds, he or she moves further and further away

from relapse. AddictBrain and RecoveryMind are yin and yang; RecoveryMind repairs AddictBrain;

6. The needed recovery skills are many and complex. However, these skills can be taught and their acquisition measured. Therefore, treatment providers and researchers can study the efficacy of this organized treatment system;

7. RecoveryMind Training defines treatment, not recovery. It does not replace twelve-step support groups and step work (a recovery management process). RecoveryMind Training is complementary to twelve-step principles. Patients who do not want to use Alcoholics Anonymous or any other support system to assist their recovery will still benefit from RecoveryMind Training but may be at a disadvantage regarding outcome.

What Is AddictBrain? What Is RecoveryMind?

AddictBrain and RecoveryMind are radical concepts. They may strike you as exaggerated or even disturbing. The treatment concepts described in this text are aimed at individuals who suffer from a significant, progressive addiction disorder. Experience has shown that once such an individual develops a serious substance or process addiction, any attempt for a gentler approach minimizes the severity of the situation and prolongs agony. A less radical approach may eventually prove to be lethal. The AddictBrain concept and its corresponding RecoveryMind care system produce sustained results. However, RecoveryMind Training is not a universal approach to addiction; there are several types of clients and patients who are not candidates for this approach. Please see Chapter Two for more information on the limits of RecoveryMind Training.

RecoveryMind Training has the power to capture recovery even if past attempts have failed. If you are unsatisfied with your results or are looking for a better way to conceptualize addiction care, then RecoveryMind Training is for you. As you read this text, I believe you will discover some of the clues to your past frustration and treatment failures. Some individuals have an unrelenting AddictBrain that cannot seem to let go, and the approach in this book might be what you need to help such a patient or client dismantle repeated relapses and maintain sustained success.

RecoveryMind Training is not an alternative to twelve-step programs. Rather, it complements the twelve-step recovery program. I think of RecoveryMind Training as a way of assisting patients out of the confusion produced by their addiction, placing them on the path to recovery. It has been my experience that RecoveryMind Training speeds the transition from addiction to recovery and provides a handle that a patient can grab onto—it decreases treatment confusion. RMT explains past behaviors in ways that are both reassuring and scientifically accurate.

In a similar way, RecoveryMind Training is not recovery itself. Rather, RMT is a way to get into recovery, to jumpstart a long change process. Recovery is a cognitive, psychological, interpersonal, and spiritual state that is different from abstinence alone. RMT challenges patients to examine their life from an unusual perspective. It encourages them to regard their illness as an external attack on their true being. RMT also views the process of recovery as one of self-exploration. This state of questioning and self-exploration, established early in the change process, will soon be deeply integrated into a sustained and satisfying addiction recovery.

Deeper into the Principles of RecoveryMind Training

What are the central tenets of RecoveryMind Training? The central concept of AddictBrain is that once addicted, an individual develops a second, unconscious series of brain thoughts and actions that attack every aspect of a person's being. The second set of values, thoughts, and learned responses is called AddictBrain. AddictBrain acts like a separate entity living inside the head and has the same central agenda of any living thing—to remain alive. Although it helps if AddictBrain does not kill its host, death can occur.

If addiction is a chronic primary, biological illness with psychological, social, spiritual, and societal contexts and correlates, how do we treat it? We know that change in only one of these areas does not conquer the disease. We have no medications that cure addiction. No sane surgical intervention exists. What we do have is a series of tools that, when applied methodically and consistently, place the illness into remission. Life-rearranging and lifelong recovery requires an intellectual, emotional, physical, and spiritual metamorphosis; with such a complete transformation, one can emerge from the hell of living with AddictBrain. RecoveryMind is a way of thinking, acting, and feeling, which is the antidote to AddictBrain.

The adjustment is more complicated and global than "changing your mind." We change our minds every day. Through the course of this book, I hope to impress upon you that the required life rearrangements are much more drastic and pervasive than a decision or change in attitude or even behaviors. RecoveryMind Training catalogs and delineates the elements of life transformation that are required to hold the disease of addiction in a state of sustained remission. When a patient asks me what he must do to recover, I often say, "You must rearrange how you view and respond to most everything in your life, *including your past.*"

As previously mentioned, RecoveryMind Training is not a substitute for twelve-step programs. Alcoholics Anonymous (AA), Narcotics Anonymous (NA), Al-Anon, Nar-Anon, and similar programs are excellent resources to maintain abstinence and engender a peaceful recovery. My patients use the techniques of RecoveryMind Training to help them start their journey in AA or NA; however, this book is not simply a manual that describes how to begin working a twelve-step program. Many such books exist and I would refer you to them for further information (see Chapter One Notes).[1-5] Rather, RMT provides techniques to open the mind and transform addictive thinking. This change brings a patient or client to a place where most patients can engage in the journey suggested by twelve-step programs.

So why don't we send people to AA (or other twelve-step programs) by itself? Why go through all the mind gyrations of RecoveryMind Training? The answer is simple. Research suggests that AA alone is less effective at moving the individual with addiction from the state of using into abstinence than treatment plus AA.[6] RecoveryMind Training provides a unified construct for that treatment. RMT catalogs each of the disparate elements of addiction treatment and weaves them together into a coherent whole. The RMT system, when combined with the AA or other support systems, produces the best long-term outcome.

What does RecoveryMind Training do? RecoveryMind trains an individual to use his objective mind to observe how AddictBrain has changed his thinking and behavior. This increases a patient's resolve to fight an enemy rather than himself or the ones he loves. All this requires training and practice while under the watchful eye of a therapist trained in this technique. Reading a book about RecoveryMind Training does not, by itself, forge a path out of the addiction jungle. Patients cannot take a correspondence course in RecoveryMind and expect to magically fall into recovery. But the insight, understanding, and practiced responses of RMT retrain the brain for recovery.

Over the years, I have had the pleasure of working with many bright, compassionate, successful people who have succumbed to this devastating illness. They wind up frustrated, bamboozled, and repeatedly tripped up by their thoughts. They relapse just as they become convinced that all is well. RecoveryMind Training has provided such people with a way of viewing the dilemma of their addictive disease that builds self-confidence, circumvents false confidence, and decreases the probability of relapse.

Addiction rearranges how one sees the world, distorting even the simplest truths. For example, most nonaddicted people agree with the statement: "I should not drive after drinking excessively." The brain of the individual with alcohol use disorder commonly rearranges this statement with exceptions ("This one time I will be fine."), justifications ("I am a better driver drunk than many are sober."), and even arrogant defiance ("The police will never detect me!"). If AddictBrain can manufacture these bold-faced lies, imagine what it can do with more subtle thoughts and beliefs. Domain D—one part of RecoveryMind Training—teaches clients to recognize distorted thinking—what I call AddictBrain thinking. As you will learn in the next section, you cannot outthink AddictBrain, but you can recognize its agenda and goals. Such recognition will help patients and clients develop a healthy skepticism about their thoughts and beliefs—especially when early in recovery. The skepticism will, in turn, motivate patients and clients to ask for help in sorting out their hijacked brain.

If education alone does not help, what will? The difference in RecoveryMind Training lies in engaging specific types of learning. RecoveryMind Training is focused on acquiring skills versus learning facts or other information, which is the difference between "learning what" and "learning how." Learning that Neil Armstrong was the first man to walk on the moon is much different from learning to whistle. Both are learning but are valuable in different ways.

Although RecoveryMind Training encourages the emotional understanding that occurs in traditional psychotherapy, it is larger than that. The core of RecoveryMind Training is procedural learning. This is the same type of learning that occurs over the two to three years a person needs to drive a car with skill and safety. It is amazing that after about two years of practice, we are able to guide a two-ton hunk of steel down the road safely at seventy miles per hour without consciously thinking about it. Recovery requires this type of learning, procedural learning, in order to subvert the automatic and subtle reactions programmed by AddictBrain. Good recovery can only be sustained when an individual integrates healthy thoughts and desires with a new set of motivations, emotional commitment, and spiritual growth. And all this has to be applied using behaviors that are as automatic as driving a car. No wonder recovery is so hard!

RecoveryMind Training defines each of these elements as Recovery Skills, which are taught and practiced to invoke procedural learning. This book is a guide to those recovery skills that need to be acquired for recovery and outlines the specific skills that need to be learned and practiced to become someone different—a recovering person. When acquired and practiced, these skills become habits and behaviors that transform patients or clients from hapless victims to successful, happy, resilient human beings.

The RecoveryMind Model

Addiction treatment found a foothold at the edge of medical care in the second half of the twentieth century when medicine, and especially psychiatry, was changing—rapidly absorbing a new model called biopsychosocial medicine.[7, 8] Addiction treatment was a perfect fit for this new model. It made intuitive sense that the damage from the illness should be matched by treatment in the same areas of humanness. RecoveryMind Training comes from this same biopsychosocial model. No other illness creates devastation in one's biology, emotions, self-esteem, and beliefs about self as well as interpersonal strife, risk of physical harm to loved ones, violence in the home, divorce, child neglect and abuse, and destruction of spirituality. Addiction is at the center of much of our crime; extensive illegal activity is often required to support the relentless hunger created by the disease.

More recently, addiction researchers are questioning the efficacy of our current treatment model. The psychiatric community also questions the biopsychosocial model.[9] Physicians and medical researchers, conceptualizing addiction as a biological brain disease, are championing drug therapy for the illness. Providers of cognitive behavioral therapy (CBT) assert that CBT has increased efficacy over other modalities. In contrast, RecoveryMind Training is decidedly inclusive in its approach. Not every patient will respond to the same treatment formula. A multifaceted, biopsychosocial,[10] spiritual approach with judicious use of medications, flexed to match each patient, offers the most opportunity when faced with such a formidable foe.

In the first section of this book, AddictBrain amalgamates several neurophysiological concepts and brain circuits under one umbrella. The brain circuits I will describe come from many different parts of the human brain. They have different origins and native functions. Although they may have no natural relatedness, RecoveryMind Training postulates that these circuits come together creating a perfect storm during the genesis of addiction.

Similarly, the treatment involved in RecoveryMind Training is a group of techniques that, when combined together, transition a client or patient from the addicted state to recovery. I do not claim these techniques are inherently interrelated except in their effectiveness to repair the damage produced by addiction. Their fit into the construct of RecoveryMind Training is a pragmatic one. Simply put, the described techniques work together.

AddictBrain and RecoveryMind are two concepts, the yin and yang of addiction treatment. Patients quickly grasp this concept in a culture with myths of good and evil, and the natural clarity is a distinct benefit of this model. A RecoveryMind restoration exists for each AddictBrain problem. The RMT path is lucid and teachable. Patients gain insight into an extremely confusing illness and start on a coherent path to recovery.

Chapter One Notes

1.   A. Mooney, A. Eisenberg, and H. Eisenberg, *The Recovery Book* (New York: Workman Publishing, 1992).

2.   Alcoholics Anonymous, *Alcoholics Anonymous,* Fourth ed. (New York: A.A. World Services, Inc., 1976).

3.   Narcotics Anonymous, *Narcotics Anonymous,* Sixth ed. (Van Nuys: Narcotics Anonymous World Services, Inc., 2008).

4.   Alcoholics Anonymous, *Twelve Steps and Twelve Traditions* (New York: A.A. World Services, Inc., 2002).

5.   P. Carnes, *A Gentle Path through the Twelve Steps: The Classic Guide for All People in the Process of Recovery,* Third ed. (Center City: Hazelden, 2012).

6.   G. E. Vaillant, "What Can Long-Term Follow-up Teach Us About Relapse and Prevention of Relapse in Addiction?," *Br J Addict* 83, no. 10 (1988): 1147–57.

7.   G. L. Engel, "The Need for a New Medical Model: A Challenge for Biomedicine," *Science* 196, no. 4286 (1977): 129–36.

8.   G. L. Engel, "The Clinical Application of the Biopsychosocial Model," *Am J Psychiatry* 137, no. 5 (1980): 535–44.

9.   S. N. Ghaemi, "The Rise and Fall of the Biopsychosocial Model," *The British Journal of Psychiatry* 195, no. 1 (2009): 3–4.

10. R. C. Smith, "The Biopsychosocial Revolution," *J Gen Intern Med* 17, no. 4 (2002): 309–10.

CHAPTER TWO

Clarifications and Limitations

As excited as I am to explore RecoveryMind Training with you, I should start by defining terms and clarifying concepts used in this book. I will also define the limits of RecoveryMind Training. Like any treatment system, it is not effective with all patients or clients. Even if you are familiar with RecoveryMind Training, I suggest you read, or at least review, this chapter.

Before we go further, I should provide a disclaimer about RecoveryMind Training. RMT integrates the latest brain neurophysiology with a practical, understandable, and an effective skill set aimed to help patients or clients recover. Since we entered the twenty-first century, there has been an informational explosion regarding brain functioning, especially as it applies to large neural circuits. In the next five to ten years, we may find much of what we hold to be true about brain functioning to be incorrect. Similarly, we may find our interpretation of the neurophysiology of addiction and how it applies to addiction treatment is actually skewed or off base. It is important, therefore, to avoid the adoption of the information contained herein as gospel or set in stone.

A Few More Definitions

Addicting Chemical or Drug

Those with the disease of addiction use all sorts of drugs, including alcohol. When I use the term **addicting drug**, I am referring to all the chemicals that have the potential to produce addiction in human beings. Although some drugs are "natural" (e.g., alcohol, nicotine, or even peyote), they are all drugs and are classified as chemicals. Many addicting chemicals are natural compounds (e.g., opium) present in plants or directly extracted from plants and are no less dangerous than chemicals synthesized in a laboratory (e.g., methamphetamine or oxycodone). I may also use the term **chemical** to refer to addicting substances because all drugs are chemicals, whether or not they are considered natural substances or synthesized in the laboratory.

Behavioral Addiction

Addiction also appears in individuals who use no external substance. **Behavioral addiction**—whether to sex, relationships, compulsive gambling, the Internet, or even compulsive shopping—produces a downhill course and eventual destruction that is, psychologically and sociologically, indistinguishable from chemical addiction. For the purposes of this book, individuals with behavioral addictions have a variant of the same illness as people who are chemically addicted. The recovery process has subtle differences in regards to the instigating factors, course of the illness, and relapse cues and triggers; however, the underlying illness is the same. RecoveryMind Training is as valuable for behavioral addiction as it is for chemical addiction.

When looking over the long term, no one with an addiction disorder limits his or her compulsion to a single substance or behavior. The combined experience of thousands of physicians and psychotherapists validates this truth. If those so afflicted state they have the disease of addiction—without qualifiers—they keep their mind open to the multi-headed hydra of their affliction. (If someone self-identifies as "an addict," this is even more evident.) Research underscores the interactive nature of multiple addiction manifestations: If an individual with addiction stops smoking tobacco, he increases the probability that his alcohol dependence will remain in remission.[1] Patrick Carnes, PhD, and his colleagues have coined the term **Addiction Interaction Disorder** to describe the interdependent and mutually reinforcing nature of the subtypes of addiction.[2, 3]

Disease

I will frequently use the term **disease** or **illness** when discussing addiction. In the previous century, a debate raged about addiction. Is it a moral failure? Is it a loss of spiritual direction? Is it a psychological or behavioral response to the hurts and harms of life? Is it a response of a culture that lacks a healthy framework or is lacking in meaning and purpose? While I firmly believe addiction has many antecedents, it is a biological disease at its core. Research in the latter part of the twentieth century affirmed that addiction has a strong genetic component. Scientists estimate that genetic factors account for between 40 and 60 percent of a person's vulnerability to addiction.[4, 5] Addiction has clear neurobiological circuits, which cause pathological behaviors that resist change. Like any illness, some individuals have a more virulent form of the disease than others do. I will discuss this further in Chapter Three.

Patients or Clients?

Many professions and institutions use the word **client** to describe the individual who is undergoing treatment. Some treatment systems and centers use the word **consumer** or another moniker. However, in this text, I will most often use the word **patient** to describe those who are under our care. This comes from decades of training and practice as a physician, and it is hard to undo this habit. I will also use the word client from time to time, as I am sure many readers are most accustomed to this term. I consider these terms interchangeable. I also believe patients must have their own investment in their care, and by using the term "patient," I am not implying that the patient has a dependent or subservient relationship with her physician, psychologist, master's level therapist, or counselor.

Clarifications

Addiction Is a Chronic and Primary Disease

During most of the nineteenth and twentieth centuries, medicine— and consequently public opinion—believed addiction was caused by something else. Drug use was a psychological response to other issues. Psychiatrists and psychologists wrote extensively on the psychological and psychiatric causes of drinking. Therapy was focused on what was called the "root cause" of the loss of control over alcohol. Theories about the origins of addiction changed and became more complex when simple approaches failed. Ultimately, when patients failed to respond to the treatment of the day, the patients themselves were described as incorrigible and unwilling to get better, and the medical community gave up on treating addiction. The treatment and care of alcoholism—or inebriety, as it was called in the nineteenth century—was dropped from medical school curricula.

Medicine instead focused on the medical consequences of addiction as a disease rather than the disease itself. Today, most medical school curricula continue this bias. Internal medicine residents become quite skilled in treating alcoholic liver disease but have little or no training in early detection and counseling of drinkers who have or are developing alcohol dependence. Attention to the extensive societal damage caused by the addictive use of drugs biased the medical community. Addiction was observed through the lens of its negative physical, emotional, and spiritual consequences. The disease—and hope for remission—was bleak when viewed from that vantage point.

This focus on the misguided and inaccurate causes of addiction, when combined with attention on the effects of the disease on the body, hid the core issue: addiction itself. It seems easier to write off the ill-timed, self-destructive behaviors as willful misconduct rather than a mysterious force running amuck in the brain.

Today we know addiction is a primary disease. It is also chronic. The chronic nature of addiction appears if a recovering individual relapses. Here is one example:

> *Jim is a forty-five-year-old who has been sober for three years. Prior to sobriety, he used alcohol and alprazolam (Xanax) daily for eight years. Employers found him to be an enthusiastic worker, hiring him with high expectations. At each new job, he started out strong and well liked by his coworkers. Predictably, however, he "snatched defeat out of the jaws of victory" and was invariably fired from each new job due to tardiness and drinking while at work. His wife became exasperated and eventually moved out. His drinking increased, and the resultant downhill spiral eventually led to treatment. After his initial treatment, he attended Alcoholics Anonymous and found a wise sponsor who led him through the steps.*
>
> *His life improved in recovery. He moved to a new job and was quickly promoted. His wife returned. When rehired at his old job, he garnered praise and promotions for his steady enthusiastic contributions to his company. Then the accident happened. As fate would have it, while riding his bicycle with friends one Saturday morning, he was struck by a drunk driver. The impact fractured his femur and ankle. His surgeon placed him on hydrocodone for pain. Jim noted that the pain was intense for about a week but seemed to improve. Even as the pain improved, a little voice in his head said, "You like those pain pills too much." He returned to his physician repeatedly, complaining of little improvement in his pain, especially the ankle pain. Jim's wife noticed his personality change. "You are acting like your old self. You are not drinking are you?" she cautiously*

*asked. Jim vehemently denied drinking but began to
suspect he was in trouble.*

*When he tried to stop the pills, Jim's mood worsened.
Not surprisingly, he soon added his old friend alcohol to
his new friend hydrocodone. When things seemed the
bleakest, Jim's wife and his AA sponsor confronted him: he
needed to enter medical detoxification and return to his
recovery program.*

In summary, Jim used alcohol and alprazolam (a benzodiazepine) as
his drugs of abuse through most of his addiction. Like many individuals
with alcohol and other drug use disorders, he had trouble getting
traction in recovery at first. Eventually he did quite well, enjoying
years of recovery. His illness remained in remission until retriggered
by a prescription for a medically necessary opioid pain reliever. It was
indeed the same illness when it returned, despite its beginning with a
different substance. The more clearly patients get this straightforward
concept—that the disease is chronic—the better prepared they will be
to manage it.

Addiction Is Not Simply a Problem with Chemicals

Addiction comes in many forms or manifestations. The most common
form of addiction is tobacco addiction; 21 percent of adults in the
United States smoke cigarettes.[6] The second most commonly abused
drug worldwide is alcohol. Despite this, addiction is not a problem
with chemicals. It is a disease of the brain and mind. The person with
alcohol use disorder who drinks to excess cannot stop once he starts. His
drinking is destructive to his health. Simple.

Addiction, however, is more complex than this example. Today, it is
very unusual for individuals who are afflicted with addiction to abuse
only one substance. Those who use tobacco are four times more likely
to be dependent on alcohol.[7] When one substance is abused, it opens
the door to additional substance use. Those addicted to stimulants

also drink alcohol. Those addicted to narcotics will use sedative drugs alongside their heroin. Once addiction takes hold, it branches out into many substances, always on the prowl to find other ways of augmenting the effect of one drug with another. As portrayed above, someone may start out abusing alcohol only to switch to hydrocodone pills after several years. Thus, it is important for the person with substance use disorder to stop using all addicting chemicals, lest the door be left open for addiction to remain alive though some other substance.

Addiction is more complex than chemical use as well. Certain behaviors can also become addictive. The person addicted to alcohol might also gamble. Another might use methamphetamine and become involved in sexual compulsion. The four behaviors that appear to be the most addictive to human beings are

1. Gambling;
2. Sexual compulsions (masturbation, pornography, compulsive use of sex workers, and compulsive affairs or relationships);
3. Shopping;
4. Compulsive attention on others (need for affection, need to be in a relationship, focusing on others, and ignoring one's own needs).

I often quip, "Addiction is a chronic disease of the mind, frequently confused with the compulsive use of substances." This quip is not meant to indicate that the compulsive use of chemicals is by default *not* addiction. Rather, it is meant to clarify that addiction is more than the chronic, out-of-control consumption of alcohol and/or other drugs. When we take careful histories or follow patients over time, we learn the illness changes; it evolves, changing its use patterns and directions. A patient with alcohol use disorder may attain strong recovery from his alcohol use, but two years later he is bankrupt from online poker. A patient may start using cocaine and make a bad situation worse by compulsive affairs. Addiction as a disease is supple, deceptive, and constantly changing. It metamorphosizes—especially when a central drug or behavior is contained—adapting to situations as they arise.

Does this mean that it is impossible to recover? Is the illness too clever, too adaptive to pin down or force into remission? Is the addicted individual doomed to a lifelong game of Whack-a-Mole? I think not. The first task in getting better from addiction is to see it for what it really is, to understand it as a multifaceted illness rather than a single abnormal behavior. How one looks at the problem of addiction is critical to recovery. Each person with addiction expresses the disease in his or her own unique manner. Manifestations of the disease change over time; therefore, cataloging the current behaviors produces a list of the current illness characteristics. Nonetheless, those with alcohol and drug use disorders need to be cautious about yet untried addictive chemicals and behaviors. To stay in recovery, the individual needs to know where his or her vulnerabilities lie.

Addiction Is Not Simply a Bad Case of Substance Abuse

This assertion is controversial. When people abuse a lower quantity of substances over a shorter time period with fewer consequences, do they have a lesser severity of the same disorder than if they used more and with more consequences? Many think this is the case. The most recent revision of the *Diagnostic and Statistical Manual of Mental Disorders, Fifth Edition (DSM-5)*, developed by the American Psychiatric Association, implies this; the same criteria are used for abuse and addiction. If one meets more of the criteria, they are diagnosed with a more severe form of the same illness.

Addiction neurochemistry, genetic research, and clinical experience point in a different direction. The work of Eric Nestler, MD, PhD,[8-11] for example, suggests that changes in intracellular transcriptional mechanisms may elicit a one-way transition into addiction and thus an irreversible change once addicted. The fact that genetics make some people more susceptible to addiction also argues against abuse being on a continuum with addiction. Clinical experience also suggests that many people who go on to develop addiction have a different relationship with substances from the start. Individuals with alcohol and drug use disorders often describe a deeper attachment and meaning to their first drug experience, remembering that event with enthusiasm decades later.

It is easy to visualize abuse and addiction as points along a continuum; you have to abuse alcohol in order to develop an alcohol use disorder. Many people have periods in their life when they abuse alcohol. A distinct number of people abuse drugs other than alcohol. Still others may abusively gamble or engage in compulsive sexual behavior. When all of these people who engage in such activities are followed over time, interestingly enough, only a portion of them develops addiction. You may say, "I know why this is. Some people stop before they become addicted." This is a reasonable but incomplete explanation. Chemical abuse is common in our society. Compulsive behaviors, especially gambling, sex, and shopping, are also on the rise. Despite this, it appears that only 10 percent of the population in the United States will develop addiction in their lifetime.[12] The definition of addiction, according to the American Society of Addiction Medicine, delineates addiction as being qualitatively different than substance abuse.[13] RecoveryMind Training agrees with the ASAM definition of addiction and disagrees with the *DSM-5*, asserting that addiction is qualitatively different—it is not a more severe form of substance abuse.

Consider Joshua, who crosses over from consistent alcohol use into addiction. When he makes this transition, his loss of control becomes hardwired, and his personality and self-concept change. He accommodates to the disruptive effects of his emerging addiction disorder. He makes excuses for his behavior; excuses that, despite being quite often patently absurd to others, make perfect sense to Joshua. His brain compensates, rearranging cause and effect in order to sustain continued addictive chemical use. Joshua loses the ability to see how his addictive behavior influences his thinking. Addiction rearranges Joshua's priorities and eats away at his self-esteem. In short, the shift from abuse to addiction is a qualitative, not a quantitative step. The disease of addiction induces a wholesale reengineering of Joshua's view of the world and his place in it. This is AddictBrain.

Early on in the progression of an addiction disorder, most people are unable to see that things are amiss. When the illness becomes severe and pervasive, the individual with addiction may experience moments of insight that rapidly slip away. Without treatment, the addicted individual's blindness to him- or herself may never go away. One of the saddest parts of my work has been to watch good people drink or drug themselves to death, asserting on their way to the grave, "I do not have a problem, Doc, not like those other people you treat!"

Substance abuse and addiction should not be viewed as a continuum; the transition from abuse to addiction is a one-way ticket. Research shows that those addicted cannot slide back the other way. Once addiction takes hold, the afflicted individual cannot return to abuse, much less return to a causal relationship with addicting chemicals. Through the years many compassionate therapists, ministers, and concerned friends have tried to counsel those suffering with addiction on how to "drink successfully" or "just cut down." Such misguided attempts eventually result in failure in the vast majority of cases. When the drug user becomes addicted, he loses the ability to self-regulate his use of a small number of nonessential chemicals. The chemicals that produce addiction do so by altering one small area of the brain, sometimes referred to as the reward center. People who develop addiction can reclaim their lives, and to do so they need only give up a tiny fraction of all life experiences—the drive to alter one's mood with substances and behaviors. The rest of life is open to enjoy.

It has always struck me as odd that we would spend any sort of effort to teach those struggling with alcohol use disorder to drink socially. What's the point? Alcohol is not essential to our species. No one would argue that we should teach heroin users to "socially shoot heroin." Similarly, I have yet to see proponents of controlled smoking of methamphetamine. Proponents of controlled drinking become indignant that abstinence is cruel deprivation. If alcohol is not a central part of one's life, what is the big deal in giving it up?

Aren't Those with Addiction Getting Better when They Learn to Control Their Use?

I have already discussed how addiction is more than "an abuse problem that gets worse." Once an individual develops addiction, he or she cannot return to casual use of addicting chemicals or behaviors. From this, it follows that "controlling one's use" is a good goal for people who abuse substances. In fact, one of the best ways of differentiating between substance abuse and addiction is the ability to control substance use over a sustained period. I am not talking about a weekend or even a month. Individuals who use heavily but are not addicted should be able to make a commitment to stop alcohol use for three to six months or more. Similarly, those consistent substance users should be able decrease from four beers most nights of the week to one beer four nights per week for a period of three months or more—if they do not have an addiction disorder.

When following substance use, the longer a time frame you use, the clearer the picture becomes. When patients come to my office asking if it is proper to diagnose them as having an addiction disorder, I believe one of the best diagnostic maneuvers is a trial of abstinence. I instruct patients to not consume any addicting substances for six months, following them in therapy during that time. We talk about how they perceive themselves, how difficult the trial feels to them, and how their family perceives them.

> *Jane came in asking if she was dependent on marijuana. Her husband was concerned about her mood and how she was withdrawing from the family. Her father had just died. She was feeling hopeless at times, and her freelance web design business was doing poorly. She agreed to stop smoking marijuana and refrain from drinking. During the course of the three months, she began feeling more intense grief from the loss of her father. She spent her time in therapy crying over her heartache and began writing a compendium of her father's fabulous quips about life. Strangely, her hunger for*

marijuana decreased. Her husband reported that his wife returned to the marriage. I instructed her not to consume addicting chemicals for an additional nine months and stopped seeing her at the end of a year. One additional year later, when Jane came in for a repeat evaluation, she stated that she drinks a glass of wine several nights per week and smokes a bit of marijuana every four months or so. When I asked why she does not smoke more often, she said, "It seems to slow me down; I do not like how I feel the next day."

Jane's story illustrates a situational abuse problem with marijuana. By using an abstinence trial, Jane and I both learned the marijuana use was not the central problem. She was able to stop. When she did so, other psychological issues opened up. As she strengthened, she did not need to close the door on chemical use forever.

Other individuals may present with a similar story and wind up with addiction. They attempt to discontinue their drug use and fail. Alternatively, they stop using drugs and some other addictive process emerges.

John, an attorney, was a daily drinker. He arrived in my office because he dropped the ball on several important items in a legal case. His senior partner told him, "That is not like you John. In all of our years together, I have never had to go around you to get things done with our clients. Get some help."

John went home and talked with his wife, Laura, who pushed him to see me. She joined his initial session and started the session saying, "John will not like me telling you this, Dr. Earley, but I have always thought he had an alcohol problem." John vehemently denied this saying that he could quit any time. I quietly jumped on the statement, suggesting that he participate in a sustained trial of alcohol abstinence. With Laura's help, John reluctantly agreed.

John returned to the first follow-up session saying he felt better, was sleeping better, and was getting along with Laura. Laura agreed. John failed to show up for the second session, but Laura came in his place asking for advice. "I know he is sneaking around drinking, but he denies it." I instructed Laura to speak her truth to John, which she did. He arrived at the next session irritable and argumentative, "This stupid abstinence trial is accomplishing nothing."

With careful motivational interviewing techniques, John began to question what would be his own personal indicators that he had an alcohol problem. He stated he valued honesty, especially in his marriage. As the trial progressed, he continued to sneak around, drinking and lying to both of us. He became ill tempered and unhappy. Eventually he exploded, pronouncing his trial a failure. With gentle external pressure from his wife and the internal conflict that came from violating his own value system, he shifted to the initial acceptance of his addiction. During his initial discovery, he related he was drinking less than before and having little pleasure from his secretive drinking. Despite this, he could not stop.

John's struggle illustrates that once addicted to alcohol, an individual cannot "just cut down." In his case, he was able to consume less alcohol, but his turmoil and conflict increased. More often, the individual may decrease use for a time while under duress, only to have his or her addiction return with a vengeance. When returning to substance use, even sporadic use, he or she spirals downhill. What starts as a walk soon picks up the pace, becoming a headlong rush of self-destructive drug use and escalating consequences. Cutting down is a futile goal and only prolongs the inevitable. When dealing with addiction, the healthiest choice is abstinence and recovery work.

Is It Important to Know the Cause of All This Destructive Drug Use?

Human beings like to know why. We solve puzzles, explore space, and contemplate the meaning of life, all in pursuit to answer the question, "Why?" We experience satisfaction when we gain insight into our motivations. As I question why I chose to drive a different and circuitous route to the office one day, I recall there is a beautiful garden along the way. Figuring out a small puzzle about my behavior produces a sense of satisfaction, "I wondered why I did that; now I know." The conscious, thinking brain is an engine of discrimination.[14] It asks why I chose the chicken and not the fish at dinner or why I like red cars and not yellow cars. This information is lumped together to define who we are: "Paul likes red cars, eating chicken, and seeing gardens along his route to work." This information is catalogued and used for decisions later in life—"I will most likely buy a red car." As humans, we value our choices; we are proud of our decisions and use our choice discriminations to answer the question, "Who am I?"

Most people, including those with addiction, believe learning why they do something is the first and most important step in changing their behavior, which is common sense. Patients come to treatment wanting to know why they have addiction in hopes of solving the riddle of their self-destructive behaviors. They ask, "Why do I drink too much alcohol? Why do I hurt my family with my affairs? What caused me to be this way?" The individual with addiction is befuddled by his or her behavior, so does it not make sense to figure it out? In the desperate struggle to conquer addiction, many of my patients have read about addiction, been in therapy, or sought spiritual guidance to better understand the inscrutable malady of addiction. Their mind is convinced that learning *why* will speed them along on the journey to recovery.

Learning why *is* a powerful tool when it comes to conscious decisions. If I learn that smaller engines with less horsepower burn less fuel, I can choose to save money and energy by purchasing a car with a smaller, lower horsepower engine. Learning why may also be of immense value in understanding unconscious decisions. For a long time, I have had a penchant for purchasing red cars. After talking with my siblings, I recalled the time when my mother bought her favorite automobile, a spiffy red convertible. She enjoyed that car immensely. After recalling this memory, I concluded that her joy had impacted me at an impressionable age. I could then use this knowledge to rethink my habit of buying red cars. I could make a more considered color choice on my next car purchase. I could choose to celebrate my mother's preference—buy red—or seek out my own color preference. Learning the why of past unconscious decisions increases opportunities for the future. Shouldn't the same be true about addiction?

On the surface, it seems that knowing why someone with addiction uses drugs should open up the choice not to use, increasing one's preferences for health. The reality is that knowing why is of little benefit in the early stages of recovery. Attempting to decipher why someone uses addicting chemicals is at best a distraction. At its worst, such a search will unintentionally accelerate the illness in a downhill direction. To recover, it is important to comprehend this simple truth. Effective recovery is facilitated by setting aside the search for "reasons why I use" in the early part of recovery, when a patient's thinking and acting is shifting from AddictBrain to RecoveryMind. Asking why will become helpful in the later stages of the journey, which I will explore more fully in later chapters of this book. In the meantime, the most powerful stand to take—and the most accurate—seems absurdist. We have to help the patient acknowledge and internalize this simple truth: "I use because I have the disease of addiction."

Not searching for why does not mean your patient or client is not firm about his or her resolve to stop addiction. These are two distinctly different mind states. Those with addiction striving to rearrange their life to health and recovery need commitment and resolve. Certainty that abstinence and recovery is the best path for today is the most desirable state.

Addiction Occurs in a Social Context

Addiction, like many chronic illnesses, occurs in a social context. This means social norms and behaviors contribute to and characterize the qualities of a given individual's disease. If a given culture places a high value on behavioral constraint, for example, addiction will attack and disrupt constraint. Out of control behaviors emerge.

One of the most striking examples illustrating the social context of addiction comes from our changing attitudes about smoking. In the United States during the post-World War II era, smoking was a pervasive, societal norm and was allowed almost everywhere. Hotels would place ashtrays in every conceivable location, including hotel bathrooms. As we learned more and more about the dangers of tobacco—through primary or secondary inhalation—our culture progressively restricted the use of tobacco to fewer and fewer locations. The increasing restrictions differentiated individuals who are tobacco dependent from those who are not. Today, those dependent on tobacco clutch their cigarettes in small glass cubicles at the airport; nonsmokers walk past, observing them like strange animals in a zoo. Smoking takes on a clandestine quality as tobacco users stand in small clusters outside public buildings, dragging on a cigarette, even in inclement weather.

The Illness Does Not Stop when the Using Stops

Addiction is a complex, lasting brain response that occurs once a susceptible individual develops a pathological relationship with certain substances or behaviors. It is crucial to remember when substances use stops the illness lives on. The long-term brain changes and rearrangements in thoughts and desires, induced by a period of alcohol or other drug use, continue to haunt the person with addiction long after he or she acquires abstinence. Many of these changes are learned responses, hardwired below the level of consciousness. For example, a recovering individual may happen upon a snippet of music from her past life. Hearing only a few notes of a tune that was paired with past substance use can induce intense urges to drink or use. Despite years of healthy recovery, the individual remains at risk for relapse when such an event occurs. Addiction rewires the brain and, in doing so, lives on long after substance use has ceased.

RecoveryMind Training emphasizes the chronic nature of addiction; it may be dormant but present for years into recovery. Also RMT teaches individuals with addiction how to continue their vigilance and when to recognize situations that have a high potential for relapse, emphasizing that addiction is a lifelong disease. The lifelong nature of alcoholism is underscored by the monumental sixty year study of alcoholics by George Vaillant, MD.[15] Recovery does become easier over time as individuals internalize recovery skills and develop life balance. RMT asserts, however, that some level of vigilance is required for the rest of one's life.

Addiction Decisions Are Not Constrained by Legal Definitions

One trap families and novice therapists fall into is confusing the biology of addiction with legal notions. People who have led their entire life within the bounds of the law often become criminals once they develop addiction. The person with alcohol use disorder racks up repeated DWIs/DUIs, sloughing off their importance. A responsible mother drives while intoxicated, her children in car seats in the back. A family man begins sharing and even selling cocaine to support his drug habit. A dedicated husband is arrested for solicitation of prostitutes once he falls into sexual compulsivity.

Family members and therapists have a tendency to overinterpret the meaning of such behaviors because of the acquired disregard for social values and legal constraints those with substance use disorders often have. They say things such as "I guess I didn't truly understand him; he really has a dark heart," and there is a strong tendency to judge, "I thought she was a dedicated mother and loved her children, but I guess I was wrong."

The truth of the matter is much simpler. One of the essential elements of addiction is that it causes an individual to violate his own moral and ethical values. Addictive drugs create compulsive use; use that overrides one's sense of right and wrong. Buying and selling illegal drugs becomes a means to an end in an otherwise moral individual. This does not mean, however, that individuals with antisocial personality traits do not become addicted. Rather, individuals with addiction all appear at first glance to have such traits. Only time in recovery will sort out a patient's true nature.

Paradoxically, an individual's most sacred beliefs and values are systematically trounced by addiction. Insightful therapists are intrigued and deeply vexed about this paradox, and it begs for psychodynamic interpretation. Early in recovery, I believe the most helpful way of viewing this dilemma is to attribute this paradox to the corrosive elements of AddictBrain. Psychodynamic or even analytic exploration should be avoided until the patient's recovery has stabilized. I will revisit this notion in Chapter Four.

Addiction Models and RecoveryMind Training

The etiology, or causation, of addiction has long been a topic of conflict and controversy. Popular notions of addiction once held that addiction was a moral and spiritual problem. Through the 1800s and most of the 1900s, many religious leaders aligned with this viewpoint, calling for a return to religious teachings as a path to abstinence. Varying amounts of moral judgmentalism were encapsulated in this way of thinking, asserting that ultimately we are responsible for our own behavior—such a viewpoint extends to substance use as well.

In contrast, the disease model of addiction asserts that addiction overrides an individual's ability to take responsibility for him- or herself during the period when the illness is active. When viewing addiction as a disease, the individual with addiction regains his or her ability to act as a moral and ethical member of society at some point, although the exact time when this occurs is different for each patient or client.

RecoveryMind Training is a subset of the larger disease model. It provides a clear description of why the "moral failing" occurs (due to the rewiring produced by AddictBrain, detailed in Chapter Four), and provides clues as to when the moral compass should be valid (when AddictBrain has quieted down). However, this does not mean such individuals should be exempt from the laws designed to maintain a stable society. It does argue that the state of their illness should be factored into legal and social sanctions.

RMT also notes that two milestones modify the degree to which personal responsibility is involved in addiction and its recovery. The first milestone occurs when the addicted individual has completed his initial withdrawal from addicting substances. At this point, the overwhelming physical drive to continue substance use decreases dramatically but by no means disappears. The second milestone occurs when the addicted individual fully accepts his diagnosis. He acknowledges and internalizes acceptance of his addiction disorder. At this point, he is much like the diabetic patient who accepts his or her plight—he or she has a chronic disease that demands lifelong care. Personal responsibility increases at these two important milestones and continues to rise with cumulative time in recovery. Said most succinctly, people with addiction are not responsible for their illness. They are, however, responsible for their recovery.

Addiction and Other Psychiatric Illnesses

A second complex controversy causes immense confusion in the psychiatry, mental health, and addiction fields, which has existed for centuries and continues until this day: Do emotional problems create addiction? This controversy surrounds the causal relationship between addiction disorders and other psychiatric and mental health problems. Unfortunately, a caregiver's training and personal life experiences greatly influence his or her point of view and approach to a patient who appears in the office. As a result, two opposing schools of thought have emerged.

In the **Mental Health Model**, depression, anxiety, thought disorders, and intrapsychic conflict produce addiction.

Mental Health Model

Emotional and Psychiatric Problems ➤ **Addiction**

Causes

In the **Mental Health Model**, depression, anxiety, thought disorders, and intrapsychic conflict produce addiction.

Disease Model

Addiction ➤ **Emotional and Psychiatric Problems**

In most cases, causes

The alternate theory is called the **Disease Model**. In the Disease Model, addiction is produced by genetic, biochemical, and neurophysiological abnormalities. Mental health problems are commonly but not necessarily produced by an addiction disorder.

RecoveryMind Model

Addiction ⇄ **Emotional and Psychiatric Problems**

Each modifies and exacerbates the other;
neither is causative or determinate

RecoveryMind Training asserts that mental health problems exacerbate and contribute to (but are not causative of) addiction. They do color its expression and often its intensity. In a reciprocal manner, addiction exacerbates and contributes to (but is not necessarily causative of) mental health problems.

What about Spirituality?

This book focuses on the science of addiction recovery, but for many people, addiction recovery is a deeply spiritual process, one that becomes more so as recovery progresses. The spiritual aspects of recovery cannot be overstated. As I am not an expert in matters of spiritual growth, this text is limited in such discussions; however, this does not mean that spiritual exploration is not critical for most people to attain and sustain long-term recovery or, that RecoveryMind Training thinks less of the spiritual nature of the recovery path. For further discussion on the psychospiritual nature of recovery, I refer you to several excellent books and articles.[16–27]

RecoveryMind Training Is Not for Everyone

When a patient or client enters your office, you can be assured of one thing: he or she does not see his or her problems in the same way as your previous client. Each is in a different place of understanding, motivation, and skills. The first thing to do with new clients is to gauge their willingness and motivation to change. One extremely helpful way of staging this motivation is the Transtheoretical Model of Behavior Change developed by James O. Prochaska, PhD, and Carlo DiClemente, PhD.[28–32] A summary of this model follows.

Table 2.1 - The Transtheoretical Model of Behavior Change

Stage	Description
Precontemplation	Not yet considering possibility of change, active resistance to change. Clients in this stage seldom change without coercion.
Contemplation	Ambivalent, undecided, vacillating between whether or not the need exists for change, wants to change but also resists the changes needed.
Preparation	Takes client from decisions made in contemplation to the steps needed to change. Increasing confidence in the decisions needed for change.

Stage	Description
Action	Specific actions intended to bring about change, overt modification of behavior and environment. Support/encouragement is essential at this stage to prevent dropout and regression.
Maintenance	Sustaining changes have begun. Consolidate gains, learn alternative coping and problem-solving strategies, and recognize emotional triggers for relapse.
Relapse and Recycling	Possible, but not inevitable, setbacks. Avoid becoming stuck and learn from mistakes to determine new cycle of change.
Termination	Ultimate stage for all changers; client exits cycle of change without fear of relapse. Some problems terminated while others are kept in remission through ongoing maintenance efforts.

Where is RecoveryMind Training useful in this continuum? Where is it not? In short, RMT is profoundly ineffective for those clients in the precontemplation stage of change. It should be used with caution and in initial small doses with patients in the contemplation and preparation stages of change.[33, 34, 35] If you introduce the concepts of AddictBrain to someone in the precontemplation stage of change, you are asking for trouble. You may be tempted to say to someone in the precontemplation stage, "You know, part of your brain—we call this part AddictBrain—is consciously plotting against you. It is trying to kill you." At that point, the patient will stand up and walk out the door, muttering to himself, "This therapist is nuttier than I am."

For RMT to be effective, patients need to have experienced repeated negative consequences and recognize their current manner of living has proved to be at least marginally self-destructive. Patients who are in the contemplation, preparation, and action stages of change are capable of recognizing their own mind has turned against them. In such cases, I recommend introducing the concepts slowly, watching the client's response. Begin by using phrases such as "Do you feel your drug use has gone out of your control despite your efforts to stop it?" Rather than trying to push AddictBrain concepts all at once, try to incorporate RMT into therapy sessions bit by bit.

At some point in the treatment process, the light seems to go on. As difficult as it is to contemplate, patients are controlled by an unforeseen force running rip shod through their life. Identifying the agent for all the chaos proves to be calming and centering. Occasionally, the patient or client might arrive at your office completely open to RecoveryMind Training. In such cases, a direct exploration of how these techniques might work for your patient is indicated. Patients might have occasional resistance to specific concepts within RecoveryMind Training. Do not try to push them all at once. Instead, know the concepts they have the most trouble with; exploring these resistance points will often prove valuable later in the therapeutic relationship.

RecoveryMind Training May Be Contraindicated in Patients with Severe Psychiatric Disorders

Individuals with all types of psychological and psychiatric diseases can develop addiction. Patients with several acute and chronic psychiatric conditions should not be treated using the RecoveryMind system. Individuals who suffer from schizophrenia and related illnesses are the most obvious example. The *DSM-5* eliminated schizophrenia subtypes— paranoid, disorganized, catatonic, undifferentiated, and residual. Nonetheless, individuals who exhibit ideas of influence are especially troubled by the AddictBrain/RecoveryMind construct. Patients with depressive illness accompanied by psychotic symptoms should also not use this treatment system until the psychotic symptoms are under control.

In many ways, RMT treats patients as if they have dissociative identity disorder (DID). Using the older term of multiple personality disorder makes this clear. Therefore, it is also contraindicated in patients with DID as it may exacerbate their symptoms. RecoveryMind Training conceptualizes addicted individuals as having two personalities: AddictBrain and their true self. When the disease is active, AddictBrain is winning. More recent research about the brain suggests that we all have cortical centers that fight for control.[36-38] This investigation supports many of the RMT concepts but also begs the question, "Are we not all a bit multiple in our personalities?"

RecoveryMind Training may also be contraindicated in patients who have any disorganized or primitive personality structure, and therapists should tread lightly with such patients. I have noted that some patients with less severe forms of borderline personality disorder do quite well with RMT, however. In these cases, the RMT constructs and clear treatment process helps some patients with borderline personality disorder organize themselves and stay on track to maintain their addiction recovery.

Lastly, patients with limitations to their intellectual capacity may struggle with some of the concepts in RecoveryMind Training. Those who are post-stroke or post-head injury with severe cognitive impairment, language difficulties, or right cortical damage may also not be the best candidates for this treatment model.

Chapter Two Notes

1. E. Stuyt, D. Gundersen, J. Shore, E. Brooks, and M. Gendel, "Tobacco Use by Physicians in a Physician Health Program, Implications for Treatment and Monitoring," *Am J Addict.* 18, no. 2 (2009): 103–08.

2. P. J. Carnes, R. E. Murray, and L. Carpenter, "Addiction Interaction Disorder," Chap. 2 in *Handbook of Addictive Disorders: A Practical Guide to Diagnosis and Treatment*, ed. R. H. Coombs (Hoboken, NJ: John Wiley & Sons, Inc, 2004), 31–62.

3. P. J. Carnes, R. E. Murray, and L. Carpenter, "Bargains with Chaos: Sex Addicts and Addiction Interaction Disorder," *Sexual Addiction & Compulsivity* 12 (2005): 79–120.

4. A. Agrawal, K. J. Verweij, N. A. Gillespie, A. C. Heath, C. N. Lessov-Schlaggar, N. G. Martin, E. C. Nelson, *et al*, "The Genetics of Addiction-a Translational Perspective," *Transl Psychiatry* 2 (2012): e140.

5. NIDA, "Drugs, Brains, and Behavior: The Science of Addiction," Bethesda, MD, 2007.

6. J. R. Pleis, B. W. Ward, and J. W. Lucas, "Summary Health Statistics for U.S. Adults: National Health Interview Survey, 2009," *Vital Health Stat 10*, no. 249 (2010): 1–207.

7. B. F. Grant, D. S. Hasin, S. P. Chou, F. S. Stinson, and D. A. Dawson, "Nicotine Dependence and Psychiatric Disorders in the United States: Results from the National Epidemiologic Survey on Alcohol and Related Conditions," *Arch Gen Psychiatry* 61, no. 11 (2004): 1107–15.

8. E. J. Nestler, "Is There a Common Molecular Pathway for Addiction?" *Nat Neurosci* 8, no. 11 (2005) 1445–49.

9. E. J. Nestler. "Cellular Basis of Memory for Addiction," *Dialogues Clin Neurosci* 15, no. 4 (2013): 431–43.

10. E. J. Nestler, M. Barrot, and D. W. Self, "DeltaFosB: A Sustained Molecular Switch for Addiction," *Proc Natl Acad Sci U S A* 98, no. 20 (2001): 11042–46.

11. E. J. Nestler, "Review. Transcriptional Mechanisms of Addiction: Role of DeltaFosB," *Philos Trans R Soc Lond B Biol Sci* 363, no. 1507 (2008): 3245–55.

12. S. Sussman, N. Lisha, and M. Griffiths, "Prevalence of the Addictions: A Problem of the Majority or the Minority?" *Evaluation & the health professions* 34, no. 1 (2011): 3–56.

13. ASAM, "The Definition of Addiction," ASAM, http://www.asam.org/docs/public-policy-statements/1definition_of_addiction_long_4-11.pdf?sfvrsn=2.

14. In Chapter Five, I will discuss how multiple brain structures are involved in addiction. In that chapter, I will also descibe in considerable depth how our brain is a discriminating engine and how AddictBrain uses this feature to its own ends.

15. G. E. Vaillant, "A 60-Year Follow-up of Alcoholic Men," *Addiction* 98, no. 8 (2003): 1043–51.

16. A. R. Krentzman, E. A. R. Robinson, B. C. Moore, J. F. Kelly, A. B. Laudet, W. L. White, S. E. Zemore, E. Kurtz, and S. Strobbe, "How Alcoholics Anonymous (AA) and Narcotics Anonymous (NA) Work: Cross-Disciplinary Perspectives," *Alcoholism Treatment Quarterly* 29, no. 1 (2010): 75–84.

17. E. Kurtz, *Not-God: A History of Alcoholics Anonymous* (Center City: Hazelden Publishing, 1991).

18. E. Kurtz and K. Ketcham, *The Spirituality of Imperfection: Modern Wisdom from Classic Stories* (New York: Bantam Books, 1992).

19. H. Dermatis, M. T. Guschwan, M. Galanter, and G. Bunt, "Orientation toward Spirituality and Self-Help Approaches in the Therapeutic Community," *J Addict Dis* 23, no. 1 (2004): 39–54.

20. M. Galanter, "Spirituality and Recovery in 12-Step Programs: An Empirical Model," *J Subst Abuse Treat* 33, no. 3 (2007): 265–72.

21. M. Galanter, "Research on Spirituality and Alcoholics Anonymous," *Alcohol Clin Exp Res* 23, no. 4 (1999): 716–19.

22. M. Galanter, "Spirituality and Addiction: A Research and Clinical Perspective," *The American Journal on Addictions* 15, no. 4 (2006): 286–92.

23. M. Galanter, *What Is Alcoholics Anonymous?: A Path from Addiction to Recovery* (Oxford: Oxford University Press, 2016).

24. M. Galanter, H. Dermatis, G. Bunt, C. Williams, M. Trujillo, and P. Steinke, "Assessment of Spirituality and Its Relevance to Addiction Treatment," *J Subst Abuse Treat* 33, no. 3 (2007): 257–64.

25. M. Galanter, H. Dermatis, S. Post, and C. Sampson, "Spirituality-Based Recovery from Drug Addiction in the Twelve-Step Fellowship of Narcotics Anonymous," *J Addict Med* 7, no. 3 (2013): 189–95.

26. M. Galanter, H. Dermatis, J. Stanievich, and C. Santucci, "Physicians in Long-Term Recovery Who Are Members of Alcoholics Anonymous," *The American Journal on Addictions* 22, no. 4 (2013): 323–28.

27. J. Grodzicki, and M. Galanter, "Spirituality and Addiction," *Subst Abus* 26, no. 2 (2005): 1–4.

28. J. Prochaska, *The Transtheoretical Model of Behavior Change. The Handbook of Health Behavior Change*, Second ed. (New York: Springer Publishing Co, 1998).

29. J. P. Carbonari, and C. C. DiClemente, "Using Transtheoretical Model Profiles to Differentiate Levels of Alcohol Abstinence Success," *J Consult Clin Psychol* 68, no. 5 (2000): 810–17.

30. S. Sutton, "Back to the Drawing Board? A Review of Applications of the Transtheoretical Model to Substance Use," *Addiction* 96, no. 1 (2001): 175–86.

31. L. Spencer, F. Pagell, M. E. Hallion, and T. B. Adams, "Applying the Transtheoretical Model to Tobacco Cessation and Prevention: A Review of Literature," *Am J Health Promot* 17, no. 1 (2002): 7–71.

32. R. C. Callaghan, L. Taykor, and J. A. Cunningham, "Does Progressive Stage Transition Mean Getting Better? A Test of the Transtheoretical Model in Alcoholism Recovery," *Addiction* 102, no. 10 (2007): 1588–96.

33. See above, n. 28.

34. J. Prochaska, K. Delucchi, and S. M. Hall, "A Meta-Analysis of Smoking Cessation Interventions with Individuals in Substance Abuse Treatment or Recovery," *J Consult Clin Psychol* 72, no. 6 (2004): 1144–56.

35. S. A. Shumaker, J. K. Ockene, and K. A. Riekert, *The Handbook of Health Behavior Change*, 3rd ed. (New York: Springer Pub. Co., 2009).

36. M. S. Gazzaniga, J. E. LeDoux, M. Gazzaniga, and J. LeDoux, *The Integrated Mind* (New York: Plenum Press, 1978).

37. M. Gazzaniga, *The Social Brain: Discovering the Networks of the Mind* (New York: Basic Books, 1987).

38. J. Jaynes, *The Origin of Conciousness in the Breakdown of the Bicameral Mind* (New York: Houghton Miffin, 1990).

CHAPTER THREE

The History and Neuroscience of Addiction

In this chapter, I will explore our evolving understanding of addiction neuroscience. By examining past beliefs, we can better understand current concepts and prejudices. Many of our current conceptions evolved out of past addiction theories formed in the eighteenth, nineteenth, and early part of the twentieth centuries. You do not need to know the information in this chapter to implement RecoveryMind Training; however, expanding your historical perspective of addiction neuroscience will help you visualize addiction as a biological illness and improve patient care.

Addiction models attempt to clarify our understanding of the disease. Unfortunately, many of the inaccurate elements of past models taint our current perception of this complicated illness. In describing the evolution of these models, I hope to remove the remnants of misperception induced by outdated notions.

I will then examine the current neuroscience of addiction with an eye toward how this scientific information can help individuals recover. The deeper your knowledge of addiction neuroscience, the better equipped you will be to fight side by side with your patients for their lives.

Addiction Models Have Changed Over Time

Public opinion about addiction and its treatment is rich and interwoven with politics, medicine, and social change. Several excellent texts have been written about the history of addiction and its treatment; please refer to them if this chapter stimulates your interest.[1, 2] Along the way, I hope to correct misconceptions about addiction as a disease. Let us start by examining a long-standing controversy in addiction: Is addiction a brain disease of neurochemistry and neurophysiology or a response to emotions, stress, psychological difficulties, psychiatric disease, and other life problems?

Is Addiction a Problem with Bad Feelings or Bad Wiring?

Throughout the history of addiction, theorists have debated very different points of view as to the cause of addiction. To understand what the fuss is all about, it is helpful—and possibly overly simplistic—to divide addiction theory into two opposing camps. I will call the first camp **Biological Theory** and the second camp **Self-Medication Theory**. Biological Theory contends that physical characteristics of certain drugs, when combined with the brain chemistry and wiring of selected people, cause addiction. Whereas Self-Medication Theory contends that addiction is caused by the accumulation of difficult feelings, past trauma or other life events, and intrapsychic conflict. Those with addiction, according to this group, attempt to decrease their internal conflict or modify disquieting emotional states by consuming mood-altering substances; therefore, addiction is an attempt to self-correct what feels conflicted or troubled. Both camps have evolved and changed over time and, to some degree, have merged in recent years. Despite increasing data that support a biological basis of addiction, public opinion has remained in the self-medication camp. When describing addiction, it seems I always hear this bottom line question, "Yes I have heard it described as a biological disease and all that, but what *caused* them to use drugs in the first place?" This tendency to see all our actions arising from cause-

and-effect, when attached to our natural tendency to find reasons for our behavior, prevents us from accepting addiction as a biological disease—one that drives its victim at a brain level deeper than the realm of choice and decision.

When pressured to choose, most people (patients, therapists, and the public) have deep-seated convictions that fall into one of the camps: Biological Theory or Self-Medication Theory. Both camps have something to teach us, so let's examine them more closely. Regardless of your belief, I urge you to keep an open mind.

Biological Theory

Prohibition

Biological Theory regards addiction as a characteristic of drugs or the brain's biochemical response to certain drugs. Supporters of this theory believe there is a physical, often predetermined problem with the brain or body that creates a vulnerability to addiction. The Biological Theory eschews the notion that emotions, trauma, and psychological difficulties *cause* addiction. One early manifestation of the biological disease model emerged from a religious and social movement that gained momentum in the 1840s: the temperance movement.[3] In the mid-1800s, many parts of the world, including the United States, increased production of distilled spirits. The increased supply led to an increased consumption of this more potent form of alcohol. Temperance groups varied on their beliefs about alcohol consumption. One influential but short-lived group was the Washingtonians. They espoused complete abstinence, or teetotalism, as the correct path but limited that belief to their members. At the opposite pole were temperance groups that preached *any* alcohol was dangerous for *anyone* who consumed it. The implicit conclusion from the temperance movement is that alcohol is the cause of inebriety (alcoholism).[4] Although temperance groups may not have agreed with it—the foundation of the movement was religious—this assertion is biological.

As the temperance movement evolved from the 1850s into the early twentieth century, its focus jelled: Anyone who used sufficient alcohol over a period of time would stumble down the predetermined path of self-destruction. They accurately recorded the steps from casual use to eventual depravity and destitution. Alcohol was the problem; therefore, the solution was quite simple. If we eliminate alcohol, society would be free from the moral, societal, and spiritual consequences of "evil spirits."

Parts of temperance evolved into the prohibition movement. Prohibition activated enormous social and legal upheaval in the latter part of the nineteenth and early part of the twentieth century. Prohibition crossed into many areas of life, affecting social values, spiritual beliefs, and eventual legal mandates. Prohibition was also an international phenomenon. In the early 1900s, the governments of Canada, Russia, Iceland, Norway, Hungary, and the United States outlawed the sale and consumption of alcohol for varying lengths of time.[5] As an outgrowth of the temperance movement, prohibition asserted that alcohol is itself a dangerous drug and, as such, it is safest to prohibit everyone from consuming it. The prohibition movement believed one-size-fits-all: any individual who consumes alcohol has the potential to fall into a progressive downhill course. Thus, all people should be prohibited from consuming alcohol.

One of the core problems with prohibition theory is seeing the problem of addiction as an emergent property of alcohol. Alcoholism was seen as a problem that lies outside the individual. It is, quite literally, a drug problem. Prohibition thinking is the earliest and simplest way of seeing the disease as strictly biological. Surprisingly, we see remnants of primitive prohibition thinking in the drug control policies of the United States today.[6] One of the central tenets of interdiction as a drug policy is the sophomoric belief that decreasing the drug supply in the United States will solve the drug problem.[7]

Confusing Physiological Dependence with Addiction

Biological theories evolved to the next stage as we moved past prohibition. Addiction was no longer seen as the unalterable fate of those who consume addicting substances. Instead, it was postulated that addiction would occur if an individual used drugs for a period long enough to induce physical dependence. Individuals who used alcohol for brief periods could discontinue its use without experiencing painful withdrawal. However, any individual who used certain addictive substances long enough to induce physiological dependence would experience withdrawal. The withdrawal would then promote further use—addiction itself.

In the first half of the twentieth century, two drugs were seen as archetypes of addiction: heroin and alcohol. Noting the severity of these withdrawal syndromes, researchers theorized that addiction is caused by the constant attempt to prevent painful withdrawal. The person addicted to heroin, "jonesing for a fix,"[8] feels like he must continue using heroin to survive. The person addicted to alcohol needs to continue drinking to prevent anxiety, shakes, delirium tremens, and seizures. The constant need for either opioids or alcohol drove the persistent desire and hunger to continue using. In short, addiction was caused by physiological dependence.

Physiological dependence to alcohol or opioid drugs such as heroin is easily measured by observation or examination of someone in the withdrawal state. However, not all drugs produce severe subjective withdrawal. Those who use opioids, alcohol, and sedative drugs experience a well-defined and often severe and measurable withdrawal after a period of sustained use. The withdrawal from alcohol and sedative drugs can prove to be life-threatening.[9]

The remnants of this line of thought remain in our addiction definitions today. The term "substance dependence" is itself a misnomer or, at the very least, confusing. Many substances that are addictive produce physiological dependence—the aforementioned alcohol, sedatives, and opioids. Other drugs that create fulminant addiction (e.g., cocaine and amphetamines) do not cause physiological dependence. Thus, the term "dependence" only serves to obfuscate. The confusion appears in the *DSM-IV*, which used the word "dependence" when defining addiction. To make matters worse, the *DSM-IV* used the criteria of physiological dependence—notably tolerance and withdrawal—when defining alcohol dependence (alcohol addiction). Luckily, this confusion is partly corrected in the *DSM-5*. People with binge-type alcohol addiction may be dying from their intense loss of control and may never experience withdrawal, yet they are just as ill as the person with addiction who is a daily drinker. Patients who are addicted to cocaine arrive in my office every day—thin, pale, with an electric disorientation and drug obsession—vehemently asserting they are not addicted to cocaine because they do not use it every day.

I have included the following table that contrasts physiological dependence with addiction.

Table 3.1 - Physiological Dependence versus Addiction

Physiological Dependence	Addiction
Is a characteristic of drugs.	Is a characteristic of people.
Occurs in all individuals who consume certain drugs for a certain length of time.	Occurs in 10 percent of the population.
If craving occurs, it does so during the drug withdrawal timeframe (in nonaddicted individuals).	Craving is tied to many emotional and cognitive triggers, occurring long past the withdrawal time.

For clarity, some addicting drugs produce physiological dependence and some do not. Physiological dependence is a characteristic of drugs, not of people. And most importantly, physiological dependence is not addiction. Despite how far we have come in our understanding of addiction, our past confusion between physiological dependence and addiction lives on in our current culture. Regretfully, this confusion extends to parts of the medical field to this day.

An Increased Number of Drugs

In the first half of the twentieth century, the pharmaceutical industry synthesized and extracted an increasing number of drugs that affect the central nervous system. For example, the first of the barbiturate class of drugs (pentobarbital, secobarbital, butalbital, etc.) was synthesized in 1902. During World War II, the Germans synthesized methamphetamine, and chemists for the Allies synthesized amphetamine. Both sides prescribed these amphetamines to soldiers to assist with combat fatigue. In the 1950s, meprobamate was synthesized; and the first of the benzodiazepine drugs, diazepam, was synthesized in the 1960s. Medicine had an increasing number of chemical tools to adjust brain functioning. Although many of these drugs were abused, widespread misuse of prescription drugs in Western society was yet to come.

The 1960s changed our worldview, promoting the notion that the use of mind-altering chemicals is a personal choice, not one that should be directed or supervised by medical personnel. Our culture was experimenting with an increasing number of mind-altering drugs. Marijuana, lysergic acid diethylamide (LSD), and hallucinogenic plants were used in social settings and to expand our self-awareness and rethink humankind. Some of these drugs have moved into a central place in the drug use culture—notably marijuana—while other drugs have moved to the sidelines. In the early 1970s, many Western cultures began experimenting with psychostimulants as well. Cocaine and amphetamines entered the mainstream.

With many of the drugs introduced during this period, a notable difference in physiological dependence was observed: users of cocaine, methamphetamine, hallucinogens, and marijuana may experience symptoms upon the discontinuance of those drugs, but the withdrawal symptoms were milder and did not follow established syndromes. Prevailing scientific and medical thought during the social upheaval of the 1960s held that a drug could not be addicting if it did not produce a known physical withdrawal syndrome. Users of this panoply of "new" drugs did not experience classic withdrawal syndromes. Thus, our culture and our scientists were lulled into a false belief that using these drugs could not be associated with addiction.

Perhaps the most disturbing consequence of the confusion between physiological dependence and addiction appeared during the cocaine epidemic of the 1970s and 1980s. In the 1980s, a leading textbook of psychiatry declared that cocaine, when used in moderation, was a nonaddicting drug.[10] This incorrect conclusion was published despite the fact that America and the United Kingdom had already experienced a cocaine problem in the early 1900s.[11]

Brain Research Reconsiders Addiction

At the end of the 1970s and in the early 1980s, brain researchers described a different and alarming story. When animals were allowed free access to psychostimulants, especially cocaine, they would use the drug with an ever-increasing hunger and often to the point of exhaustion or death.[12] Research then expanded to take into account these new animal models of compulsive drug use. Psychostimulants, especially cocaine, redefined our theories about how addiction works in the brain.[13] The most important of these theories is the discovery of a unitary reward center. Better defined as the mesolimbic dopamine reward system, several diminutive clusters of neurons (nuclei) are organized in the brain of nearly every higher animal species. These interconnected nuclei, when fired, drive the organism to repeat the inciting event.

Self-Medication Theory

Self-Medication Theory of addiction began during the same era as Biological Theory. Starting in the late 1800s, the concepts and teachings of Sigmund Freud's psychoanalysis permanently changed how we understand ourselves and others, creating what George Makari appropriately labeled a "revolution in mind."[14] Psychoanalytic thought laid the groundwork for a totally different approach to understanding all behaviors, including addiction. Alcohol and other drug use, from a psychoanalytic, and subsequent psychodynamic, perspective is viewed as an attempt to self-regulate the internal conflicts of the psyche.

Emerging from psychodynamic psychiatry, Self-Medication Theory posits that an individual's drug of choice is unconsciously selected in an attempt to self-regulate distressing intrapsychic and emotional states.[15] Edward Khantzian, MD, states that individuals with drug use disorders are "predisposed to addiction because they suffer with painful affect states and related psychiatric disorders."[16] The analytic approach to addiction suggests the process of addiction arrests the development of one's personality; when caught in an addictive process, he or she remains fixed in a regressed state of personality development.

Self-Medication Theory has a strong face value; that is, it seems to fit personal experience and has less objective scientific validation. However, that does not mean self-medication theories of addiction are of no inherent value. In our current era of brain biology, psychoanalytic theories are difficult to study and nearly impossible to prove with controlled studies. Thus, Self-Medication Theory has fallen from favor, replaced by volumes of neuropharmacological addiction research. In RecoveryMind Training, many elements of Self-Medication Theory are used in the later stages of addiction treatment and recovery. See Chapters Four and Ten for further discussion on the use of psychodynamic and self-medication theories in the treatment of addiction.

Is addiction a problem of bad feelings or of bad wiring? My conclusion is that the preponderance of data supports the concept that addiction is caused by bad wiring; it is a biological illness. Individuals with a wide spectrum of life experiences, emotional health, and socioeconomic backgrounds are susceptible to this devastating illness. As the neuroscience of addiction moves forward, emerging data support the notion that abnormalities at the level of neurons and even the genetic control of receptor production lead to addiction vulnerability. There is a general consensus that 40 to 60 percent of the variation in the incidence of alcoholism comes from genetics.[17, 18] Emotional states and our management of them have a distinct role in the treatment of addiction. RecoveryMind Training asserts that maladaptive feelings drive drug use and, at the same time, addiction and pre-addiction experiences create painful feeling states, notably shame. Complex emotional experiences exacerbate and color the quality of each individual's addiction experience; repairing the intrapsychic conflict of the addicted state is essential for a robust recovery.

Why did I spend so much time on this issue? Let's look at three common questions for the answer:

- **Is it an esoteric point we should set aside until scientists get back to us with their confirmatory conclusion?** No. Knowledge that the illness has strong genetic and biological characteristics has practical issues when caring for families.

- **Does information about the biology and genetics of addiction have any practical value in the day-to-day care of patients who suffer from addiction?** Absolutely. Children of alcoholics who swore they would never develop addiction should be heartened by information about addiction genetics. Knowing biological truths makes it easier to accept that addiction is a lifelong illness. Understanding the biological and genetic nature of the disease can ameliorate the crippling effects of self-blame and shame.

- **Should we think of addiction solely as a biological illness?** No. Everyone has many factors that drive substance use, especially in the initial stages. People use alcohol or other drugs in an attempt to manage anxiety, depression, and other problems. Knowing these difficulties helps chart the course of therapy of a given patient.

Several drawbacks come from relying solely on the biological nature of addiction. Inquisitive patients and families have a hunger to know the causative agent in addiction. It is all too easy to hope that knowing this information will make the journey from the depths of addiction to a joyful recovery easier, faster, or more substantive. In reality, knowing the answer is a bit of a booby prize. This knowledge, by itself, is as valuable to recovery as the trinket inside a box of Cracker Jack. However, there is a more precious reason to know and understand addiction neurophysiology: how individuals with alcohol and drug use disorders conceptualize their addictive disease is crucial to sustaining recovery. This is one of the potent effects of RecoveryMind Training—it provides such a framework for recovery. To establish a backdrop for future work with patients or clients, we need a cohesive and lucid model, which necessitates a deeper dive into addiction neuroscience.

The Neuroscience of Addiction

Our knowledge about neuroscience and especially human neuroscience is expanding at an accelerated pace. In the last twenty-five years, there has been an explosion of information that often provides startling insights into the brain and its myriad responses and functions. Much of this explosion has been brought about by the use of new and innovative recording and imaging techniques that record the brain as it executes thoughts, plans actions, and interacts with language and ideas. The imaging techniques are labeled with acronyms, such as PET (positron emission tomography), fMRI (functional magnetic resonance spectroscopy), MRS (magnetic resonance spectroscopy), EMT (electromagnetic tomography), or MEG (magnetoencephalogram). Each of these provides a slightly different portal into the inner workings of the brain; some do so in near real time. Before the invention of this collection of sophisticated imaging technology, science had a limited view of brain functionality; the most accurate techniques came from single and multicellular recordings of the brain's electrical activity. Such recordings have been limited to studies in lower species, including rats, cats, and primates. One notable exception has been limited recording of the human brain during surgery for brain tumors and severe seizure disorders.

How Complicated Is My Brain Anyway?

The human brain is a staggeringly complex organ containing eighty-six billion neurons—roughly twelve times the population of Earth.[19] Each neuron has from hundreds to several thousand synapses, or interconnections. Each of these synapses has hundreds of receptors and chemical modulators. This organizational structure leads to about 86,000,000,000,000 (about 10^{13}) potential brain responses, a number greater than the number of stars in about 250 galaxies. Our current study techniques use either a needle in a haystack approach (e.g., single cell or multi-cell electrical or biochemical recordings) or make expansive and overly generalized conclusions of brain functioning by looking at the metabolism of literally millions of cells (e.g., fMRI studies). With either approach, it is amazing that we are able to estimate what we are thinking.

Using widely varying experimental approaches from different disciplines of study, brain research has begun to coalesce, producing startling insights into brain functioning—despite the astounding complexity of the subject. Functional imaging (e.g., fMRI) is especially valuable in this regard. For example, we now know the human brain is best thought of as a group of specialized components and fewer general purpose computers[20] with a limited number of parallel computation processes.[21] It is beyond the scope of this chapter to explain how each of these experimental tools work and, more importantly, their limitations in understanding complex brains. For more information about the use of these newer techniques in addiction research, please review the articles I have referenced.[22-28]

Addiction Is a Maladaptive Learned Response

The evolution of the brain is the defining characteristic of our species. Our brain is enormously flexible and adaptive. It has allowed us to adjust to our environment, changing our living habits and food acquisition skills. Our curious and constantly learning brain has propelled us to the top of all animal species and, in doing so, allowed us to become masters of our planet—although our benevolent mastery has certainly been called into question lately. We learn new techniques and pass these on to our children using oral and written traditions. We build and create, producing art and beauty for those who live on past our death. Our cultures are varied and nuanced. As a species, we have become quite adept at reading the emotions of others, detecting the subtleties of human interaction with just a glance. Our brain works especially fast in areas that are critical for survival.[29]

One of the central tenets of this book is *when an individual develops addiction, all this wonderful machinery is recruited by addiction, hijacked toward its own ends*. How does this occur? To understand addiction, we must have a passing familiarity with our instinctual brain. All life forms have basic instincts wired into their brains. Instincts are driven by a brain system that has been dubbed "the reward center." More recent research has suggested a more accurate term: the **incentive salience area**. This system prioritizes life-sustaining behavior. The basic instincts tied to the incentive salience center are

1. Maintaining adequate hydration and water access;
2. Ensuring an adequate food supply;
3. Maintaining shelter from cold and excessive heat;
4. Ensuring safety and preserving one's personal life from predators (seen most dramatically in the fight or flight response);
5. Ensuring safety for our family, tribe, or communal group;
6. Engaging in sex to continue the species;
7. Nurturing and protecting our young.

When an event related to any of these high priority or life critical behaviors occurs, the brain jumps into action. Brain centers that regulate these seven essential functions have an immense amount of control over our day-to-day lives. This is especially true if any of these important basic drives are challenged.

As we grow in life, we have many experiences—some minor, others major. We decide on the importance of our experiences based upon hardwired priorities. For example, if we live in a nomadic tribe with limited access to water, we learn how to protect our water supply and find scarce water in an arid environment. We develop rituals based upon the supply of water and teach these rituals to our children so they, too, can survive. These rituals become priorities for the continuation of life. Such priorities command a response; we cannot disregard thirst for too long.

Addicting chemicals create a false high priority event, a signal that commands the same priority as our basic instincts. Using the previous example, once addicted, the brain becomes more skilled at seeking alcohol or other drugs. We learn to protect our supply, ensuring that alcohol and/or other drugs are available, even in a scarce environment.[30] We develop rituals based upon drug or alcohol supply. Drugs appear to have become a priority for the continuation of life. Such priorities command a response; we cannot disregard them once addicted.

Addicting chemicals interact with deep brain centers, the same centers that control instinctual drives that sustain life. These centers reside below the areas of the brain that create conscious thought. This instinctual area of the brain attaches a high priority to drugs that have the capacity to promote addiction; this prioritization is one of the crucial differences in the brain of an individual who is prone to develop addiction, setting him or her apart from a non-addiction-prone individual. The addiction-prone individual experiences something different when he or she uses these substances.

Many patients say, "I knew I was in trouble from the moment I first used X." X could be cocaine, alcohol, narcotics, sex, or gambling. The critical difference is the instinctual response that sets the drug use as dissimilar from all other past experiences. Other patients describe a gradual shift in their priorities and values. They begin with casual alcohol use, for example, and, unbeknownst to their conscious mind, priorities change. Alcohol use gradually grabs the center stage, and patients discard non-alcohol-related activities. Its use incentivizes continued use, creating a series of signals that are marked as salient or important. Those addicted to alcohol experience increasing reward from their alcohol use and less and less with other activities. Discontinuing alcohol commonly causes dysphoria, which drives further use.

Reward drives learning. The unconscious mind of individuals with addiction disorders carefully catalogs information about the surroundings of chemical use, or the addictive behavior, and attaches special significance to those surroundings. The "special significance" to the using environment causes them to return to their "favorite watering hole"—the bar where they stop for a drink on the way home from work. It is not the fixtures, the furniture, the ambiance, or a bar's feng shui that keeps such establishments alive; it is the mind's assertion that "this place is important, wonderful, and meaningful to me in an inexplicable way." This assertion comes from alcohol-induced reward attached to the bar. Crack cocaine smokers attach meaning in this manner, as well. Bizarrely and despite the crime and squalor, crack houses commonly induce the same kind of nostalgic longing in the person addicted to crack cocaine. This sense of meaning and purpose is produced by the reward and the learned significance that occurs in the addicted individual's brain. It is one part of AddictBrain. Decoupling this false sense of importance is a critical part of the recovery process. Left uncorrected, the individual with addiction retreats to a life that feels hollow and empty. An example might illustrate this more clearly.

> *Let's say you have decided to go on a four-day backpacking trip. On the second day, you become lost, slowing down your progress, but find your way back to the trail and are over a day behind your original route. In planning for the trip, you brought just enough food for the four days—to conserve pack weight, of course. Your brain responds by increasing the priority of the food you have left. You ration your meals. Along the hiking trail, you find yourself foraging for food. What started as a pleasant backpacking trip becomes an exercise in survival. The grand sights you were planning to see along the trip become less important now.*

You repeatedly search your backpack in vain for a leftover
morsel of food from previous hikes, despite knowing exactly
what you packed at the beginning of the trip. Basic survival
instincts take over whenever and wherever they are needed
to ensure your continuing survival.

Being addicted is like running out of food but more like running out of food every day. Addicting chemicals hijack the neural circuits in the brain, creating a persistent urgency to use, which causes addicted individuals to ensure alcohol or other chemicals are available, focus day-to-day energy on protecting their supply, set priorities on continued access, and push aside the pleasures of everyday life. Just as one cannot "decide to not make food a priority" when starving, those addicted cannot simply *decide not* to use.

In order for a chemical or set of behaviors to be addictive, they must stimulate the reward center. As you will learn later in this chapter, only a limited set of chemicals we consume during the course of our lives induce addiction. If a chemical does not stimulate the reward center, it will not induce addiction. Consider penicillin, for example. Doctors have used penicillin, and its derivatives, daily for the past seventy years. Despite this, no one has ever developed penicillin addiction.

In a similar manner, only certain behaviors are addicting. I have never seen, nor heard of, anyone addicted to sharpening pencils. Pencil sharpening induces very little response in the reward center of the brain. However, other behaviors can become addictive. With its intermittent reinforcement—the more intermittent the better—gambling is based upon winning money or other objects that can be construed as prizes, which is addicting to some. The driver for gambling addiction is the trigger of the reward response in the brain. By the way, casinos have perfected the stimulation produced by gambling addiction. They know the more intermittent, unpredictable, and multi-sense of the reward, the greater the human reaction. Sexual behaviors also have the potential for becoming addictive. As discussed previously, our sexual response is hardwired; it ensures the continuation of our species. If there was no reward, we might decide to paint the house rather than make love to our spouse. Connecting sex with money or taboo behaviors augments the potential for the sexual behavior to become addictive.

If the Brain Is So Elegant It Must Be Coordinated, Right?

As more and more stories appear about the brain and its numerous and complex functions, science writers are increasingly describing the human brain as "elegant." With all its complexity, we might be tempted to ask, "How do those billions of neurons work together so seamlessly and efficiently?" The direct answer to this question is simple: They don't. Many of the problems we experience as human beings, in fact, arise out of the problems from the brain's construction.[31]

At the center of this design problem is evolution. The sole purpose of each species brain is ensuring survival of the animal. As each increasingly complex species appeared, the continuance of life did not permit a redesign of their brains from the ground up. The brain that evolved to ensure the survival of a reptile is less helpful to the chimpanzee. Parts of the reptilian brain were retained as they evolved into amphibians. Amphibian brain structures remained as they evolved into birds and mammals. And all these evolutionarily older parts remain in the brain of *Homo sapiens*. This evolutionary perspective of the brain—first described by Paul D. MacLean, MD[32]—explains much about the idiosyncratic nature of our thoughts and actions. Evolution prevented a *tabula rasa*[33] redesign of our brain from the ground up. Neural centers from the reptile or amphibian that produce a stereotypical survival response remain in the brain of the chimpanzee—and even *Homo sapiens*. The very brain components that helped our evolutionary ancestors survive cripple us today with brain inefficiency. Older circuits that produce stereotypic responses have to be manipulated or suppressed by newer overlying complex systems in our more sophisticated brains. The result is a kludge or Rube Goldberg apparatus.

To manage this complex kludge, more evolutionarily recent and complex brain centers have to spend an enormous amount of time modulating and suppressing older circuits from our biological ancestors. This makes the brain inefficient and, more importantly, engenders conflict. Human beings struggle with internal battles about their intentions, decisions, and actions. "Should I eat that piece of cake or walk away from the table at the end of the meal? Should I go with my feelings in that meeting, or should I do my best to negotiate an outcome that would be best for all participants?" We experience these brain conflicts as clashes between urges and principles, impulses and carefully laid plans, and selfish desires and our ethical values.

The layer upon layer nature of our human brain has so many opposing and conflicted circuits that some theoreticians have remarked that it is a wonder we are able to function at all.[34] As you will see in future chapters, AddictBrain takes advantage of this complexity for its own ends. AddictBrain creates conflicts in deep brain centers that challenge the fiber of those so afflicted. In fact, AddictBrain exaggerates normal everyday conflicts, keeping its victims confused and off guard. The result of this conflict is simple: AddictBrain wins at its host's expense.

Finding the Biological Center of Addiction

The search for the brain basis of addiction began in the 1950s when two brain researchers, James Olds and Peter Milner, discovered a specific area of the brain they later labeled "the pleasure center." Olds and Milner, placing electrodes in various areas of the rat brain, stumbled upon one that resulted in intense reinforcement.[35] That is, the animals would press a lever over and over to obtain short, low intensity electrical stimulation. The experimental design placed rodents in an operant training box,[36] also known as a Skinner Box. The electrodes were affixed to the rat's skull in a manner that provided electrical stimulation, limited to discrete locations within its brain. In the box, a lever was affixed to one wall. When the rat pushed the lever, the dose of electric current simulated the discharge of nerve cells in that conscripted area. Using this experimental design, Olds and Milner noted that rats showed no tendency to press the stimulation bar when electrodes were placed in most areas of the brain. One small area was a notable exception.

When the electrodes were placed in several areas of the hypothalamus, especially the mesolimbic pathway, the rats would repeatedly press the bar at high frequencies for prolonged periods of time.[37] When left connected to this lever-pressing system, the laboratory rats would self-administer stimulation to this one specific brain location in preference to food and water. The rats would continue pressing the lever to the point of exhaustion or even death. Electrodes placed in the same location in human beings produce similar experiences.[38, 39] The conclusion of these researchers was that the electrical discharge produced intense pleasure. This location in the brain—better localized to the mesolimbic pathway and the nucleus accumbens—was called the "pleasure center." The early work of Olds and Milner provided clues for subsequent research on the neurobiology of addiction; the rat behavior was strikingly reminiscent of human behavior once an individual becomes addicted.[40]

Most clinicians and researchers from the 1950s to the 1970s believed the driving source of addiction was the addicted person's constant hunger to use his drug to ward off drug withdrawal. These beliefs were challenged by the social climate in the 1970s. Cocaine use was escalating; increasingly, social researchers were identifying drug use patterns in cocaine users that were quite similar to alcohol and heroin addiction. Interestingly, individuals who developed an addictive pattern of cocaine use did not exhibit classical physiological withdrawal upon stopping or in between cocaine binges. This led to considerable confusion regarding the drug cocaine; was it addictive or not? Even as late as 1980, the

Comprehensive Textbook of Psychiatry stated that "taken no more than two or three times per week, cocaine creates no serious problems."[41]

Sociologists depicted a different pattern, however. Cocaine use, especially the smokable form of cocaine known as crack, devastated lives and drastically increased violent crimes in the United States during this period.[42] Although cocaine and crack cocaine did not produce the same withdrawal phenomena seen in previously studied drugs, its addictive qualities were undeniable. An improved paradigm for the brain basis of addiction was needed.

Partly in response to the increased experimentation with stimulant drugs, researchers designed experiments around the stimulant drugs amphetamine and cocaine. They administered extremely small doses of these drugs to localized areas of the rat brain. Experiments demonstrated that rats would continuously administer stimulant drugs in a pattern that was indistinguishable from the addictive behavior of human beings. Addiction theory added a positive reinforcement model (seeking pleasure from drugs) to the existing negative reinforcement model (attempting to decrease the pain of withdrawal).[43] A more complete picture of addiction evolved in the 1980s as cocaine use became an expanding epidemic, encompassing a wider spectrum of American society.

The Positive Reinforcement Theory of addiction also began to question Self-Medication Theory. Animals who had not been subjected to any stressors or traumas would seek certain drugs of abuse. The social backdrop of this era shows striking similarities: In the 1960s, the United States was in a time of self-examination of meaning and values. Some may argue that in the 1970s our culture moved to hedonistic self-centeredness. Our social makeup mirrored expanding concepts about addiction. Addiction was no longer limited to a response to depression, oppression, trauma, loss, or even the negative effects of drug withdrawal. Addiction had something to do with pleasure seeking gone awry.

The animal research in the 1980s, when combined with the human phenomenology of cocaine addiction, led to the "dopamine depletion hypothesis."[44] In this hypothesis, rising levels of dopamine in the neural circuits first described by Olds triggered the euphoria of drug use. The subsequent depletion of dopamine from intense binges resulted in the drug hunger and craving so characteristic of the binge cycle seen in cocaine addiction.[45] Dopamine moved to center stage. The theories of addiction research and its clinicians moved from the "negative reinforcement" model of addiction to the "positive reinforcement" produced by drugs and in an extremely small, primitive but powerful area of the brain described as the mesolimbic dopamine circuit.

Despite the caution by several laboratories,[46] clinicians began describing addiction simply as an abnormality of the reward (and thus pleasure) circuits in the brain. A more balanced view suggested that both negative and positive reinforcement played a hand in the genesis and maintenance of the addicted state.[47] The area of the brain known as the ventral tegmental area (VTA), the mesolimbic pathway, and the nucleus accumbens were seen as the major players in altering the reward response and driving addiction in those so afflicted.

Beginning with the work of Olds and Milner, expanded by research into the negative reinforcement properties of substance withdrawal, and finally the discovery of the reward center established a solid brain-based theory of addiction. By the end of the twentieth century, addiction neuroscientists asserted, "Addiction is best conceptualized as a disease of brain reward centers that ensure the survival of a species."[48]

One other small but important area of confusion remained. In the laboratory, the effects of addictive drugs were labeled as reward behaviors. Scientists could not interview the rats and ask them if they felt pleasure, instead they recorded their behavior as identical to other reward behaviors.[49] In the treatment community, this reward response became confused with the human notion of pleasure. We assume when something is rewarding (i.e., it drives the animal to repeat the previous sequence of events) then it is pleasurable. Newer research suggests that reward is not synonymous with pleasure. The decoupling of reward and pleasure is one of the central tenets of RecoveryMind Training.

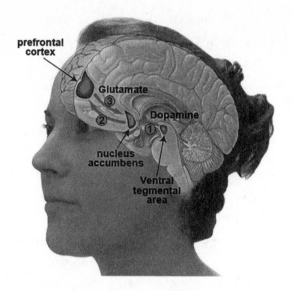

**Figure 3.1 - The ventral tegmental area, nucleus
accumbens, and the prefrontal cortex** (Image courtesy
of NeuroScience, Inc. www.neuroscience.com)

The last twenty years of addiction research have consolidated the position of Biological Theory. At the center of the research from the 1990s and 2000s was the notion that abnormalities in the reward center, either from genetic or environmental origins, created a vulnerable state in the brain. This vulnerable state was then exploited by drug use, which caused further deterioration in goal seeking and the addiction-related behaviors. Research confirmed a whole litany of drugs of abuse stimulated the reward center. In 2005, a unifying hypothesis of the neural circuitry of addiction was postulated by Eric J. Nestler, MD, PhD.[50] Additional work postulated molecular biological mechanisms felt to be at the core of the lifelong irreversible nature of the human addiction experience.[51, 52] The neurotransmitter dopamine is the central signaling chemical in the reward center. More recent research suggests that multiple subtypes of dopamine receptors are involved in the genesis of addiction, including the dopamine D_3 receptor.[53, 54]

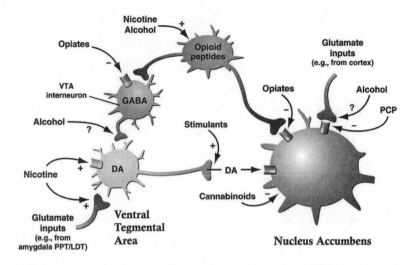

Figure 3.2 - Addicting drugs and their interaction with the ventral tegmental area and nucleus accumbens (Adapted from E. J. Nestler, "Is There a Common Molecular Pathway for Addiction?" Nat. Neurosci 8, no. 1445–49 (2005))

Despite advances in neuroscience, addiction is not caused solely by bad circuits—a literal interpretation of Biological Theory. Human beings begin using addictive substances and relapse due to any number of reasons, ranging from experimentation, stress, and reemerging trauma to environmental exposure to drug cues, as well as a broad spectrum of emotional experiences and memories. Individuals relapse over loss and grief, anger and hurt, and, surprisingly, accomplishments and joy. For the purposes of this book, Biological Theory is helpful when describing the causation or etiology of addiction, but the self-medication hypothesis continues to be useful when teaching individuals relapse prevention techniques and other recovery skills.

More than One Biological Theory

As research into the brain circuitry has expanded in the last twenty years, researchers have increased their focus on how brain changes induce the intensely driven, yet complex, nature of the addiction drive. In the past twenty years, models have divided into three basic camps:

- The opponent process theory, first described by Richard L. Solomon, PhD,[55] and later proposed as a model for addiction neurophysiology by George F. Koob, PhD, and Michel Le Moal, MD, PhD (among others)[56, 57]
- The aberrant habit learning addiction theory championed by Barry Everitt, PhD, Trevor W. Robbins, PhD, and several others[58, 59]
- The incentive sensitization model of Kent Berridge, PhD and Terry E. Robinson, PhD[60–63]

The **opponent process model** asserts that the rewarding effects of a drug or addicting behavior drives initial drug use, but continued use decreases the proper functioning of the brain's reward system. As his addiction progresses, the individual attempts to correct this decrease in natural rewards by increasing the frequency and amount of alcohol and/or other drug use. In between uses, those with addiction develop withdrawal symptoms, stress, and a chronic dysphoria that appears to be repaired by continued use. This removes the brake from continued use, and the user soon finds him- or herself in a vicious cycle of addiction. To see the opponent process model in action, all you have to do is sit beside someone in acute withdrawal and listen to her anguish and yearning.

The **aberrant learning model** posits that drugs of abuse "enhance positive learning and memory about the drug while inhibiting learning about the negative consequences of drug use."[64] Aberrant learning shifts the thoughts and behaviors of those addicted toward continued use as a result of learning. At the same time, faulty learning keeps them from properly assessing the damage created by their use. Although individuals with addiction become poor judges of their own situation, they retain their critical analysis of others. For example, I worked in therapy with a physician who was addicted to alcohol (we will call him Dan). He said this:

> I started smoking pot in college. I never drank much, and
> my father was an alcoholic and wound up drinking himself
> to death. I told myself I would never do that. Then, when

my marriage began to deteriorate, I decided smoking marijuana would help me relax. After coming home from a hard day at work, I would smoke weed and go listen to music with my headphones on, blocking the outside world. As time progressed, these moments became the best time of my day.

When I asked whether smoking marijuana caused problems in his marriage, Dan stated

No, it is not making things worse. I find I have more patience with my wife after I smoke pot. For a while, I was thinking about divorce but I think weed has mellowed me out—now I can tolerate her tirades.

Then I asked his wife to join the session. She was a lovely woman who was in marked distress over his distancing through marijuana use. She described the situation like this:

He arrives home quite irritable. He goes out to the garage and smokes pot every evening while I make dinner. Then he comes in from the garage, grabs a plate, and goes to the den to put on his headphones. We never sit together and have dinner anymore. After a while, he leaves the den and comes at me with a litany of complaints. At first, I thought I was the problem. I should be more patient and interested in his day. After a while, I came to the realization that every conversation was a veiled invitation to his caustic tirades. I never thought I would say this but I am considering divorce.

I gently brought this information to Dan, indicating that his wife sees him as more difficult now because he smokes pot so often. With surgical precision, he let me know of every one of his wife's faults and how they, not he, were the root cause of their marital distress. This illustrates the inability to learn the negative consequences about substance use—a good example of the aberrant learning model.

The **incentive salience model** states that the nervous system, with repeated drug use, increases its reactivity to the drug experience. It further states the drug-induced changes hijack functions of adaptation that are part of the brain's natural adaptation to changing environments and situations. The changes, postulated to occur due to incentive salience, sensitize the brain to drug- or alcohol-related phenomenon. This, in turn, causes the individual to attach salience to the process and circumstances of drug procurement and use. These stimuli become increasingly relevant, attractive, and desired. Because such stimuli take center stage, drug seeking continues. Drugs of abuse are powerful and unforgiving instructors. Ask anyone addicted to cocaine to describe his first significant cocaine high—watch the look of wonderment on his face and excitement in his voice. You will observe the bodily manifestations of incentive salience.

Each model describes part of the clinical and biological effects of addiction. In many ways, these theories are complementary and, at least phenomenologically, mutually inclusive. Current research cannot champion or eliminate any of these three presiding theories, but recent work has suggested that the opponent process model might have a bit of an edge.[65, 66]

In Chapter Four, I will discuss the phenomenon of AddictBrain and how addiction rearrange one's thoughts, goals, memories, and behaviors to keep addiction alive. I will follow this discussion with additional information on the neuroscience of AddictBrain in Chapter Five.

Chapter Three Notes

1. W. L. White, *Slaying the Dragon: The History of Addiction Treatment and Recovery in America* (Bloomington: Chestnut Health Systems/Lighthouse Institute, 1998).

2. S. W. Tracy, *Alcoholism in America: From Reconstruction to Prohibition* (Baltimore: Johns Hopkins University Press, 2005).

3. Ibid.

4. Many names were used for alcoholism during this century, including intemperance, inebriety, and dipsomania.

5. See above, n. 1.

6. P. Cohen, "Re-Thinking Drug Control Policy: Historical Perspectives and Conceptual Tools," in *Palais des Nations, Symposium The crisis of social development in 1990's* (Geneva: United Nations Research Institute for Social Development (UNRISD), 1993).

7. A. Cloud, "Cocaine, Demand, and Addiction: A Study of the Possible Convergence of Rational Theory and National Policy," *Vanderbilt Law Review* 42 (1989): 725–88.

8. The phrase "to Jones" or "Jonesing" appeared in the mid-1960s. Its origin is unclear. The Oxford English Dictionary states it comes from Jones Alley in Manhattan, an area where the drug trade flourished. An interesting discussion of the word appears in the 2003 New York Times: http://www.nytimes.com/2003/05/11/magazine/the-way-we-live-now-on-language-jonesing.html.

9. In contrast, the withdrawal from opioid drugs is not life threatening in a reasonably healthy person. The individual with opioid addiction may feel like he or she is going to die during withdrawal (or may even want to die) but death is an extremely rare complication of opioid withdrawal.

10. F. H. Gawin and H. D. Kleber, "Evolving Conceptualizations of Cocaine Dependence," *Yale J Biol Med* 61, no. 2 (1988): 123–36.

11. D. Musto, "Americas First Cocaine Epidemic," *The Wilson Quarterly* 13, no. 3 (1989): 59–64.

12. R. Pickens and W. C. Harris, "Self-Administration of d-Amphetamine by Rats," *Psychopharmacologia* 12, no. 2 (1968): 158–63.

13. R. A. Wise and M. A. Bozarth, "A Psychomotor Stimulant Theory of Addiction," *Psychol Rev* 94, no. 4 (1987): 469–92.

14. G. Makari, *Revolution in Mind: The Creation of Psychoanalysis* (New York: Harper, 2008).

15. E. J. Khantzian, *Treating Addiction as a Human Process* (Northvale, NJ: Jason Aronson, 1999).

16. E. J. Khantzian, "The Self-Medication Hypothesis of Addictive Disorders: Focus on Heroin and Cocaine Dependence," *Am J Psychiatry* 142, no. 11 (1985): 1259–64.

17. T. Foroud, H. J. Edenberg, and J. C. Crabbe, "Genetic Research: Who Is at Risk for Alcoholism?" *Alcohol Res Health* 33, no. 1–2 (2010): 64–75.

18. NIAAA Staff, "The Genetics of Alcoholism," *Alcohol Alert* 60, July 2003 (2003): 1–3.

19. S. Herculano-Houzel, "The Human Brain in Numbers: A Linearly Scaled-up Primate Brain," *Front Hum Neurosci* 3 (2009): 31.

20. N. Kanwisher, "Functional Specificity in the Human Brain: A Window into the Functional Architecture of the Mind," *Proc Natl Acad Sci U S A* 107, no. 25 (2010): 11163–70.

21.   H. V. Georgiou, "Estimating the Intrinsic Dimension in fMRI Space Via Dataset Fractal
       Analysis - Counting the 'Cpu Cores' of the Human Brain," *arXiv:1410.7100* (2014): 27.

22.   J. S. Fowler, N. D. Volkow, C. A. Kassed, and L. Chang, "Imaging the Addicted Human
       Brain," *Science & Practice Perspectives* 3, no. 2 (2007): 4–16.

23.   N. D. Volkow, J. S. Fowler, G. J. Wang, J. M. Swanson, and F. Telang, "Dopamine in Drug
       Abuse and Addiction: Results of Imaging Studies and Treatment Implications," *Arch
       Neurol* 64, no. 11 (2007): 1575–9.

24.   S. J. Gatley, N. D. Volkow, G. J. Wang, J. S. Fowler, J. Logan, Y. S. Ding, and M. Gerasimov,
       "Pet Imaging in Clinical Drug Abuse Research," *Curr Pharm Des* 11, no. 25 (2005):
       3203–19.

25.   N. D. Volkow, J. S. Fowler, G. J. Wang, and J. M. Swanson, "Dopamine in Drug Abuse and
       Addiction: Results from Imaging Studies and Treatment Implications," *Mol Psychiatry* 9,
       no. 6 (2004): 557–69.

26.   N. D. Volkow, J. S. Fowler, and G. J. Wang, "The Addicted Human Brain Viewed in the
       Light of Imaging Studies: Brain Circuits and Treatment Strategies," *Neuropharmacology*
       47 Suppl 1 (2004): 3–13.

27.   N. D. Volkow, J. S. Fowler, G. J. Wang, and R. Z. Goldstein, "Role of Dopamine, the
       Frontal Cortex and Memory Circuits in Drug Addiction: Insight from Imaging Studies,"
       Neurobiol Learn Mem 78, no. 3 (2002): 610–24.

28.   M. Buhler, and K. Mann, "Alcohol and the Human Brain: A Systematic Review of
       Different Neuroimaging Methods," *Alcohol Clin Exp Res* (2011).

29.   M. Gladwell, *Blink: The Power of Thinking without Thinking*. 1st Back Bay trade pbk. ed.
       (New York: Back Bay Books, 2007).

30.   My patients tell me that they can arrive in a new city, even in a foreign country, and
       simply ride around in a cab to find drugs. When they arrive in a neighborhood where
       drugs are available for purchase, they instinctively know it. They get out of the cab and
       walk around for a bit, sensing who to approach. They are rarely wrong—almost always
       successful at procuring drugs to protect their supply.

31.   D. Linden, *The Accidental Mind: How Brain Evolution Has Given Us Love, Memory,
       Dreams, and God* (Cambridge, MA: Belknap Press of Harvard University Press, 2007).

32.   P. D. MacLean, *The Triune Brain in Evolution: Role in Paleocerebral Functions* (New York:
       Plenum Press, 1990).

33.   *Tabla rasa* loosely translates into English as "clean slate." In this case, I am refering to
       scrapping old designs and rebuilding the computational networks of the brain from
       scratch.

34.   M. L. Minsky, *The Society of Mind* (New York: Simon and Schuster, 1986).

35.   J. Olds and P. Milner, "Positive Reinforcement Produced by Electrical Stimulation of
       Septal Area and Other Regions of Rat Brain," *J Comp Physiol Psychol* 47, no. 6 (1954):
       419–27.

36.   B. F. Skinner, *Science and Human Behavior* (New York: Macmillan, 1953).

37.   See above, n. 35.

38.   R. G. Heath, "Electrical Self-Stimulation of the Brain in Man," *Am J Psychiatry* 120
       (1963): 571–7.

39.   R. Heath, "Pleasure and Brain Activity in Man. Deep and Surface
       Electroencephalograms During Orgasm," *J Nerv Ment Dis* 154, no. 1 (1972): 3–18.

40. J. Olds, "Self-Stimulation of the Brain; Its Use to Study Local Effects of Hunger, Sex, and Drugs," *Science* 127, no. 3294 (1958): 315–24.

41. B. J. Grinspoon L. "Drug Dependence: Non-Narcotic Agents," in *Comprehensive Textbook of Psychiatry, Third ed.*, eds. A. M. Freedman, H. I. Kaplan, B. J. Sadock (Baltimore: Williams and Wilkins, 1980).

42. J. A. Inciardi, *The War on Drugs: Heroin, Cocaine, Crime, and Public Policy* (Palo Alto, CA: Mayfield Pub. Co., 1986).

43. M. Gold, A. Washton, and C. Dackis, "Cocaine Abuse: Neurochemistry, Phenomenology and Treatment," in *Cocaine Use in America: Epidemiologic & Clinical Perspectives*, eds. E. H. Adams, N. J. Kozel (Rockville, MD: NIDA Research Monograph, 1985), 130–50.

44. C. A. Dackis and M. S. Gold, "New Concepts in Cocaine Addiction: The Dopamine Depletion Hypothesis," *Neurosci Biobehav Rev* 9, no. 3 (1985): 469–77.

45. C. Dackis and C. O'Brien, "Neurobiology of Addiction: Treatment and Public Policy Ramifications," *Nat Neurosci* 8, no. 11 (2005): 1431–6.

46. K. C. Berridge and T. E. Robinson, "Parsing Reward," *Trends Neurosci* 26, no. 9 (2003): 507–13.

47. G. F. Koob and M. Le Moal, "Plasticity of Reward Neurocircuitry and the 'Dark Side' of Drug Addiction," *Nat Neurosci* 8, no. 11 (2005): 1442–4.

48. C. A. Dackis and C. P. O'Brien, "Cocaine Dependence: A Disease of the Brain's Reward Centers," *J Subst Abuse Treat* 21, no. 3 (2001): 111–7.

49. Drug induced reward behaviors are very similar to other reward responses in animals. The only notable differences are intensity and priority. The response to addicting drugs is more aggressive than natural rewards. In addition, the response to addicting drugs overrides natural rewards. Animals given free access to cocaine will disregard food, water, and sex, often using to the point of exhaustion or death.

50. E. J. Nestler, "Is There a Common Molecular Pathway for Addiction?" *Nat Neurosci* 8, no. 11 (2005): 1445–49.

51. E. J. Nestler, "Review. Transcriptional Mechanisms of Addiction: Role of DeltaFosB," *Philos Trans R Soc Lond B Biol Sci* 363, no. 1507 (2008): 3245–55.

52. E. J. Nestler, M. Barrot, and D. W. Self, "DeltaFosB: A Sustained Molecular Switch for Addiction," *Proc Natl Acad Sci USA* 98, no. 20 (2001): 11042–6.

53. D. Erritzoe, A. Tziortzi, D. Bargiela, A. Colasanti, G. E. Searle, R. N. Gunn, J. D. Beaver, *et al*, "In Vivo Imaging of Cerebral Dopamine D_3 Receptors in Alcoholism," *Neuropsychopharmacology* 39, no. 7 (2014): 1703–12.

54. C. A. Heidbreder, E. L. Gardner, Z. X. Xi, P. K. Thanos, M. Mugnaini, J. J. Hagan, and C. R. Ashby, Jr., "The Role of Central Dopamine D_3 Receptors in Drug Addiction: A Review of Pharmacological Evidence," *Brain Res Brain Res Rev* 49, no. 1 (2005): 77–105.

55. R. L. Solomon and J. D. Corbit, "An Opponent-Process Theory of Motivation: I. Temporal Dynamics of Affect," *Psychol Rev* 81, no. 2 (1974): 119.

56. G. F. Koob and M. Le Moal, "Drug Addiction, Dysregulation of Reward, and Allostasis," *Neuropsychopharmacology* 24, no. 2 (2001): 97–129.

57. G. F. Koob and M. Le Moal, "Neurobiological Mechanisms for Opponent Motivational Processes in Addiction," *Philosophical Transactions of the Royal Society of London B: Biological Sciences* 363, no. 1507 (2008): 3113–23.

58. B. J. Everitt, A. Dickinson, and T. W. Robbins, "The Neuropsychological Basis of Addictive Behaviour," *Brain Res Brain Res Rev* 36, no. 2–3 (2001): 129–38.

59.   M. M. Torregrossa, P. R. Corlett, and J. R. Taylor, "Aberrant Learning and Memory in Addiction," *Neurobiol Learn Mem* 96, no. 4 (2011): 609–23.

60.   T. E. Robinson and K. C. Berridge, "The Neural Basis of Drug Craving: An Incentive-Sensitization Theory of Addiction," *Brain Res Brain Res Rev* 18, no. 3 (1993): 247–91.

61.   K. C. Berridge, "The Debate over Dopamine's Role in Reward: The Case for Incentive Salience," *Psychopharmacology (Berl)* 191, no. 3 (2007): 391–431.

62.   K. C. Berridge and T. E. Robinson, "What Is the Role of Dopamine in Reward: Hedonic Impact, Reward Learning, or Incentive Salience?" *Brain Res Brain Res Rev* 28, no. 3 (1998): 309–69.

63.   K. C. Berridge, T. E. Robinson, and J. W. Aldridge, "Dissecting Components of Reward: 'Liking', 'Wanting', and Learning," *Curr Opin Pharmacol* 9, no. 1 (2009): 65–73.

64.   See above, n. 59.

65.   D. Caprioli, D. Calu, and Y. Shaham, "Loss of Phasic Dopamine: A New Addiction Marker?" *Nat Neurosci* 17, no. 5 (2014): 644–6.

66.   I. Willuhn, L. M. Burgeno, P. A. Groblewski, and P. E. Phillips, "Excessive Cocaine Use Results from Decreased Phasic Dopamine Signaling in the Striatum," *Nat Neurosci* 17, no. 5 (2014): 704–9.

What Is AddictBrain?

Do I contradict myself?
Very well then I contradict myself,
(I am large, I contain multitudes.)
WALT WHITMAN

Addiction is such a complex illness; it befuddles patients and caregivers alike. As such, it is easy to give up hope of ever understanding the disease and the way out of the addiction maelstrom. RecoveryMind Training and the AddictBrain concept can offer a way out of this confusion. AddictBrain is a thought model, or a framework, of the mind that develops once it has succumbed to the ravages of addiction. RecoveryMind Training gathers the current hodgepodge of treatment approaches into a cohesive whole. The combination of the AddictBrain concept and RecoveryMind Training is powerful. This combination has a sole purpose: deconstructing the effects of addiction and constructing a new life in recovery.

But before we chart a course forward into RecoveryMind Training, we must take a hard look at how our current models of addiction treatment fall short. People who have limited experience with friends or relatives with addiction see the solution as a straightforward task: just stop drinking. Their use of alcohol, other drugs, or addictive behaviors has increased over a series of months or years, and now it handicaps or threatens their life. If they stop, all will return to normal, yes?

In reality, the recovering person must learn how to stop a complex cascade of thoughts, emotions, predicted responses, and drives. As with all things, the devil is in the details. But what does this really mean? In what ways are people altered? What types of thoughts are relatively intact, and which are grossly disturbed? How is motivation changed? How are their goals and value sets different? How is experience or learning altered? What types of memories have been injected deep into the neural circuits of the brain, and what are the consequences of these memories in his or her future recovery? These questions are the subject of the next two chapters.

Addiction produces a rich and multifaceted set of neural changes that confuse and befuddle the conscious mind. We call the sum of all these effects **AddictBrain**. The remainder of this section examines the physical, intellectual, emotional, and spiritual losses that are the components of the AddictBrain concept. More importantly, I will discuss the things addiction puts into the mind: an array of feelings, thoughts, ideas, and behaviors whose single aim is self-preservation.[1] Self-preservation here does not refer to the welfare of the individual. It refers to the preservation of an autonomous pattern of thought, a foreign invader that seizes more of an individual's personality and soul over time. AddictBrain is interested in its own self-preservation—the continuance of the addicted state. AddictBrain does this by reprogramming the mind to ensure its own preservation. The individual with addiction becomes a hapless victim; he or she is "along for the ride." We do know, in fact, that preservation of the individual is not the goal of AddictBrain because addiction is often fatal. What addiction puts into the brain is more important than the loss of brain functioning produced by the toxic effects of substances.

Origins of the AddictBrain Model

I have been working for over thirty years with patients who suffer from addiction and all its manifestations. Early on in my work, I wondered how seemingly normal individuals from all walks of life and with varied backgrounds appeared to regress into the same self-destructive and truly dumbfounding behavior. Psychiatrists, psychologists, and social scientists from all fields of study have their own, often well-researched, theories on why addictive behaviors occur. What struck me was that every individual—whether he or she is addicted to alcohol, cocaine, or gambling—repeated the same self-abusive and destructive sequence of behaviors. Every victim of the disease would become obsessed with using, stop other life activities, alienate loved ones, and have obsessions and compulsions to find the time, place, and money to continue his or her slow suicide. Formerly honest and ethical individuals would cross their every moral and ethical boundary to continue their habit. They would compromise their physical, emotional, interpersonal, and spiritual values blindly in an all-consuming need to feed their addictive hunger.

Clinicians would write about this destructive process, metaphorically shaking their heads with concern about the damage wrought by addiction on patients and their families. When I entered the field of addiction medicine, the prevailing thought was that addiction was an erratic and unpredictable disease. As a scientist and physician, giving up on understanding a disease—no matter how complex— troubled me. Was addiction capricious and unknowable? Little did I know that my addiction training would soon be turned on its ear.

I was fortunate to have amazing mentors. None were more brilliant and out-of-the-box as Thomas Butcher, PhD. Dr. Butcher eschewed cultural norms—I can still see him waving his hand dismissively when addressed as Doctor, saying, "Call me Tom." When he returned to my office, after previously vanishing from sight for a number of years, one of my new staff members warily poked her head into my office and said, "Dr. Earley, I hate to bother you, but there is a very nice man out front who says he knows you." She was quiet for a moment, bit her lip, and then added, "He looks like he might be homeless." Arriving in an ancient Volkswagen Beetle, Tom quietly walked in, still lost in thought with holes in his tennis shoes, his long, wavy hair askew. As he arrived in my office, I remembered his quixotic smile. It was as if life was singularly amusing, and he knew why. Tom was a genius.

Dr. Butcher taught me to visualize the mind—once addiction takes hold—as engaged in a game of espionage. It is full of double agents, double crosses, stealth attacks, and, at its core, committed to a mission deadly to its host. Addiction is like living in a neighborhood with constant covert actions. Its double agents trick its victim into thinking all is normal; however, hidden in the mind's neighborhood are deeply subversive, self-annihilating drives, operating beyond one's ability to recognize or comprehend. Most importantly, the espionage continues for years into abstinence and recovery. While in the throes of his or her addiction, the patient remains the unknowing victim of a brain bent on destroying its host.

AddictBrain and RecoveryMind Training evolved from Dr. Butcher's initial training. Dr. Butcher's thinking, revolutionary at the time, shunned conventional norms. He knew the person struggling with addiction, an unsuspecting victim of a hidden and complex malady, could not solve his or her problems by insight alone. However, he taught me that curiosity was an important tool for the patient and the therapist when battling the disease. He spoke of *the disease* in a new and radical way. He encouraged patients and therapists alike to see addiction as being distinct from one's true self. He stressed the importance of differentiating the individual from their addictive thoughts and labeling maladaptive concepts and urges as arising from the dark force of "the disease." He pointed out that, when addicted, a person's many thoughts cease being his or her own. This frightening notion, that AddictBrain is literally "not us" rather a foreign invader, is at the core of RecoveryMind Training. Importantly, this notion opens the door to a way of understanding addiction that is powerful and regenerative.

Among the things Tom taught me, none was more powerful than listening to the patient with curiosity and an open mind. I would listen to my patient's validating phrases he heard from others, such as "An addict alone is in bad company" or "An alcoholic at home alone is behind enemy lines." And a phrase, attributed to author and comedian, Mark Lundholm always stayed with me: "First thought wrong." Such phrases helped me listen with a different set of ears. One day, a new patient arrived in my office, desperate for help. These sentences stood out from a longer tale of wholesale destruction:

> *It slowly dawned on me that I might have an alcohol problem. I decided to quit. I managed to stop for five days. When I finally gave in on day six, I wound up drinking myself into a stupor. That was when it really got bad, days of barely holding on, alternating with ferocious binges that seemed bent on killing me.*

I began visualizing addiction as a foreign intruder, a mind virus, and an insidious interloper that so subtly and skillfully alters the course of one's life—so much so that its victim never sees it coming. Most importantly, it dawned upon me that when its victim tries to contain his or her illness, AddictBrain fights back.

At first glance, the moniker AddictBrain might seem negative. Patients who are reluctant to accept the depth of their disease might have problems using the term AddictBrain. Ultimately, I felt this term was the best for two reasons. One, it is clear. Two, it does not mince words or try to make nice of a dark force.

Over the ensuing years, I added Tom's seminal teachings to this evolving thought experiment. The more I used the tools in this book, the more quickly my patients were able to peel back their façade of self-sufficiency and self-control. These efforts helped construct the antidote to AddictBrain: RecoveryMind. Finally, after coming to the conclusion that the best framework for treatment is that it involves internalization of a complex set of skills, I dubbed the treatment process: RecoveryMind Training.

AddictBrain Is Not Simply Drug Toxicity

It might be tempting to consider AddictBrain as the product of the toxic effects of drugs on a susceptible brain. This would be an unfortunate underestimation of such a formidable force. Many drugs, when consumed over prolonged lengths of time, produce a marked deterioration in brain functioning and compromise the brain's ability to make clearheaded choices.[2] Sustained alcohol use over many years, for example, impairs executive functioning and impulse control.[3, 4] Although brain toxicity is often a consequence of addiction, AddictBrain is much larger than brain damage. The AddictBrain concept emphasizes how addiction entrains the brain, reengineering thoughts, reprioritizing an individual's goals and values, and increasing impulsive reactions by damaging the circuits of reflection and contemplation. The most enduring consequences of addiction arise from learning. AddictBrain underscores how aberrant new learning occurs when a susceptible individual falls into the grip of addiction. The new learning creates AddictBrain, an efficient machine driven to continue addictive thoughts and behaviors regardless of the consequence to its host.

Addiction—and the total effect on the brain, AddictBrain— is similar in some ways to a primitive drive that has gone awry. Our primitive drives are central to survival, and the higher centers of our brain are highly attuned to them, learning quickly to preserve life and perfect our instincts for self-preservation. Our brains are amazing organs, always learning and changing. When addiction takes over an individual's deepest drives, it mimics survival mechanisms. As I will discuss in the next chapter, the neural circuits of addiction work in a manner similar to our basic instincts. The rest of the brain stands up and listens, just as it would with any primal drive. Once addiction sets up house in the brain, the individual quickly adapts, becoming more facile and efficient at sustaining this "false primitive instinct" over time. Those afflicted with addiction feel an urgency to maintain the addiction, often at the cost of the real instincts of self-preservation.

The key concept of AddictBrain comes from this double whammy: a primal drive that cannot be ignored combined with the brain's learning and adapting in order to sustain the illness. The brain is not a passive hapless victim to the effects of addicting chemicals. It responds, learns, and refines a set of skills that perfect the seeking, acquiring, and consumption of chemicals or behaviors—be it alcohol or other drugs, sex, shopping, or gambling.

It may seem counterintuitive to consider the mind as learning and adapting to "improve" addiction, but that is exactly what it does. The brain is a learning machine. Stop and consider several examples for a moment. What happens if a person with alcohol use disorder goes to a party where no alcohol is served? In such a situation, the alcohol-dependent individual would cleverly, and often automatically, have a drink before the function or smuggle alcohol into the alcohol-free event or both. The invention of the hip flask comes from this "addiction-preservation response." Consider Emil, addicted to opioids, whose primary drug of choice is hydrocodone.

> Emil is planning to go to Costa Rica for a vacation with his wife. Emil's wife, by the way, knows he has a problem but tries her best to look the other way. Weeks before the vacation, Emil is panicked about running out of hydrocodone on the trip. He tries to stockpile pills by buying more from a friend who sells them. Emil goes on the Internet to see if he can purchase hydrocodone pills in Costa Rica because he knows he often runs out earlier than planned. He searches out a place to hide the pills in his suitcase where his wife will not find them and (heaven forbid) throw them out. He spends hours planning for continued drug use during his vacation rather than deciding where to go or what to see. As an individual in the clutches of his illness, he has developed a primitive instinct to continue using hydrocodone. As an adaptive, learning member of the species Homo sapiens, he puts intense effort into maintaining his supply at all costs.

AddictBrain has changed Emil, shifting his priorities and establishing single-minded efforts to hoard pills and hide them from his wife.

All this robs Emil and his wife of the pleasure of travel and vacation, doesn't it? This is just one example of the how addiction steals pleasure and lies to the mind—ensuring that what little pleasure remains must come from alcohol and/or other drugs.

All of Emil's careful, well-planned activity appears to others to be conscious and, more importantly, a choice. Such behaviors drive the underinformed to come to the conclusion that people choose their self-destructive addiction behaviors. Emil's wife, if she found him hiding pills in his suitcase, might accuse him of choosing to stockpile his drug and making his drug use more important than their conjoint vacation. His use has long since passed the point of choice. And she is right; using opioid drugs is now more important than the vacation itself. A better way to think of the response to the intense addiction drive is to compare it to our built-in drives, such as the drive to sustain an adequate food intake.

Consider how much of our day and our culture is focused on food. We have restaurants, fast food, and daily food rituals that sustain and simplify our need for continuous sustenance. To control the darker side of the compulsion to eat, society has diets, health magazines, and radical surgical procedures for weight loss. Addiction and our drive to eat have much in common. Eating food is sanctioned and integrated into our culture. Using drugs is commonly illegal and looked upon as a scourge. Eating is necessary for survival, but many people develop severe medical consequences from their loss of control over food. Using alcohol is not necessary for survival; however, approximately 10 percent of drinkers will develop severe social and medical consequences at some point in their life from their loss of control over alcohol use. Both are primitive drives with complex behaviors that result from and continue that drive. Once the addiction drive is engaged, asking the addicted individual to stop using is similar to asking the hungry person not to eat.

One other key component of AddictBrain is how it unconsciously controls its victim. Most of the time, AddictBrain hides below consciousness, manipulating the organism toward its own ends and wreaking havoc for those so afflicted. AddictBrain rewires much of the functioning of the central nervous system by changing the reward center, motivation center, many aspects of learning, and the conscious, interpretive circuits of the mind. These combined effects of AddictBrain control the individual at the level of his or her automatic response system, below the level of conscious choice and free will. This is how "choice" is removed from the picture once addiction takes hold.

It is true that each person makes a conscious choice to consume addictive substances at first. After a certain period of use—the length varies from person to person—the susceptible individual crosses an invisible wall and cannot return to using addictive substances by choice or with conscious control.

Addiction is more complicated than a hunger to "get high." The maladaptive brain response is the real enemy of recovery, which alters many brain circuits. Thus, no one approach will extricate the many parts of AddictBrain's neuronal rewiring. It is part of our nature to intrinsically trust what comes from our own thoughts and beliefs; however, AddictBrain comes from inside. For individuals struggling with addiction, AddictBrain thoughts *feel* like their own. It is difficult to accept that one's own beliefs are faulty and go against one's own intuitions, even when they originate in AddictBrain.

In order to move addiction into remission, we, as practitioners, must help our patients and clients accept that their beliefs are often incorrect in any area that even indirectly intersects with addiction. Recovery introduces the concept that others may know best, despite deeply held convictions to the contrary.

AddictBrain Uses a Four-Pronged Attack

AddictBrain attacks the brain and derives its power in four distinct ways. Let's look more closely at the four centers of control for AddictBrain.

AddictBrain Hijacks Our Instincts

Addictive drugs (alcohol, nicotine, opiates, stimulants, etc.) flood the reward mechanisms in the brain. While this initially produces pleasure or even euphoria, it is soon replaced by a hunger to repeat the process. Conventional rewards (e.g., food, the completion of a desired goal, or the love or acknowledgement by one's family or peers) fade in importance. What started as an intensely enjoyable experience is eventually replaced by "wanting."[5-7] With continued use, pleasure fades, but the false promise of future reward escalates. The growing hunger for the addictive chemical or behavior increases the frequency and intensity of the addiction over time. The individual with addiction is trapped in unfulfilled desire: false hopes of pleasure combined with the vicious downhill spiral that comes from chasing the increasingly elusive goal.

AddictBrain Redirects Motivation to Ensure Its Survival

The expanding drug hunger places the attention and focusing systems of the brain on high alert. Addiction behaviors and chemical use are seen as critical, which neuroscientists call **signal salience**; drugs confuse the mesolimbic dopamine circuit (see Chapter Three), falsely signaling a novel event. This triggers the brain to be on high alert.[8] This response activates learning mechanisms in the brain; the mind is primed to learn quickly and accurately. Each drug use retriggers the attention focusing centers in the brain as if the event is new and important—creating false meaning in the drugs and the rituals associated with their use.

AddictBrain Establishes Stereotypical Responses for Continued Use

Once activated by the focusing areas of the brain in the frontal cortex, the learning centers of the brain acquire knowledge that promotes continued access to the addictive chemicals or behaviors. Much of this learning is automatic, below the level of conscious intent and volitional control. The repeated use of chemicals or enactment of the addictive behavior rewires the brain to further habitual use.[9, 10] When brain activity is preferentially reprioritized by addiction, all other learning and growth activities are moved to a secondary position—they become less important than drug use. The afflicted individual literally learns how to be more efficient and effective in procuring alcohol or other drugs or reenacting an addictive behavior. Their learning is automatic and appears effortless to the conscious mind. The cascade of drug use, automatic effortless learning, and reprioritizing intensifies AddictBrain's grip on its victim.

AddictBrain Rearranges Reality to Prevent Detection

The last concept of AddictBrain describes how it evades detection in its victim, despite its wholesale rearrangement of self. This concept explains the most baffling attribute of addiction: it is the only disease that tells you that you don't have it. One way of conceptualizing AddictBrain's "stealth mode" is by using the analogy of a computer virus. Most of us who use personal computers have, unfortunately, been targets of a computer virus. Computer viruses implant themselves within your operating system, sending false emails, stealing important data, and changing the functionality of the computer. AddictBrain is like a computer virus in that it is an autonomous process, running in the background—virtually undetectable. Oftentimes, computer viruses run for weeks or months without us knowing they are present. They hide their tracks and evade attempts at detection by virus protection software. Their agenda is distinct from your activity and intent with the computer.

The human brain is millions of times more intricate and complex than our laptop computer. As a result, we would expect AddictBrain to be eminently more sophisticated than a computer virus, and it is. It operates with elegance, persistence, and ruthlessness. Over time, it systematically destroys the intent, meaning, and direction of one's life.

Self-survival is critical to the concept of AddictBrain. Human beings, like all animals, have amazing, hardwired circuits that ensure self-survival. Try as we might, none of us can hold our breath until we turn blue. The self-preservation circuit that guarantees regular breathing overrides all conscious attempts to override control. AddictBrain, because it becomes part of this same neural circuitry, inherits this self-survival mechanism from its host and makes it its own. Oftentimes, we have seen the conflict between survival of the human being and AddictBrain—the mind virus that lives within.

> *Stan was a patient I met many years ago, referred by the liver transplant team at our local university. Our practice provided addiction evaluations for patients on the liver transplant list for many years. Stan was a forty-year-old man; he arrived at my office jaundiced, edematous, and short of breath from his failing liver. He completed a battery of psychological and neurocognitive tests. Despite his failing liver, his neurocognitive testing was intact. Psychologically he suffered from no psychiatric illness, with the glaring exception of his alcohol dependence. Our team was asked to evaluate whether his addiction status was stable enough for him to receive the precious resource of a transplanted liver.*
>
> *I asked Stan my usual addiction evaluation questions. When, in the course of the evaluation I arrived at the battery of questions related to addiction, I asked this simple question, "Do you now or have you ever in the past had a problem with alcohol?" He replied somewhat indignantly, "No." I reviewed collateral data from his family and his medical support team, and that information told a completely different story. He drank compulsively and*

addictively for almost fifteen years of his life. Despite his failing liver, he was unable to stop drinking alcohol. His statement about alcohol was "Everyone deserves a drink every now and then, just to relax."

I asked questions about what his medical team thought of his continued alcohol use. He let me know in no uncertain terms that his physicians, including those on the transplant team, were overly alarmist. Yes, he drank alcohol daily; it was his right. The last day he abstained completely from alcohol was over ten years ago. I was unable to convince him that in its current state, his liver was unable to metabolize even the smallest amounts of alcohol. He disagreed with me, stating, "You have the same point of view as the transplant team, a bunch of doctors who think they know everything."

Finally, in a last ditch desperate maneuver, I let him know that his unwillingness to discontinue alcohol would prohibit him from being eligible for a liver transplant. He considered his response for a moment and then replied, "I think I will be able to talk them out of this overly rigid and incorrect understanding about my use of alcohol." Four months later, Stan's family called to tell me that he had died.

This case vignette, as unusual as it might appear, has much to teach us. Stan's AddictBrain had rearranged Stan's reality to protect its survival. Despite his lack of any diagnosable psychiatric illness—with the exception of alcohol dependence—he suffered from a condition we have termed "psychotic denial." His inability to see his situation made way for his own imminent demise. This denial of his addiction was psychotic in proportion and placed him completely out of contact with reality. His AddictBrain was operating so efficiently and so covertly that it tricked him into thinking its thoughts were accurate and his own. More dangerously, he knew he was right, and his doctors were wrong. He believed, with every fiber of his being, that he could correct the misaligned thinking of the entire transplant team. His AddictBrain, intent on its own survival, committed murder.

Every person with addiction does not suffer denial to such an intense and self-destructive level. However, every person with addiction does have the same covert, unconscious agenda. Perhaps the cruelest aspect of this mind virus called AddictBrain is how it convinces individuals that its agenda is their own. Stan could not even consider stopping drinking so that he might be potentially eligible for a liver transplant, but this doesn't mean that Stan was not physically capable of stopping drinking. I'm making a point here that Stan's brain, driven by the ruthless AddictBrain agenda, could not for a moment grasp the simple truth that alcohol was destroying his liver and, thereby, destroying his life.

More AddictBrain Dirty Tricks

Despite its complexity and baffling nature, AddictBrain manhandles its victim in exceptionally consistent ways. Let's review some of the most common "dirty tricks" that arise when AddictBrain rewires the mind.

Urgency and Impulsiveness

AddictBrain hijacks our basic drives. Let's consider one such drive, hunger. Assume you are at your job, working hard, focused on the task at hand. You are hours from breakfast, your blood sugar level is dropping, and multiple body signals indicate the need for sustenance. The dropping blood sugar signals the hypothalamus, a part of your brain that regulates core survival behaviors. As the low blood sugar continues or increases over time, you become distracted. Unconsciously, you reach for a snack that you had stashed in your desk drawer. It is no longer there. The drive remains unfulfilled, but in an effort to complete the task at hand, your conscious mind refocuses on your work.

You may repeat this cycle several times until your hypothalamus finally overrides your determination, forcing you to scan the environment for food to ameliorate your dropping blood sugar and rising hunger. The experience is urgency. Try as you might, when hunger rises, it becomes more difficult to focus on the conscious task at hand. Anyone who has sat in a school classroom just before lunch knows you do not learn when you are "starving." When hunger becomes severe, you may—despite your determination—stop work, impulsively stand up, and walk about your environment seeking food. These basic instincts are life preserving, and they prioritize behavior and prevent us from starving to death. They ensure the survival of our species.

When AddictBrain sets up shop in an individual's hypothalamus, the hypothalamus then inherits these basic drives. The needs and drives of addiction, once established, feel urgent. As it progresses, even if that person tries to hold it at bay with his conscious mind, he is tripped up by impulsive drives to relapse. The urgency and impulsiveness ultimately override his concerted efforts at limiting his use of chemicals or corralling addictive behaviors.

Relapse Is Inevitable

A second, especially damaging AddictBrain trick is called "Relapse Is Inevitable." When an individual who has developed an addictive disorder progresses far down the road into his or her addiction, hardwired patterns of alcohol and other drug use emerge. The brain has learned, above all else, how to efficiently acquire and consume alcohol and/ or other drugs. Despite conscious efforts to quit, the well-worn neural pathways continuously trip up AddictBrain's well-intentioned victim.

As multiple relapses pile up, the afflicted patient begins to experience hopelessness; relapse seems inevitable—maybe not today or tomorrow—but some time in the future. Repeated episodes of relapse construct a self-fulfilling prophecy. Such an individual returns to a profound, heavy truth that has invaded the core of her being: the more one relapses, the more one relapses. Individuals who have the most intense forms of this distorted belief may need to remain in an environment that physically blocks relapse for a long time (measured in months or years), waiting for hope to replace their sense of impending doom.

You Get the Opposite of What You Desire, but You Do Not Realize It

People begin using potentially addicting drugs for many reasons. Alcohol is called a social lubricant. Many people have an alcoholic drink at a party to loosen up, and a small percentage of them wind up addicted. Benzodiazepine medications reduce anxiety quite effectively for almost anyone who takes them. What makes those individuals with substance use disorders different is what happens over time; the desired effect slips away without them realizing it.

Over decades I have met new alcohol-dependent patients in my detoxification unit, shaking and agitated, filled with the restless anxiety of withdrawal. When conducting their intake history, patients told me they began drinking to help with an anxious life situation or to moderate social anxiety. Observing their shakes and tremors, I thought to myself, *So how is alcohol working for that anxiety now?* Alcohol did help with their anxiety for a time, no doubt about it. Over a longer period, however, alcohol stops working. This is cruel—and a consequence of addiction. When I ask why they have been drinking more recently, most patients say, "Why, to take care of my continued anxiety!" This adds insult to injury. Over time, the anti-anxiety effect of substance use slips away, but AddictBrain continues its empty promise of help. The hapless victim is in truly delusional thinking that her substance use is curing, when in truth it manufactures her misery.

Loss of Self

The next AddictBrain trick is called "Loss of Self." In the latter stages of addiction when all excuses and denial finally slip away, it becomes easier for a victim to acknowledge he does indeed have the disease of addiction. In such moments of despair, he loses his true self. AddictBrain's actions feel automatic, effortless, and fundamental—his true fate. In this state, he says, "I am my addiction; there is little else." The thoughts and actions produced by AddictBrain seem to be the center of the client's identity. Although the self-destructive thoughts and actions are, at times, crazy and unfathomable, he accepts his illness as all there is left of his true self. The inevitable conclusion of someone so afflicted is that addiction's darkness and evil have taken over that individual's true identity. This leads him to be convinced that his inner core is "bad," and it is imperative for the patient to break himself of this false belief. The loss of self is nothing more than an AddictBrain trick, designed to lock in continued use.

Shameful Not Sick

Different cultures have varying views of addiction. Some see it as a failure of morality and some see it as a sign of degenerate behavior. Others see it as a spiritual failing. Despite our increasing understanding that addiction illnesses are primary brain diseases, a pervasive judgment of inadequacy, lack of willpower, and personal defects subtly or not so subtly colors how our society views addiction. Almost everyone has some degree of negative feelings or conclusions about those who become addicted. It may be as subtle as "she seems to persistently make bad choices" or as stark as "he is a depraved person." Individuals with alcohol or other drug use disorders commonly have the worst self-judgmentalism and self-castigation. Shame is powerful and pervasive in us all.

RecoveryMind Training asserts that AddictBrain uses this harsh self-judgment to its own ends. Shame and inadequacy only serve to exacerbate substance use. When faced with a sense of moral failure, social and spiritual bankruptcy, and repeated bad choices, AddictBrain quietly whispers, "Drinking alcohol will make this feel better," or "Taking drugs will ease the pain," or "Escaping into sex or gambling will help you forget who you have become." Having robbed one's self-esteem, AddictBrain skillfully uses that theft to further the self-destruction of its victim. This viscous cycle locks the individual in a downward spiral.

Going Silent

Addiction is also a fickle disorder. For a time, it feels constant, gnawing at one's insides, persistent and undeniable. At other times, the drive seems to disappear completely. During these times, the person with addiction is tempted to see herself as cured. Nothing could be further from the truth. The false sensation that addiction has been removed is best visualized as "silent running" like a submarine deep in the water. During such periods, the individual with addiction must take the stance that her illness has not been eradicated. It lies in wait patiently, only to spring back up at a later date—often when it is least expected.

AddictBrain often goes silent after a dose of treatment. The patient feels better, garners hope, and learns recovery skills. These skills can make AddictBrain go silent, waiting for a chink in the recovery armor. Each patient should learn their illness can and will go silent. When it reemerges, she doubles up on her recovery skills, tells others about AddictBrain's reemergence, and relies on her support system to help her through the rough patch.

Loss of Values

One of the best indicators of addiction disorders comes from examining a client's values and comparing those values with the client's current behavior. Addiction exhorts its victims to cross moral and ethical boundaries they hold dear. A mother or father may say, "It is very important that my children are safe." That same parent, once addicted, will drive his or her children around town after drinking alcohol or using other drugs. If a therapist has good rapport with an addicted patient, he or she can tease out a list of past values. It is striking how the values individuals hold dear are invariably the ones they violate most flagrantly once addicted. A patient who says, "I was brought up to be honest and forthright" becomes devious and dishonest. Another who says, "I learned from a young age to be conscientious about my work" becomes sloppy and negligent in her or his occupation. And so on. I often think this is part of AddictBrain's plot: The systematic destruction of everything its victim holds dear in order to maximize shame. The shame, in turn, fuels continued use.

Some individuals who arrive in a therapy office or treatment center are too defensive to examine their values transgression. They vociferously report high moral standards and honesty. Such individuals remember their past values and cling to the possibility that they still adhere to them. In such cases, a therapist must judiciously and respectfully help the client differentiate between *remembering* one's past values and *acting* on them accordingly. Once they have slid into the abyss of addiction, most people have long since left their moral and ethical standards behind. In Chapters Ten and Twelve, I will discuss techniques that deepen a patient's acceptance of lost or discarded values and moral standards. Remember, this is critical to an enlightened recovery: AddictBrain loves confusion; RecoveryMind demands clarity.

AddictBrain and the Theories of Self-Medication

Self-Medication Theory posits that individuals take psychoactive substances in an attempt to fix difficulties with emotions. Someone with addiction uses alcohol or benzodiazepines in an attempt to manage anxiety. The cocaine user consumes the drug to fix the need for excitement and to repair anhedonia. The person addicted to narcotics is racked with emotional pain that immediately and sweetly disappears when opioids are ingested. Self-Medication Theory feels correct based upon first principles. A therapist trained in psychodynamic theory—

from which Self-Medication Theory is derived—hearing these complaints might be fooled into attempting to correct these symptoms, hoping that it will thwart alcohol or other drug use. This inevitably fails.

Although RecoveryMind Training asserts that Self-Medication Theory has its place in treating addiction, once addiction takes hold, the individual's use is most often driven by neurophysiology. An anxious person addicted to alcohol experiences increased nervousness during inevitable periods of alcohol withdrawal. The person addicted to cocaine feels empty, flat, and depressed for prolonged periods because of the cocaine crash and post-acute withdrawal. By a spiteful sleight-of-hand, AddictBrain gives the addicted individual the exact opposite of what he or she desires.

As you will see in the second section of this book, RecoveryMind Training asserts that the concepts of Self-Medication Theory are valuable when treating addiction, but they must be used judiciously and with exquisite timing. When the person with addiction enters treatment and cannot stop active substance use, the therapist's first task is helping the patient differentiate between the initial drivers for substance use and what happens in addiction: anxiety is worse, pain increases, and anhedonia has returned displacing the initial relief provided by substances. If addictive use is only seen as a symptom of something else, abstinence will never get the attention needed for recovery.

The therapist should abstain from psychodynamic formulations and self-medication hypotheses and stay on solid ground, helping the patient come to the realization that symptom reduction from addicting substances has long since stopped working. Once the individual with alcohol and other drug use disorders is in solid remission, the therapist can carefully approach the domain of psychodynamic formulations. When the patient has a proven track record in recovery and desires additional growth, the psychodynamic approach and Self-Medication Theory can prove to be quite helpful, expanding self-understanding.

Recent neuroscience research shows that genetic and biochemical factors are more potent when predicting who will develop addiction. The complex origins of addiction are not, however, a "one is 100 percent right and the other is 100 percent wrong" situation. Issues of personality style, disorders of personality, past trauma, loss or grief, and other psychiatric disorders, especially anxiety and mood disorders, are important in coloring the presentation and characteristics of an individual's addiction. Finally, the concepts in Self-Medication Theory become critical when maintenance of a strong recovery and relapse prevention are reached. I will discuss this further in Chapters Twelve and Fourteen.

AddictBrain and Personality

Perhaps the most interesting aspect of AddictBrain is how it interacts with the personalities of the afflicted. Most theoreticians believe we, as humans, are genetically wired with aspects of personality. Anyone who has spent time with toddlers has noticed how certain qualities of personality appear to be hardwired. To that, we add our habits and life experiences, which shape the innate qualities forming our personality. Using terminology developed by C. Robert Cloninger, MD, we have temperament and character—what we are born with and how our temperament is molded by life events, habits, and interpersonal interactions with others, respectively.[11-13] Temperament, according to Cloninger, has to do with our inclinations to think and act in a particular way. His work defined temperament as something we are born with. Character, on the other hand, is a way of building habits and thought patterns based upon our temperament. Using a computer analogy, our temperament is our hardware, and our character is our software.

RecoveryMind Training also borrows from the work of Glen Gabbard, MD,[14] and Edgar P. Nace, MD,[15] who, when studying personality characteristics of healthcare professionals, assert that all traits have healthy (adaptive) and maladaptive characteristics. Combining this with Cloninger's classification, our temperament produces healthy and maladaptive character traits throughout our lives. Using one of Gabbard's examples, guilt can produce conscientiousness when it is expressed in healthy ways. When expressed in unhealthy ways, it produces feelings of helplessness.

AddictBrain uses temperament and character toward its own ends. It rides on the back of one's existing personality, exaggerating the maladaptive elements of that individual's personality that promote continued addiction. At the same time, it diminishes aspects of one's personality that promote recovery. Curiosity is one such trait, which helps us question and explore. Once an individual with a curious nature becomes addicted, AddictBrain bends this character trait to its own ends. The curious individual might explore different abusable drugs and routes of administration. His or her curiosity would give way to impulsiveness—the maladaptive side of curiosity. In this way, AddictBrain does not introduce a new or different temperament in its victims. Instead, it exaggerates the maladaptive elements of what is already present, using them to ensure its own survival.

With this knowledge, we can visualize the most natural and effective manner of working with patient personalities. By looking at a patient's temperament, RecoveryMind Training encourages the growth of the adaptive and healthy components of each character trait. Using the example of curiosity described above, RMT would engage the patient's curiosity to explore what has happened to him through the course of his illness. The therapist would find ways of engaging his curiosity about recovery. In such an individual, the therapist might ask him to write several paragraphs about which parts of recovery he thinks might work best for him. The individual might explore what recovery would look like at some point in the near future. The patient's curiosity, once engaged, would explore recovery as naturally as it explored addiction. The therapist might also explore how the patient's curiosity has caused trouble in the past and find ways of redirecting it away from addiction.

It is important to note that AddictBrain's maladaptive responses, once ingrained, are tenacious. It would be foolhardy to think that simply practicing healthy responses wipes out previous, well-ingrained, maladaptive ones. Experience has shown that the maladaptive responses to character traits remain active for years into recovery. This is where personal vigilance, spending time with others in recovery, working the Twelve Steps, and soliciting feedback from friends and a sponsor enter recovery. RecoveryMind Training lays down an alternative, healthy track heading in a different direction from the sickness of AddictBrain. It does not and cannot remove these tendencies directly.

In Summary

AddictBrain is the primitive drive to consume addicting chemicals or behaviors, combined with the learning, brain adjustments, and reality distortion produced by the addict's adjustment and learning response. It is a newly engineered, artificial instinct that is as demanding as one's innate instincts, as if honed through years of evolution. It hijacks primitive control centers, shifts motivation toward continued use, sets up its own learning and stereotypical responses, and operates in a stealth mode similar to a computer virus. It is bent upon its own survival. AddictBrain exaggerates the maladaptive characteristics of individuals' personalities toward its own ends. RecoveryMind, then, is a compendium of skills that unwind and repair damages to the individual, as well as his or her family and social network, caused by AddictBrain.

Chapter Four Notes

1.   J. Y. Huang and J. A. Bargh, "The Selfish Goal: Autonomously Operating Motivational Structures as the Proximate Cause of Human Judgment and Behavior," *Behav Brain Sci* 37, no. 2 (2014): 121–35.

2.   A. Bechara, "Decision Making, Impulse Control and Loss of Willpower to Resist Drugs: A Neurocognitive Perspective," *Nat Neurosci* 8, no. 11 (2005): 1458–63.

3.   G. Fein, L. Klein, and P. Finn, "Impairment on a Simulated Gambling Task in Long-Term Abstinent Alcoholics," *Alcoholism: Clinical and Experimental Research* 28, no. 10 (2004): 1487–91.

4.   A. G. Schindler, M. E. Soden, L. S. Zweifel, and J. J. Clark, "Reversal of Alcohol-Induced Dysregulation in Dopamine Network Dynamics May Rescue Maladaptive Decision-Making," *The Journal of Neuroscience* 36, no. 13 (2016): 3698–708.

5.   K. Berridge, "Motivation Concepts in Behavioral Neuroscience," *Physiology and Behavior* 81, no. 2 (2004): 179–209.

6.   K. C. Berridge and M. L. Kringelbach, "Affective Neuroscience of Pleasure: Reward in Humans and Animals," *Psychopharmacology (Berl)* 199, no. 3 (2008): 457–80.

7.   K. C. Berridge, T. E. Robinson, and J. W. Aldridge, "Dissecting Components of Reward: 'Liking', 'Wanting', and Learning." *Curr Opin Pharmacol* 9, no. 1 (2009): 65–73.

8.   T. E. Robinson and K. C. Berridge, "The Neural Basis of Drug Craving: An Incentive-Sensitization Theory of Addiction," *Brain Res Brain Res Rev* 18, no. 3 (1993): 247–91.

9.   S. E. Hyman, "Addiction: A Disease of Learning and Memory," *Am J Psychiatry* 162, no. 8 (2005): 1414–22.

10. S. E. Hyman, R. C. Malenka, and E. J. Nestler, "Neural Mechanisms of Addiction: The Role of Reward-Related Learning and Memory," *Annu Rev Neurosci* 29, no. 1 (2006): 565–98.

11. F. De Fruyt, L. Van De Wiele, and C. Van Heeringen, "Cloninger's Psychobiological Model of Temperament and Character and the Five-Factor Model of Personality," *Personality and Individual Differences* 29, no. 3 (2000): 441–52.

12. C. R. Cloninger, D. M. Svrakic, and T. R. Przybeck, "A Psychobiological Model of Temperament and Character," *Arch Gen Psychiatry* 50, no. 12 (1993): 975–90.

13. D. H. Angres, "The Temperament and Character Inventory in Addiction Treatment," *FOCUS: The Journal of Lifelong Learning in Psychiatry* 8, no. 2 (2010): 187–98.

14. G. O. Gabbard, "The Role of Compulsiveness in the Normal Physician," *JAMA* 254, no. 20 (1985): 2926–9.

15. E. Nace, *Achievement and Addiction: A Guide to the Treatment of Professionals* (New York: Brunner/Mazel, 1995).

CHAPTER FIVE

Neuroscience and AddictBrain

The concepts described in Chapter Four, buttressed by the science described in the next two chapters, illuminate addiction's deep-seated disruption of the fundamental nature of human beings. The result is AddictBrain. This clear and concise addiction construct will serve as the foundation for the chapters in the second half of this book where I will particularize RecoveryMind Training.

Patients are often surprised and occasionally astonished at how well the AddictBrain concept fits their internal experience, saying, "It's like you are telling me what is going on in my head—even better than I could describe it myself!" You will gain trust and patient confidence as long as you do not attempt to push the AddictBrain concept before a patient or client is ready to hear it. Also be aware: the AddictBrain model does not describe every patient's experience; no model can cover the entire landscape of every patient's internal world. However, the AddictBrain concept helps most patients and therapists recognize their common enemy and join forces on the road to recovery. When you implement the concepts from Section One of this text, you will visualize the contortion and distortion of the thoughts, beliefs, and actions produced by addiction. The resultant clarity of your vision will jumpstart your treatment plan and coalesce your approach. This is one of the central advantages in RecoveryMind Training.

As I explained in Chapter Three, neuroscience is a rich, complex, and rapidly expanding field. Do not be discouraged if some of the concepts I discuss are difficult to grasp in their entirety. Reread sections that puzzle or confound you; I promise your efforts will be rewarded by a newfound wonder about the mind and a deeper respect for addiction as an illness.

Patients with alcohol or other drug disorders offer up unusual and even bizarre descriptions of their experiences. Instead of discarding them as the toxic byproducts of an addled brain, I carefully catalogued and examined them—all in an effort to refine RecoveryMind Training. The same can be said for observing patient behaviors. Rather than writing off the unusual and at times unfathomable and maladaptive behaviors to the toxic effects of addiction, those, too, were catalogued. As outlandish and surreal as the thoughts and behaviors of those afflicted with addiction may seem, RecoveryMind Training teaches that nearly every thought, feeling, and behavior can be assigned to an organized, methodical, and self-destructive neurological process called AddictBrain. It is not substance toxicity that kills those with alcohol or other drug disorders; it is a clever, surreptitious AddictBrain that destroys its host.

The neuroscience concepts covered in this book are wide-ranging; therefore, I have split this information into two chapters. Chapter Five will cover general brain systems and concepts. Chapter Six will dive deeper into neuroscience research specific to addiction, relating it to the AddictBrain concept along the way. Many of the neurobiological concepts will be juxtaposed with examples from clinical experience. For example, when discussing the AddictBrain phenomenon of "wanting," I will provide examples of the thoughts and behaviors seen in everyday clinical experience that arise from this internal brain process. It is my hope that tagging the major components of AddictBrain with clinical examples will clarify the neurobiology and deepen your understanding of the plight of your patient or client.

How to Use the Information in This Chapter

This chapter will touch on many of the important constructs or models that conceptualize the complexities of the human brain. Each individual construct cannot, on its own, describe the human mind in its entirety. Presented here are the best constructs available at the time of this writing that build a clinically useful treatment model. Our incomplete understanding prevents me from asserting that the model accurately explains *every* aspect of brain functioning in addiction; however, I believe RecoveryMind Training is the best we have today, sure to be expanded and modified as science moves forward.

The more the addiction physician or therapist understands how the brain works, the better he or she can use the AddictBrain/RecoveryMind model to build a deeper appreciation of the knotted conundrum of addiction—a brain illness that often seems hopelessly complex. With continuing research, many of the brain models discussed here will be connected to RecoveryMind Training. In the meantime, I hope a careful reading will fill you with wonder as you learn about the human mind.

In this chapter, three constructs will be examined:

- The Triune Brain
- Our Faulty Memory System
- The Nature of Consciousness

The Triune Brain

The human brain is not a singular integrated computer. Instead, it is a combination of multiple computing centers, each vying for control and attention of the organism as a whole. In addition, each of these computing centers functions in radically different ways that leads to the amazing—and occasional vexing—complexity of our species, *Homo sapiens*. One important way of understanding the "multiplicity" of our brain comes from the work of Paul D. MacLean and his concept of the three-part or Triune Brain.[1] MacLean, an evolutionary biologist, noted that when he compared primitive brains with species higher on the evolutionary chain, higher species retain—and use—the vestiges of the brain structures inherited from their primitive ancestors. Although we like to think of ourselves as more rational and sophisticated than a lizard, in truth some behaviors—and all our reflexive actions—are as atavistic as that of our reptilian or amphibian ancestors!

In an attempt to bring clarity to the multiple, redundant circuits in the brain, MacLean postulated that the human brain was divided into three overarching systems, the **R-complex** (Reptilian brain), the **Limbic Area**, and the **Neocortex**. Of these, the reptilian brain is the oldest. As evolution produced more sophisticated control systems, the limbic area[2] came onto the scene. Limbic structures can modify the output and color the input to the reptilian brain, but they cannot turn it off or completely override its effects. Similarly, once the neocortex evolved, it had the capability to change the actions and alter the interpretation of the older limbic and reptilian areas, but the neocortex could not override their hardwired firing patterns. MacLean described our brains, evolving from the thrust of three separate periods of evolution, as creating a byzantine and frequently conflicted command and control center. When thinking about the triune brain concept, it is important to remember that sensory input moves through each of these separate structures, and each independently controls our motor output. Using this model alone, we can begin to understand why the mind of earlier *Homo sapiens* had complex reactions to the external world and why we so often feel conflicted about our thoughts, beliefs, and actions.

Let's explore this in more detail. Evolution, through selection of the fittest, changes characteristics of living organisms with the constant goal of increasing the probability of survival. Survival as a prime directive often creates attributes that are strange bedfellows,[3] and at times it creates seemingly illogical biological adaptations. This also holds true for the evolution of the brain. Neuroscientists believe the structure of the brain in our remote ancestors began as a series of inputs (sensory events) that produced stereotypical, reflexive outputs (behavioral events). To improve adaptability to the environment, evolution increased the mass and complexity of the brain in the area between sensation and action—input and output, respectively.[4] This increasing complexity honed the survival of the reptilian species.

At some point, the organizational structure of the reptilian brain reached the end of its ability to adapt, and another system was needed. We see the same thing today in our computer systems. One operating system, such as CP/M or MS-DOS, comes to the end of its usefulness. Newer operating systems arrive, such as Windows or Mac OS, replacing their antiquated counterparts. In the hardware world, the desktop computer is replaced by the laptop to allow humans to use computers in an increasingly mobile society. Soon the laptop is replaced by the tablet or smartphone. Many of us eventually discard our desktop computers, moving to computing platforms that fit our changing needs.

The evolution of the human brain is different from emerging computing technology in one critical way. Because the brain cannot go offline or be discarded while waiting for the latest and greatest upgrade, current brain control systems cannot be set aside while evolution (or God, Allah, or your Higher Power) reengineers a better design. The old systems must remain in place, sustaining the organism. New and better technology can only build on top of the old. David J. Linden, PhD, lucidly describes in his fine book *The Accidental Mind*, stating, "During the course of evolution, the brain has never been redesigned from the ground up. It can only add new systems onto existing ones."[5] The problem with adding new structures on top of the older, more deeply wired neuronal foundations is that we continue to respond to the dominating effect of older brain structures, even as new ones appear. Linden emphasizes that the brain "has very limited capacity for turning off control systems, even when these systems are counterproductive in a given situation."[6]

Let's turn our attention to the human brain divided into the three sections delineated by MacLean. Keep in mind the overwhelming power of addiction as you review these brain subdivisions. I will apply and amplify MacLean's model to AddictBrain later in this chapter.

The Reptilian Brain

The primitive, reptilian brain, including the brain stem and the cerebellum, evolved in the Triassic Period, or 248–206 million years ago. During this period, the first dinosaurs and flying animals appeared on Earth's singular landmass, Pangaea. The oldest reflection of our predecessors' entire central nervous system remains within our brain to this day. MacLean called this primitive remnant the R-complex. Today, it is often referred to as the reptilian brain. The reptilian brain controls some reflexive, nonvolitional muscular activities, balance, and life-sustaining functions, such as the speed of your heartbeat and breathing. Our reptilian brain repeats the same behaviors over and over again with a very limited ability to learn from past mistakes. Its "thinking" is characterized as rigid, obsessive, compulsive, ritualistic, and, most importantly, self-preserving at all costs. Our reptilian brain remains active during sleep, maintaining essential life-support functions.

One important component of the R-complex is the mesolimbic dopaminergic system. It prioritizes life-sustaining activities, promotes goal-directed behaviors, and reinforces learning.[7] Drugs of abuse literally hijack this life-sustaining area of the brain, rearranging priorities and establishing new goals focused on continued acquisition and use of those substances.[8] We can best understand the power of addiction and how difficult it is to attain and maintain recovery by recalling how Linden's describes the brain as having a "limited capacity for turning off control systems, even when these systems are counterproductive in a given situation."

Examples of the R-complex in action are many. When a sudden, unpredictable event occurs—a person unexpectedly appears from around the corner while walking down a dark street—we feel an urge to yell, attack, or run away. This action is part of the self-defense system of the "fight or flight" reflex in our reptilian brain. Our heart beats rapidly, equipping us to engage the unknown enemy or run the other way. We may even take a quick few steps before we recognize our neighbor walking his dog.

The Limbic Area

The Paleomammalian brain, or limbic area, was the next brain system to evolve. It is not an organized system but rather a loosely connected group of structures that manage our drives and emotions. To a large extent, each division of the limbic area operates autonomously and occasionally in conflict with other limbic subsections.[9] To help keep you from thinking of it as an integrated system, I will refer to this portion of the triune brain as the "limbic area" and not the "limbic system." It is the second oldest part of our triune brain, evolving mostly during the rise of the dinosaurs in the Jurassic Period, 206–144 million years ago. Structures contained in the limbic area are the hippocampus, amygdala, anterior thalamic nuclei, septum, habenula, limbic cortex, and fornix.

The limbic area in humans is involved in emotion and appraising the importance of external and internal stimuli. Recent research dispels the simplistic notion that our emotions arise solely from this area;[10] however, the limbic area is intimately involved in regulating feeding, fighting, fleeing, and sexual behaviors. The limbic area is the most complex brain structure in primitive mammals. Said another way, what we call "feelings" are the highest forms of thought in simple mammals. In humans, the limbic area attaches a positive or negative quality, also known as valence, to current events and memories. Emotions help prioritize experiences, and the stronger an emotion we have, the more likely we are to remember the experience associated with it.[11]

Each time we recollect a past story or situation, the limbic area chimes in with its information. The memory circuits of our temporal lobe and hippocampus provide us with the details of that memory: *I was driving down the road on a spring morning. The sun was out. I was about age twenty-two. I was alone in the car.* When recalling such an incident, the limbic area adds richness, flavor, and emotional valence—whether you feel positive or negative—to the recall of the memory: *The wheels hummed gently on the road, and the sun felt warm on my face. Although I was alone in the car, I felt contented and happy to be alive.*

As you can see, the limbic area adds important qualities to factual recall. The limbic area also does this for current events, such as *I squint my eyes at the computer screen,* painfully *reviewing each sentence for clarity and content.* It prioritizes our experiences, causing us to seek positive situations and avoid painful negative ones. Memories that primarily arise in the limbic area are timeless; we cannot locate them in time, making it difficult to dredge up factual details about an impression that arises from this set of brain structures.

The Neocortex

Elements of the neocortex were present in the earliest mammals. However, the enlarged cerebral cortex, or neopallium as we know it today, evolved fifty-five to twenty-four million years ago in the Eocene to Oligocene Epochs. These epochs saw the spread of mammalian species to the newly formed temperate grasslands. The expansion of mammals during the Oligocene Epoch was accelerated by the adaptive advantages of the neocortex. Organized in a distinctly different fashion from its predecessors, changes in the structure and organization of neurons in the neocortex of *Homo sapiens* improved the computational complexity and speed of interneuronal communication during their emergence later in evolution.

The cortex is the highly convoluted mass that appears on the surface of the brain. In human beings, the neocortex takes up two thirds of the total brain mass. Monkeys and chimpanzees share a similar cortex with man. One difference between *Homo sapiens* and our predecessors is the presence of a larger cortex. Our human cortex also has a more complex organizational structure and newer types of associative neurons. This is especially true in the front of our brain, called the prefrontal cortex, which manages the executive functioning specific to our species.[12]

In the past fifteen years, we have learned more about the specialization that occurs within the cerebral cortex. We have begun to map specific parts of our neocortex to specific functions. Such neurological information is now part of the lingua franca; you may hear a wife tell her husband to "stop being so left-brained" when she wants him to stop being literal. The full extent of lateralized functions is greatly exaggerated in the popular literature, almost to the point of absurdity. However, we do know that the right brain is more spatial, abstract, musical, and artistic, while the left brain is more linear, rational, and verbal. Neuroscience has also tracked multiple areas of the cortex working together to perform complex functions, such as recalling a past event, organizing it into a sequential story, and using language so others can understand and even visualize our experiences.

When humans develop addiction, the neocortex trips them up in many ways. Driven by the reptilian brain and the limbic area, the neocortex may remember minute details about a favorite alcoholic beverage. It also may remember how the sunlight illuminated the wall, the music that was playing, and even the crisp smell of autumn in the air the first time a person used cocaine. By recording these events in vivid detail, the next time that person hears that particular music, sees the sun playing on the wall in that peculiar way, or smells that cool sharp autumn air, she is triggered. She recalls her past drug use with fondness and yearning. Although our conscious cortex asserts we are the captains of our fate, the self-control originating in the neocortex goes off-line when addiction takes over. Even worse, the neocortex waylays itself by providing rich addiction-related memories to the limbic system, which in turn trip up its own self-control mechanisms.

Let's apply our understanding of Maclean's triune brain to human behavior. When considering Maclean's model—that the brain is organized in three evolutionary layers—we expand our understanding of the human mind: we do not have one brain; we have many—or at least three. Different parts of this command-and-control organ operationalize a wide variety of actions, ranging from controlling heart rate to composing a symphony. Some of these appear to be under our control (composing a symphony) and others are not (our heart rate). This model also explains why our evolutionarily older brain structures dominate the more recently evolved areas such as the neocortex. Newer parts of the brain can modulate but cannot override basic commands emanating from our reptilian brain. This makes intuitive sense; you would never want to be able to decide to stop your heartbeat. If you could do so, casual experimentation might prove fatal. Table 5.1 summarizes some of the differences in the three centers.

Table 5.1 - Comparison of MacLean's brain areas

	R-complex (Reptilian brain)	Limbic Area	Neocortex
Evolutionary Age	Oldest (early reptiles)	Pre-mammalian evolution	Late mammals and primates
Numbers of neuronal interconnections	Few	Moderate	Many
Complexity of thought	Low	Medium	High
Ability to dominate other brain activity (signal priority)	Highest	Medium	Lowest
We sense activity in this area as	Urges, drives, or unnoticed regulation of the body	Emotions or like/dislike	Ideas, words, and complex human interaction

What Does the Triune Brain Concept Teach Us about AddictBrain?

One important area within the reptilian brain that is outside conscious control is the mesolimbic dopamine circuit. Discussion of this area will take center stage in Chapter Six. The neurons that make up this circuit are a central driver in addiction; to date, all drugs of abuse stimulate this circuit. Looking at Table 5.1, you can see the activation of circuits in the reptilian brain dominate and overwhelm the limbic area and neocortex. This, in part, explains the overwhelming and uncontrollable aspects of addiction.

Several other important AddictBrain concepts arise from MacLean's noteworthy model. Addiction is best described as an illness characterized by periods of remission and relapse. During abstinence, those afflicted make a solemn vow—a conscious decision in the neocortex—to remain abstinent from alcohol or other drugs. Many succeed in their endeavors for a time, only to be tripped up by deeper, unconscious drives (the reptilian brain) and emotions (the limbic area). A corollary of this concept is that willpower alone, which originates in the neocortex, is doomed to failure over time—the neocortex cannot override the reptilian brain.

Overcoming AddictBrain requires a complex group of thoughts, actions, and planned maneuvers that may appear counterintuitive or downright foolish. One common aphorism in many twelve-step fellowships is "You conquer by surrender or win the war by admitting defeat." A straight-ahead, forward attack based upon concentration, determination, and willpower alone is rarely successful. Recovery requires a type of mental jiujitsu rather than a frontal attack (willpower from the cortex); such maneuvers sidestep the push from the R-complex through a process that is called surrender in the parlance of twelve-step recovery.

The triune brain model also provides clues on the interaction between conscious thought and AddictBrain. Because our deeper drives begin at a subliminal level, awareness of a craving often shows up in our conscious mind as a seemingly random thought. In fact, the conscious awareness of many cravings is the result of persistent, low-level, subterranean activity in our reptilian brain. RecoveryMind Training teaches clients to pay special attention to such random thoughts that appear out of nowhere; they may be signals of unrest from deeper brain structures. Conversely, reading or talking about drug use or watching a movie with a protagonist who is alcohol dependent may stimulate memories, associations, or emotions that inadvertently and unconsciously reactivate drives to use. Memories in the neocortex about past use signal the limbic and reptilian brain, activating feelings and urges that drive individuals to repeat these past patterns—in this case, relapse.

One important healing experience in treatment and recovery is the telling of one's story. The teller has a feeling of exculpation, a release of the darkness inside. Once told, the patient can be guided from a narrative filled with distortion, justification, and faulty logic to a proper accounting of the truth of addiction's destruction. Over the years, I have noted these stories can have two diametrically opposing effects on the listener, one of which can prove to be troublesome.

On the one hand, the listener remembers his or her own past and develops an empathic connection with the speaker. The listener may recall a forgotten piece of his or her past and, in its recollection, have a deeper understanding of his or her own addiction journey. On the other hand, these stories may have a quite different effect. As the teller recounts explicit scenes or events, the listener's association circuits fire, dredging up more exacting images or even video sequences of past using events (addiction memory). Despite their negative nature, these memories can reactivate craving circuits and desires. The memories induce feelings of regret, recalled pain, shame over past behaviors, and "drug romancing." The last component of the recall is the most treacherous. Oddly enough, the more painful the past event, the more powerful the relapse urge. The counterintuitive collusion of "And then I did something that I can barely speak of . . ." and "Why do I feel an urge to use now?" is deeply vexing. A therapist overseeing the telling of a patient or client's addiction story should be attentive to the inadvertent activation of alcohol or other drug cravings in the teller and, if enacted in a group setting, other group members.

So, how is this conflicting, and downright disorienting, experience explained to those early in recovery? When we apply MacLean's model of the triune brain, the explanation is straightforward: The storyteller induces memories in the listener's mind. These memories are pulled up from the temporal lobes of the neocortex. The amygdala and other components of the limbic area add emotional content to the factual experience. If the recall is associated with a past powerful chemical use experience, the R-complex produces strong urges to repeat the past using event. The urge signals the anterior cingulate gyrus to rivet attention to the recalled past. Once started, the storyteller is "on a roll." While this is occurring, the frontal lobes of the neocortex react to the activation of craving and attempts to control the thoughts and actions that could lead to relapse. A deep and disturbing cognitive dissonance is produced by the scuffle between the memory and its associated urges, and the anguish that arises from a past regrettable addiction experience. At times, this cognitive dissonance piles on top of all the aforementioned thoughts, feelings, and urges, pushing the newly recovering individual closer to relapse. Therapists should respond with normalization and support when this occurs.

Our Faulty Memory System

Those suffering with addiction have difficulties putting their illness in proper perspective. A clear understanding of the course of one's illness is important to gain that perspective. Patients encounter many obstacles while reconciling their past, one of which is the inherently faulty recording and memory circuitry in the human brain. On top of each of our natural inborn inaccuracies, people with alcohol or other drug use disorders have additional challenges that stand in the way of the truth. The following is a list of the sources of faulty memory in addiction.

- The neurotoxic effects on memory caused by many drugs of abuse
- Psychological repression of the painful using experiences
- AddictBrain's attempts to rearrange memories to prevent detection
- The normal inborn twists in how memory is recorded and recalled

Many drugs of abuse are neurotoxic. These include the stimulants (methamphetamine, and to a lesser degree, cocaine), alcohol, and some hallucinogens. If a patient displays signs of drug toxicity, you can count on his or her learning and memory system being faulty as well. Psychological repression is also problematic when helping patients take stock of their addiction-related behaviors. Patients who have a previous history of psychological or substance-related trauma and are easily hypnotizable[13] have more difficulty recalling and cataloging the breadth and depth of their disease. Delicate psychotherapy skills are required when uncovering addiction-induced trauma in patients who suffer from the effects of other past traumatic events. Most importantly, patients are unable to comprehend their past completely because AddictBrain actively reorganizes and rewrites past events, which I will discuss further in Chapter Six.

As if these troubles were not enough, normal human recall is built on a shaky foundation. Everyone who is older than the age of fifty-five has noticed a failing memory; it is hard at times to recall a name or phone number. But our memory problems are much deeper than that. In truth, people of all ages have gross misrepresentations of the past, especially in autobiographical memory. In *The Seven Sins of Memory*, Daniel Schacter, PhD, summarizes research in this area.[14, 15] Problems with memory are universal and built into our species. Several of the seven intrinsic memory problems are especially relevant to addiction, including transience, misattribution, confirmation and stereotypical biases, and persistence.

- **Transience** is the degradation of memories over time. Memories of autobiographical events are modified and distorted each time an individual recalls them causing repeated deterioration in his or her accuracy.
- **Misattribution** is a phenomenon where true memory becomes distorted by additions of false information. In such a case, the memory of the past substance-related events might become misattributed and distorted, often by unrelated events. For example, let's consider Joe, a person with alcohol use disorder

who is married to Amy. Joe and Amy fight, in large part due to Joe's addiction disorder. He arrives in treatment after a particularly destructive binge. His brain remembers the highly destructive binge, but his memory misattributes what happened before the binge. He mistakenly believes that a particularly difficult fight occurred prior to the binge and blames his behavior on his wife's hostility. Upon further discussion, his therapist uncovered that Joe's drinking started first. His wife, frustrated with his return to drinking, complained to him about it. This resulted in a familiar verbal altercation that propelled Joe deeper into the bottle. Joe unconsciously misattributed the sequence of events, proffering his marital conflict as the cause rather than the victim of his drinking.

- **Confirmation and Stereotypical Biases** occur because individuals attach unconscious feelings, stereotypes, and belief biases when they encode information in their memory. Often they consider their points of view as being similar to those previously held. This distorts a person's memory in predictable ways, but the toxic effects of many abusable substances that impair cognitive flexibility exacerbate this. Consider the son who grew up in a household with a father who drank six vodka tonics every evening. As an adult, the son may decide to "drink limit" himself to one or two beers per night. After twenty years of controlled drinking, he slowly increases his consumption and develops alcohol addiction. His long habit of "two beers a night" produces bias that prevents him from recognizing the change in his pattern of use. He reports, "I limit myself to one or two beers a night, like I always have."

- **Persistence** is the unwelcome recall of unwanted or painful memory experiences. Many patients and clients suffer direct trauma from their addiction. When the memories of such events recur, the individual is triggered to relapse, either from the pain associated with the memories or the paradoxical excitation of craving described previously.

One central task in treatment is a careful review of the patient's using history, cataloging all available events related to the patient's using history and then placing them in an appropriate context. The myriad problems with memory make this a challenge for the patient and his therapist. Once collected, the patient has a compendium of his illness. The more accurate the history, the clearer the illness becomes; this, in turn, increases a commitment to recovery and creates reasons to avoid relapse. Each of the noted problems obstructs a healthy recovery perspective. Correcting memory faults is crucial, and I will discuss the techniques RecoveryMind Training uses to assist this process in Chapter Ten.

Faulty Memory and AddictBrain

The faulty nature of our memory system keeps individuals from remembering important details. "Did I start drinking after I heard of my brother's death or was I already imbibing?" All addictive substances exacerbate the transience of memory collection and distort recall.

Misattribution is particularly problematic when putting together one's past—especially when unhealthy or risky substance use is involved. What is often labeled "blaming others" is partly related to memory misattribution. Schacter describes it this way: "A strong sense of general familiarity, together with an absence of specific recollection, adds up to a lethal recipe for misattribution."[16] Consider someone with an alcohol use disorder recounting a particularly disturbing bout of drinking that resulted in a driving while intoxicated conviction. Because she often drank heavily with one friend who is also a heavy drinker, she misattributes her friend's presence at this event as well. She places the blame in part on her friend's tendency to encourage heavy alcohol consumption. After careful review with her therapist, she discovers this particular binge was an episode of solo drinking, driven by her illness alone.

Most inherent memory system flaws impede the reconstruction of past substance use; however, one of Schacter's "Seven Sins," persistence, directly abets relapse. The recall of past events and situations is often beyond our conscious control. All of us, when otherwise unoccupied or quietly gazing out a window, have had the experience of a memory rising to the surface, seemingly out of nowhere. Our memory system is not like a computer. Recall is only partly under voluntary control. Also memories have a capricious quality; they percolate to the surface at irrelevant times. Memories that are reinforced by substantive emotional content can be especially erratic and tenacious in this regard. Such is the case with memories associated with past experiences related to substance use. We label such memories **Addiction Memory**; they are cousins of post-traumatic stress disorder (PTSD). Actively trying to suppress addiction memory is a futile enterprise. RMT uses a helpful technique first suggested by G. Alan Marlatt, PhD, to "surf the urge," rather than attempting to push away or resist addiction memory. A further discussion of this topic will appear in Chapter Fourteen.

Certain events overwhelm our ability to record and make sense of them. Such events are locked in implicit memory by intense firing within emotional brain circuits. If such events are obstinate and severe enough, they can create symptoms of PTSD in a susceptible individual. PTSD memories contain two to three elements: sensory information, emotion overwhelm, and, often, a distinct "video loop." When the brain is unable to move such memories from implicit to explicit memory, this causes an extreme variant of Schacter's Persistence.[17, 18] Such traumatic memories are randomly triggered, often at the worst possible time. The individual re-experiences flashbacks of pain, confusion, and emotional upheaval that are nearly identical to the original event. This is best described as a "limbic storm." Intense discharge in this brain area overwhelms rational thought. Relapse into substance use can be a reflexive response, an automatic attempt to manage this limbic storm. Individuals with alcohol or other drug use disorders who suffer from significant addiction-induced PTSD almost always need one or more rounds of focused cognitive behavioral therapy,[19] medication management,[20] exposure therapy,[21] or EMDR[22] to prevent relapse.

Consciousness

Consciousness is a vast and complicated field, and research into the nature of consciousness is still in its infancy. The study of consciousness is truly multidisciplinary—neurobiologists, philosophers, evolutionary biologists, computer scientists, and many other disciplines contribute to this complex subject. Thousands of papers[23-29] and hundreds of books[30-50] have been written on the nature of consciousness. Note that in the process of culling consciousness theory and applying it to RecoveryMind Training, I will have unavoidably oversimplified concepts or left out important lines of thought.

The History of Consciousness

The late Francis Crick, PhD, called the mystery of consciousness "the major unsolved problem in biology."[51] The study of consciousness is indeed tricky; it is something we can only validate by subjective assertion, which is to say that its presence can only be detected by someone saying it is present. We do not even know if anyone besides our self is truly conscious.

The foundation of consciousness and rational thought began with work of René Descartes, the seventeenth century French philosopher and mathematician. Descartes was skeptical of the senses, concluding that they provided questionable information about the outside world. In contrast, Descartes believed the mind was able to visualize and comprehend all aspects of thought and that all thought is conscious:[52] ". . . there can be nothing in the mind . . . of which it is not aware, this seems to me to be self-evident."[53]

Descartes's view—that the mind was entirely self-aware—established one of the first frameworks for consciousness. When functioning in the most refined manner, man was a rational being, capable of complete self-control. Today, Descartes's framework may seem foreign, but this viewpoint permeated the Western world over the ensuing centuries; people surveyed their world and their reality and assumed that all actions occurred through conscious intent. This notion that the brain was completely conscious, aware of all its thoughts and actions, continued into the late 1800s with the work of William James, MD. James, heralded as one of the founders of modern psychology, also believed the mind was made up of only conscious thought. James's *Principles of Psychology*, published in 1890 described the working brain as entirely self-aware; only simple biological processes, such as breathing, were beyond our conscious control.[54]

It was not until the last decade of the nineteenth century and the early years of the twentieth century that human mind models leaped forward in their complexity. Sigmund Freud, revolutionized what it meant to be human—Bernard Baars, PhD,[55] clarifies that Pierre Janet, MD, PhD, and Jean-Martin Charcot, MD, were important to this revolution as well. Freud introduced a radical notion for the time: our brain acts, at times, in ways that are not accessible to conscious thought,[56] and we do not always act strictly under volitional control. Our mind is capable of thoughts that are beyond our access. We are at times the hapless victim of our attitudes and behaviors. Everything from the briefest of reactions to decades of family strife are manufactured and maintained by our unconscious brain.

Our recent ancestors did not think of themselves in this way. When we compare our understanding of what it means to be human with the understanding of our relatives from as little as three previous generations, it is as if humans today view themselves in a completely different light. Today, we acknowledge that each of us has unconscious thoughts, scattered liberally through our day and night. We may have habits, such as reaching for our coffee cup and taking a sip without previous perceived intent; automatic thoughts, or thoughts or memories that appear without any volitional effort; and sleep that is filled with complex and nuanced dreams that may be filled with meaning.[57]

What Is Consciousness?

Let's start by looking at the conundrum of consciousness by reviewing definitions. Much of this information comes from Dr. Adam Zeman's fine book: *Consciousness: A User's Guide.*[58] The word "conscious" has many definitions. It is, unfortunately, used to describe a whole host of human activities, which makes a highly complex topic even more obtuse. In an effort to bring order to the chaos, I will survey the multiple meanings of the word "conscious," using Dr. Zeman's classification.

The first and simplest meaning of "conscious" is as a synonym for "awake." We say, "He has come out of the coma and is now conscious." We may even use this term in the morning, observing our partner before her first cup of coffee, saying, "Are you conscious yet?" Here we are describing whether someone has the potential for self-awareness without implying that any is present. Interestingly enough, two very small areas of the brain render us conscious in this way: the reticular formation, located in the brainstem, and the intralaminar nuclei of the thalamus (the thalamus has two intralaminar nuclei, one on the left and one on the right side). We can have large sections of our cerebral cortex removed and remain conscious if we use this definition. However, both of these small brain areas—together about the size of a pencil eraser—must be functioning for us to be awake.[59, 60]

A second meaning of the word "conscious" denotes being aware of something, as in "He is aware of his surroundings." Gerald Edelman, PhD, proposed that this type of sensory integration is the most fundamental form of consciousness and labeled it *primary consciousness.*[61, 62] When scanning our environment and using our senses, the brain integrates this information with memories, creating an internal map. Several authors argue that animals, especially vertebrates, evolved this basic form of consciousness during the rapid expansion of life in the Cambrian period 540 million years ago.[63]

Sensory or primary consciousness forms the foundation for more complex forms. Note that when we notice, it is just the first of a cascade of events that occurs when something falls under our mental gaze. Being aware of the color orange, for example, creates associations that quickly accelerate into memories and associations. Upon seeing a certain shade of orange, we might think of pumpkins, which then trigger thoughts about fall, which in turn recalls memories of Halloween or the Thanksgiving dinners of our youth. In this manner, something as simple as awareness of a color extends its tendrils into emotions, memories, yearnings, and regrets from our past.

The third use of the word "conscious" arises in the term "self-conscious," meaning "prone to embarrassment." Most of us recognize and understand the term self-conscious when used in this manner. It is of little relevance in this discussion.

The fourth meaning of "conscious" means "recognizing oneself." At a very early age, children learn to recognize themselves and differentiate their being from others. This type of consciousness appears to extend down into the animal kingdom, where primates can easily detect themselves in mirrors and understand the difference between observing themselves in the mirror and recognizing others.[64] Recognizing oneself is an important prerequisite to understanding others as distinct entities, conscious or not.

A fifth meaning of "conscious" means "being aware that we are aware." We not only know something, we know ourselves to be beings who carry knowledge. We know that we know. This type of consciousness shows up in our everyday language. You may describe yourself as someone who likes pizza. I might describe myself as someone who dislikes crowds. When we make such statements, we are intuiting that we are autonomous and self-aware beings. Researchers call this phenomenon "Theory of Mind." We extend this type of consciousness to others when we say, "Sally knows she is not the kind of person who enjoys going outside of her comfort zone." When making this statement, we are using our abilities to intuit a self-aware quality in Sally. I will further discuss the Theory of Mind in the section entitled the Default Mode Network.

Zeman goes into more detail with these and several other meanings of the word "conscious." Suffice it to say that the many definitions of this word—for a whole array of mental events—reflect on how poorly we understand the phenomenon of consciousness. In this text, focus will be placed on the fourth (recognizing oneself) and fifth (being aware that we are aware) previously described. As you will soon learn, AddictBrain derails these types of consciousness, misdirecting self-awareness and simultaneously asserting that nothing is amiss.

Are Other Animals Conscious?

Consciousness feels magical or even spiritual. Some thinkers extend consciousness to other animals, our planet, or the entire universe. Most of us attribute some level of consciousness to animals other than *Homo sapiens*. Because most of our pets are vertebrates, we can safely say they have primary consciousness as described previously. Owners may ascribe a higher awareness to their pets, claiming their four-legged companions are conscious while citing the fifth definition. Most of us believe dogs have more consciousness than a fish. We attribute the "embarrassment" type of consciousness to our dogs, as they sulk away with a knowing look of contrition when caught stealing food from the table. Some owners point to their pets' remarkable personality as evidence their pets have the fifth and highest form of consciousness: being aware that they are aware.

We do not truly know the level of consciousness in other animal species due to our inability to communicate with them in a meaningful way. On the other hand, when human babies begin talking, we confer on them a rising level of consciousness. Language, including thinking with words, is different from consciousness but appears to be intuitively intertwined with it. We assume the capabilities of language impart a higher level of consciousness on those who possess such skills. In fact, psychologist Julian Jaynes proposed that consciousness arose out of our facilities for language, and without it, we would quite literally be unconscious beings.[65]

Many of us feel that consciousness has spiritual or religious dimensions. The emergence of self-awareness appears in the Book of Genesis, the first book of the Hebrew Bible and the Christian Old

Testament. Some physicists and physics buffs see the entire universe as conscious. One theory posits that consciousness is an inherent property of everything in the universe, integrated into matter at the deepest level by quantum mechanics.[66] Our mystical attachments to consciousness confer a degree of the sacred upon the organisms in which we infer it exists. Thus, we have more problems hurting a chimpanzee than killing a cockroach, presumably due to their different levels of consciousness.

The Limits of Consciousness

The brain processes thousands of signals all at once. Computer scientists—many of whom are interested in consciousness—call this parallel processing. While typing this page, my ears hear the clack of the keys. My skin sensors note that most of my body is warm but my fingers are cold. My eyes are watching the computer screen and noting the location of my fingers as they stumble across the keyboard. All the signals are consistent with the task at hand—writing these words. At the same time, my conscious mind is solely focused on the concepts I attempt to convey, pausing occasionally to search for the best word or phrase then moving back to the idea within this particular paragraph.

Suddenly, my auditory system picks up the sound of a truck barreling down the street. First, my unconscious auditory processing detects that there might be something amiss in this particular noise. Deeper structures in the brain send signals to my thalamus that distract me from my writing. Because consciousness can only hold a few items in our attention at a time, I drop my focus on the ideas contained in this text; my attention quickly shifts to the truck noise. It sounds loud and fast. My auditory processing circuit determines if something is indeed amiss. Is it simply a vehicle that is too large for the street? Is my car—parked on the street—safe? The truck rumbles by, and my attention refocuses on the writing at hand.

Despite the wonderment of associations developed by our consciousness, it has limits as to its extent and sustainability. For example, we cannot focus on a single element for more than a few minutes. Sustained attention is friable. Some argue that our ability for sustained attention has withered as society has created more and more intrusive technologies. These limits also extend to the number of items we can hold in our conscious mind. Even at our best, cognitive psychologists report that we cannot hold more than four to seven items in our working memory at one time.[67]

The illusion that our consciousness has depth comes from the rich associations and memories and the emotional content that emerge out of conscious deliberation. Even when we are deep in thought, our mind wanders off track, down side alleys, and away from our central train of thought. We forget what we are thinking and daydream for a moment about unrelated items. After a few seconds, we pull the initial thought out of our recent memory and return to the task at hand. Our consciousness is capable of discarding these interruptions when stitching the threads of consciousness together into a flowing sequence. This makes our conscious cogitation appear to us as a seamless and continuous story of importance, rather than the jagged and continuously interrupted helter-skelter set of brain firings that it really is. The rich nature of this interconnection and our ability to construct an imaginative whole out of the thoughts that reach our conscious mind causes us to overestimate how deep and wide consciousness is. In fact, consciousness is a tiny—but important—island in our big brain.

The Default Mode Network

Let's turn our exploration to one more aspect of the human mind, a brain process called the **Default Mode Network (DMN)**. I have previously discussed how the nervous system in animals has evolved over millennia. Figure 5.1 depicts the increase in complexity from simple animals, such as the earthworm, to an amphibian and to our own species, *Homo sapiens*. To better understand the default mode network, let's first delve into the evolution of brain systems across the animal kingdom.

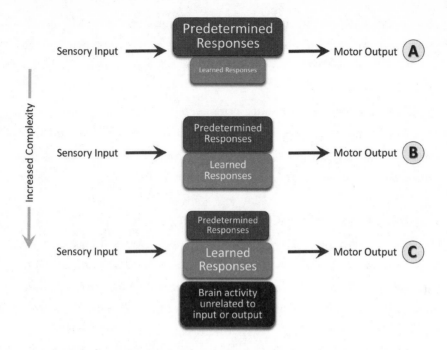

Figure 5.1 - Increasing complexity of the nervous system in animals

Section A of Figure 5.1 depicts an elemental nervous system. It collects sensory input (heat, cold, touch, pain, the proximity to food, etc.), and from this information it creates motor output (avoiding heat, retracting from pain, moving toward food). Throughout their life, animals with this type of nervous system rely heavily on the nerve connections they are born with. Hardwired responses are rapid and predictable, but the response is rigid. However, as Section A indicates, even primitive animals have a limited capacity to learn.[68]

Animals with more sophisticated nervous systems (depicted in Section B of Figure 5.1) learn throughout their life. They do not have to rely almost entirely on innate, hardwired behaviors depicted in Section A. A lioness spots a gazelle grazing on the plain. Its nervous system processes the sensory input, recognizes food, and begins calculating how fast to run. Thanks to her training as a cub, she swiftly separates the gazelle from the pack. Her nervous system sends signals to her muscles to begin the attack and alter her approach to create the most successful hunt. Increased processing power between sensory input and motor output leads to a more successful adaptation to a changing environment.

Note the nervous systems portrayed in Sections A and B are simply computers that gather input, massage those signals, and then produce a motor response. They are limited to two types of signal processing: responses hardwired at birth and learned adaptation to the environment.

Over the course of eighty-three million years, a third type of brain activity evolved: thoughts, ideas, and concepts appeared that were not related in any way to sensory input or motor output. It is unclear when this occurred, but the highest thoughts of human beings are the product of this dissociation. Like other mammals, the human brain, represented schematically in Section C of Figure 5.1, learns from the environment, constantly adapting to changing conditions. However Section C depicts a third type of nervous system activity. Consciousness and, more specifically, the default mode network are the products of this third brain type of brain activity.

In the 1930s, Hans Berger, the inventor of electroencephalography, or brain wave recording, discovered that our brain remains active whether we are active, resting, awake, or asleep.[69] Lower centers of our brain control our blood pressure, breathing, and other functions that keep us alive. Animals use the very same centers to perform the exact same life-sustaining tasks. Our brain's overall metabolic rate does not dramatically change when it moves from a resting state to intense mental effort.[70] The types of signals change, but they never stop. But what is the brain doing when we are not actively pursuing a goal, when we are awake but at rest? Eric Klinger, PhD, best summarizes the contents and seeming importance of this human state:

> Human beings spend nearly all their time in some kind
> of mental activity, and much of the time their activity
> consists not of ordered thought but of bits and snatches

of inner experience: daydreams, reveries, wandering interior monologues, vivid imagery, and dreams. These desultory concoctions, sometimes unobtrusive but often moving, contribute a great deal to the style and flavor of being human. Their very humanness lends them great intrinsic interest; but beyond that, surely so prominent a set of activities cannot be functionless.[71]

Our functional comprehension of these "bits and snatches" began in the late 1990s when neuroscientists built a new tool for peering into the working brain. The functional magnetic resonance imagery scanner (fMRI) tracks nerve cell activity based upon the use of oxygen in various locations within the brain; however, fMRI cannot accurately detect brain activity in real time. To overcome this problem, scientists had a subject in the scanner repeatedly perform a task, alternating with periods of "rest." They could detect a "signal" related to an activity under study by averaging the signals of multiple trials. Researchers eventually noticed that during periods without goal-directed activity, the brain fell into a predictable pattern. When not focused on a specific task—during "rest"—several interconnected but widely dispersed brain areas fell into a characteristic repeatable pattern of activity confirming earlier EEG data that the brain changes its activity pattern but never really goes into an idle state.

Struck by the consistency of the brain activity patterns that occurred *between* experiments, several laboratories began studying the brain at "rest." The network of brain centers that activated when a subject was not engaged in purposeful activity became known as the default mode network.[72] Multiple widely dispersed regions of the brain were connected in this default-firing pattern when not purposefully engaged. Thus, these regions were said to make up the default mode network. Our understanding evolved rapidly in the ensuing years. Research into the DMN has been described as "among the most rapidly growing neuroscientific topics of the new millennium."[73] The results of hundreds of published papers suggest the default mode network is responsible for quite a bit of conscious thought.

When we stop focusing on a specific task, we fall into a stream of consciousness and often become inattentive to the outside world. We are "lost in thought." The DMN is an extremely flexible neural network. It pulls in data from the past, adds emotional states (both real and imagined), and performs multiple, widely varying simulations about the future. Humans spend between 30 and 50 percent of their daily life engaged in such thoughts.[74] Interestingly enough, infants have little, if any, DMN activity; the network develops as a child matures from an unaware baby to a fully conscious adolescent.[75]

But what is the purpose of the default mode network? Research has suggested two seemingly disparate hypotheses about the DMN, summarized by Randy Buckner, PhD.[76] The first is that the DMN broadly monitors the environment without focus on any particular sensory event or events. A second, arguably richer proposition is that the DMN manages "internal mentation." Several large groups of research support this second hypothesis. The internal mentation hypothesis states that the default mode network is responsible for

- Self-reflective thoughts and judgments that comprise autobiographical memory;
- Envisioning and creating "what if" scenarios about the future;
- Theory of Mind—attributing consciousness to self and others;
- Making moral decisions, especially if those decisions involve ethical dilemmas.

The brain regions involved with the DMN are activated to a different extent based upon the activity of the DMN, as seen in Figure 5.2.

The first of these components is **autobiographical memory**. Autobiographical memory recalls past events and specific circumstances complete with their attached emotions. Each time we pull up such memories, we rebuild them to incorporate later information, our interpretations of the event, and our place in them. Our tendency is to expand our role in past events, as if we were the central actor in every recalled scene. As a memory ages, we shift from being a participant to observing the event as a spectator. When in the default mode network, we revisit and mull over past events, subjecting them to these distortions.

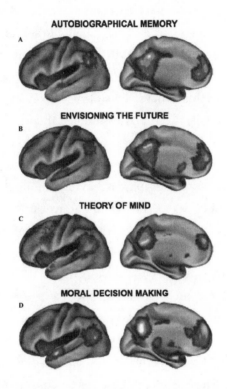

Figure 5.2 - Brain regions and activities of the Default Mode Network (From Bruckner, R.L., J.R. Andrews-Hanna, and D.L. Schacter. 2008. *Ann. N.Y. Acad. Sci.* **1124**: 1–38. © The New York Academy of Sciences.)

The default mode network produces a second type of experience: **envisioning the future**. Psychologists Dan Gilbert and Tim Wilson use the term "prospection" to refer to our ability to pre-experience the future by simulating it in our minds.[77] To illustrate this concept, Gilbert and Wilson use the example of someone knowing chocolate pudding would taste better if cinnamon was added to it instead of dill, although the person has never actually made such a comparison. This comes from the ability to construct a simulacrum of the future without experiencing it. Such mental pre-enactment has obvious evolutionary advantages; for example, an accomplished hunter-gatherer human living 15,000 years ago was most likely able to use prospection to think through the risks of hunting wild boar by himself, knowing how difficult it was in a previous outing when he was among a team of four men. This aspect of the DMN is thought to be partly driven by the brain's hedonic and attentional circuits.

The third aspect of the DMN is **Theory of Mind (ToM)** or "mentalizing." R. Nathan Spreng, PhD, Raymond Mar, PhD, and Alice Kim, PhD, describe this process by stating, "A key aspect of successful social navigation involves our possession of a theory of mind, that is, an understanding that the behavior of others is motivated by internal states such as thoughts, emotions, and beliefs."[78] ToM allows us to create an internal map of others, using past behaviors, thoughts, conversations, and expressed emotions to create an active simulacrum of others inside our head. We then interact with this person in our mind using prospection and make predictions about future interactions with him or her. In this manner others "live in our head." We create overarching beliefs about others, such as *Jane overreacts to her current husband because she was hurt in her previous marriage*. Even more importantly, we attribute conscious intent to those who live in our head, for example, *Because she knows how sensitive she is, she often chooses to withdraw*. As we think about Jane, we see ourselves as conscious as well; that is, *I should think about how to help her with this marital problem. We both value our deep friendship*.

The fourth putative aspect of the default mode network is its role in **moral decision-making**. The DMN is activated, for example, when experimental subjects deliberate whether it is acceptable to push one person off a boat to save five other people. It appears the DMN is activated the most intensely when moral dilemmas are personal as opposed to abstract. Such predicaments involve prospection, empathy, and Theory of Mind, and preliminary research shows decreased brain activity in several areas of the DMN when psychopathic individuals consider moral dilemmas, compared with empathetic controls.[79] Several researchers argue that more intense moral dilemmas engage emotional centers and decrease activation of the brain's memory circuits.[80]

Rumination is an all too human problem that is housed in the default mode network. The first two elements of the DMN are implicated in pathological rumination.[81] Thus the evolutionary benefits of the DMN may have an unwanted side effect: the propensity for ruminative depression. Malfunctions of the DMN are implicated in many brain diseases, including autism spectrum disorders and Alzheimer's disease,[82] as well as mental illnesses such as depression and schizophrenia.[83]

The most likely overall function of the default mode network is that of a "life simulator."[84, 85] When our focus on a current task falters, our minds smoothly fall into default mode. In this state, our minds wander across past events, often rearranging what happened (i.e., autobiographical history). We create future scenarios using internal representations of our friends, family, bosses, and others around us (i.e., envisioning the future). We consider others as individuals who act with conscious intent in ways that are consistent with our concepts of them— correct or not (i.e., Theory of Mind). We attempt to resolve interpersonal dilemmas using all the aforementioned tools (i.e., moral decision-making). This process weaves its way throughout our day, consuming one-third to one-half of our day without us even realizing it.

AddictBrain, Consciousness, and the Default Mode Network

Research into consciousness is in its infancy, especially when we consider its complicated nature. Our understanding of addiction is a bit further along, but research here too is only beginning. As a result, we can only make educated guesses about how addiction and consciousness interact. Because addiction changes so many brain functions, it seems self-evident that AddictBrain interacts with consciousness circuits as well. Based on clinical evidence, I postulate that this occurs in several ways. First and foremost, AddictBrain operates at lower levels in the brain. Human beings do not have the proper brain wiring to manage the powerful perturbations in brain functioning that occur while actively addicted. Individuals with alcohol and other drug use disorders attempt to use justifications that are readily at hand to rationalize the unusual and aberrant thoughts, drives, and events that occur during periods of substance use. If an individual is depressed, he or she may believe "I drink to feel better." An anxious person purports that he or she drinks to relieve anxiety, failing to comprehend that the extended alcohol use induces anxiety rather than reducing it.

As previously described, the consciousness circuits in the mind weave a coherent story out of an extremely chaotic existence. We experience our consciousness as a deep and wide expanse even though it is but a fraction of our brain functioning. We trust what our inner voice says even when it is incorrect. This leads to the **arrogance of consciousness**: We assert with a quiet confidence that we know what is *really* happening at any given moment. In fact, what we know is but a story manufactured by our consciousness that is often inaccurate but rarely in doubt. AddictBrain loves this delusion; it lets consciousness pontificate on false cause and effect while it stealthfully furthers its own agenda—continued destruction through substance use.

Let's dive further into how the default mode network might be distorted by addiction. The first element of the DMN, autobiographical memory, participates in the AddictBrain concept in at least two ways. When one recalls memories, they are reprocessed and placed back into storage. During this process, the remembrance of the event changes subtly, and the individual's role in the event changes—he or she tends to become the central actor. Painful memories become self-inflicted wounds; shame increases with each recall and reprocessing.

> Josie was a "hard partying woman," drinking to excess and using cocaine whenever she could get it. As her illness progressed, her behavior deteriorated. At parties with her friends, she would, on occasion, proposition men. One night, Errol, the husband of her best friend Lynn, approached Josie with a not-so-subtle proposal, which began a six-month affair. Josie was convinced she broke up her best friend's marriage.

Josie arrived in treatment with her head full of shame about past behaviors. None was more poignant than her affair with her best friend's husband. She was convinced Lynn would never speak to her again. After treatment, she cautiously approached Lynn to make amends. Propped up by her sponsor, she made a long stumbling apology for her reckless behavior. Lynn listened with a stone face. Josie sunk deeper in her chair. Finally, Lynn looked calmly into her eyes and said, "Josie, don't you remember our long talks about my marriage? I had been trying to get out of it for years. While I do not condone what you did, it set me free. Why would I be mad at you for helping get me out of jail?"

Slowly, Josie recalled snippets of her past conversations with Lynn. Despite what Lynn said, she continued to feel guilty for years. As her shame improved, her memory of Lynn's past unhappiness returned. Yet she could not shake the sense that she was a culprit rather than liberator because she violated her own moral code.

Therapists have long noted the antidote to this malady: each person with an alcohol or other drug use disorder needs to recognize that he or she does not produce all the world's pain and strife. This requires a corrective anamnesis of each individual's life story; the recovering individual gets "right-sized" as one of the world's billions of troublemakers. Hints as to the goal of the reparative history come from the work of William Dunlop, PhD, and Jessica Tracy, PhD. They assert that self-stories should aim at positive self-change in recovery—"I have a lot to do to get better"—rather than attempting to project an aura of stability—"A lot happened, but I am fine now."[86]

The second element of the default mode network is swept up into addiction as well. Once addicted, deeper areas of the brain—MacLean's R-complex—add the procurement and consumption of substances to the list of items that are essential for survival. When the default mode network envisions the future, continued use is deeply integrated into that vision. When applying prospection to an upcoming vacation, for example, someone with a drug use disorder immediately focuses on protecting access to his or her drug of choice. Travel logistics, possible activities, and potential fun and relaxation fall by the wayside, coloring the desirability of any planned activity. Traveling in winter to a warm, serene secluded beach on a Caribbean island will feel like a horrorshow to the person addicted to hydrocodone who needs to be near his supply.

When the DMN of a person with alcohol use disorder envisions the future, it is filled with scenes that center on drinking—despite his or her verbal attestation "I can quit at any time." Early in recovery, the longing for substances alters prospection, making a sober future seem bleak and lifeless. This distortion is particularly tenacious; it is not unusual for individuals with decades of sobriety to say, "When I retire I might start drinking; I hate to think I will never taste wine again."

The third element of the DMN, Theory of Mind, seems to be intertwined with AddictBrain as well. When people with alcohol and other drug use disorders "mentalize," they project their drug obsession onto other people because drinking remains front and center in their thoughts. Patients often resist asking family members to discontinue alcohol consumption during the first year of their recovery, saying, "It's not fair that they have to stop just because I have to." When they do ask, their spouse or significant other quickly responds, "That's a great idea; I will stop right away," leaving them nonplussed or incredulous. Individuals with alcohol and other drug use disorders are shocked by the number of people who do not drink or are indifferent to drugs; they often suspect that nonaddicted people are dissembling or yet to be initiated into the club of heavy substance use.

Individuals with alcohol and other drug use disorders also experience deterioration in the ability to construct Theory of Mind. Repeated use of alcohol and other drugs blunts many cognitive processes, especially those involving the frontal lobes of the cortex. Over a period of months or years of substance use, the person with alcohol or other drug use disorders increasingly misunderstands how his or her actions affect friends and loved ones, loses the ability to construct internal representations of others (ToM), and often believes he or she is the catalyst for much of what occurs around him or her. These behaviors are residual from childhood called phenomenalistic causality, a term described by psychologist Jean Piaget.[87] Long into recovery, many recovering individuals continue this misattribution, feeling as if they are the cause of all the problems occurring in their families or support systems. These defects of meaningful empathic connection produce an apparent indifference to others that is often confused with sociopathy.[88] In Domain C and E of RecoveryMind Training, I will discuss the importance of building emotional awareness and interpersonal skills to begin the repair of Theory of Mind.

Another important aspect of the default mode network is resolving moral decisions. The realignment of basic needs—alcohol and/or other drug use becoming a basic need—colors the moral decision process of the DMN. The moral code of every person with an alcohol or other drug use disorder shifts when the necessity of alcohol or other drug use escalates. Shifting values can make their moral judgments sociopathic, causing them to pilfer drugs from medicine cabinets, steal money from family and friends, and engage in other antisocial and criminal behaviors. Procuring drugs becomes more important than maintaining relationships; one's moral compass drifts way off course. Friends and family see behaviors deteriorate and, more importantly, ongoing moral judgments are severely eroded as well. AddictBrain deeply perverts the moral decision-making process of the DMN; considerable therapy and time in recovery is needed to realign healthy moral judgment.

Our Conscious Mind Is Not a Unity

Several researchers have suggested the cortex is organized into a series of social networks, each of which is constantly vying for control of conscious thought. Multiple computational centers operate in parallel. Using priority mechanisms that are, to date, unclear, a singular nidus of neuronal activity takes hold of consciousness for a brief moment. It holds on to conscious thought until another one of the processes takes over. The brain is constantly involved in a game of "King of the Hill"—at the top of the mountain lies conscious awareness. This concept was advanced during the rise of computer programming and is best articulated by Marvin Minsky, PhD,[89] and Michael Gazzaniga, PhD.[90] Dr. Gazzaniga's social network model of the brain also has import when discussing the AddictBrain concept. In this model, multiple computational centers are working in parallel on interpreting and reacting to the environment. In contrast, consciousness is seen as a thin veneer of short-lived attention to a singular task or thought. What we perceive as conscious thought is the current computational thread that has successfully bid for our attention.

When I train therapists or general audiences about the human mind, I highlight the concept of the triune brain and relate it to how difficult it is to be a human being. Addicted or not, each of us has multiple conflicting agendas. Dr. Minsky put it this way:

> The brain is . . . a great jury-rigged combination of many gadgets to do different things, with additional gadgets to correct their deficiencies, and yet more accessories to intercept their various bugs and undesirable interactions—in short, a great mess of assorted mechanisms that barely manage to get the job done.[91]

We live in a crowded, busy, and conflicted internal environment— our own mind. We are barraged by hundreds of thousands of simultaneous sensory inputs—the sound of a jet in the distance, your neighbor's car driving by, an occasional bird singing his springtime courtship ritual, the sound of the fan in the next room—combined with thousands of biological processes—the growling belly of hunger, aches and pains, the urge to scratch that itch, a full bladder. Even as I write this paragraph, I am harangued by thoughts of what I might eat for lunch, when my wife will return home from her exercise class, what I have to do next week at the office, and a vague unease that comes from making too many commitments. While all this is going on, somehow I expect my mind to stay on track to complete this book and communicate effectively to my readership.

Although we think of our consciousness as an inseverable unity, it is not. The neurophilosopher, Patricia Churchland[92] challenges this belief, stating the following:

> Our sense of self is a brain construct, it is something your brain does. But the parts are dissociable. Our autobiographical memory, spatial orientation and placement of the body, our collection of ongoing experiences and the knowledge of what we can and cannot do are parts of this sense of self. Each of these parts are woven together into a unified construct, our "sense of self."[93]

Perhaps the most difficult part of being human is managing all our conflicted thoughts and emotions and reconciling our primitive drives with societal ethics and framework. Most patients with alcohol and other drug use disorders suffer from serious emotional disturbances, including those that occurred before the onset of chemical use and the many others produced by addiction itself. The interior battles in those suffering with addiction are immense, and they often feel insurmountable.

Addicted or not, our kludge brain rests at the core of our conflicts and emotional battles, while at the same time, it is—remarkably—the towering miracle of living a life of ineffable fullness, rich in meaning, joy, and pathos—and ending all too soon.

Much of Our Decision Process Is Unconscious

Human beings like to believe they make their own decisions; therefore, they control their own life. We prefer to see ourselves as aware and in charge of well-considered decisions. Neuroscience makes it increasingly clear, however, that many of our thoughts—therefore our eventual "decisions"—are indeed unconscious in nature. The Eureka Effect, a neurophysiological problem-solving process is one good example of this. Everyone has been stumped by a problem, given up on it, and then been surprised some time later when the answer inexplicably pops up. This *ah-ha* moment is universal; the correct answer suddenly appears, clear and implicitly correct. Mark Jung-Beeman, PhD, has studied this universal phenomenon and has determined that it occurs in a sequence of stereotypical steps.[94, 95]

First, you apply yourself to a vexing problem with concentrated effort. You become frustrated and give up on an immediate solution. At some later point when your mind is wandering with no conscious attention to the past problem, you are startled by a revelation—the answer to your previous conundrum. Although you are surprised by the result—it seems to have come out of nowhere—you intuitively recognize the answer as correct. Clearly, some of our best thinking occurs outside our conscious mind. The process of solving difficult solutions—sleeping on a problem or thinking in the shower—involves a complex interplay between the executive frontal lobes and the right hemisphere of the brain. With this process, we achieve insight by giving up; we are as far from voluntary effort as one can get. The problem that stumps conscious effort is solved by an unconscious event. The more we understand brain neurophysiology, the better we see the limitations of conscious choice.

Addiction and the Non-Unity Mind

The human mind is made of many conundrums. Addiction, too, develops outside conscious observation. AddictBrain is one of the many voices vying for attention in the head of a person with alcohol and other drug use disorders. As the illness progresses, AddictBrain gains strength, controlling thoughts, decisions, and actions. Over time, AddictBrain is increasingly the source of the "great ideas" that pop into the consciousness of a person with a drug use disorder. A clinical example might illustrate this process.

> *Frank is a married man who has had a long struggle*
> *with oral opioids. He has used heroin by insufflation and*

injection in the past. In an attempt to "get his life together," he makes a vow to limit himself to opioid pills, primarily oxycodone and hydrocodone. His life slowly improves; he marries and gets a better job, escaping his old using friends, especially his source who worked with him at the old company. He maintains himself on a tightly regimented dose of hydrocodone. He begins to call it "my medicine" because he functions well as long as he maintains a uniform dose. Soon, he and his wife are pregnant. Frank makes a vow to himself to get straight once and for all. He stops taking the pills.

As he and his wife approach delivery, Frank is excited about the future but troubled by the financial burden of a new family member. He needs to find a way to supplement his income. He broods about the future. One morning he is struck with a "great idea." He can moonlight at his old job for the extra cash he and his wife need.

Everyone reading this knows what happens next: Frank is reintroduced to his supplier at his old job. Working two jobs increases his stress and soon using opioids magically appears in his head as a good idea. Frank relapses shortly before his child is born.

AddictBrain pokes and prods the mind looking for ways to divert everyday decisions to its own ends. The unconscious problem-solving that occurs in the right cortex is hijacked by AddictBrain, similar to how it hijacks every other brain function to its own ends. This concept is best illustrated by a pithy recovery saying, "My best thinking got me here."

Gazzaniga's Interpreter

The final line of research I will discuss in this chapter explores how the brain constructs a coherent picture of the self from myriad sensations and actions. Science long ago identified the five senses—touch, sight, sound, smell, and taste. In the early 1800s, proprioception was identified and later became known as the sixth sense,[96] which often gets overlooked. **Proprioception** is the brain's ability to understand the relevant relative position of our body parts and the power that is required for controlled movement. In the past twenty years, science has come to understand that the brain has specific centers for each sense. Each of the sensory centers collects and processes information simultaneously. Borrowing a term from the world of computer science, our brain uses "parallel processing." My eyes register the color and shape of text on the screen. This information travels to my visual cortex where the shapes and colors are categorized. From here, the neuronal firing patterns travel to the occipitotemporal area where they become letters and words.[97] At the same time, my ears hear the hum of my computer and the muted roar of an airplane off in the distance. My sensory cortex detects the positions of my fingers, and my motor cortex produces just enough movement in the right places to type. I am only aware of the meaning that results from this effort.

Other higher processing centers (e.g., language construction and deconstruction) also use parallel processing. When I pause my typing and reflect on all this activity, despite the thousands of parallel processes that are occurring in my brain, I only sense language. When I step back a bit further and reflect upon myself performing this task I sense a unified whole, not a cacophonous multiplicity of sensory inputs, motor outputs, language construction, etc. Thankfully, I cannot perceive the millions of calculations that go into each bit of sensory processing and motor action. But how do we create the sense of a unified self, the thing we mean when we point a finger at our chest and say, "This is me"?

Dr. Michael Gazzaniga has spent much of his career exploring this phenomenon.[98–102] He has said he fell into the big question of self-identity after working with a small group of patients who had a specific brain surgery for epilepsy. Based upon extensive research, he posited the existence of a unification agent he dubbed the "interpreter."

Dr. Gazzaniga studied patients with epilepsy who had undergone a corpus callosotomy: surgically cutting the massive band of fibers that exchanges information between the right and left hemispheres of the neocortex. Individuals consented to this surgical procedure in the 1960s as a definitive effort to control frequent and debilitating seizures. The result for most patients was a dramatic decrease in the number and severity of their epileptic events; however, strange side effects emerged:

> In the first months after her surgery, shopping for groceries was infuriating. Standing in the supermarket aisle, Vicki would look at an item on the shelf and know that she wanted to place it in her trolley (cart)—but she couldn't. "I'd reach with my right for the thing I wanted, but the left would come in and they'd kind of fight," she says. "Almost like repelling magnets."[103]

At first glance, it seemed as if the two halves of the cortex were separate entities, vying for control of the brain's intentions. The left and right hemispheres of the cortex had lost communication when the corpus callosum was severed. After the surgery, the loss of communication between the two halves of the brain was played out though conflicted behaviors. In Vicki's case, the left arm—controlled by the right hemisphere—acted independently and at times in conflict with the right arm—controlled by the left hemisphere.

Dr. Gazzaniga, his mentor Dr. Roger Sperry, and other colleagues extensively studied these patients after surgery. In one experiment, for example, when the word *walk* was visually presented to the patient's left visual field, which is controlled by the right side of the brain, he got up and started walking. When he was asked why he did this, the left brain— where language is stored and where seeing the word *walk* was not available to conscious comprehension—quickly manufactured a reason for his action: "I wanted to go get a Coke."[104] It soon became clear that the right hemisphere of the brain lacked language; it could not "speak" or construct an internal dialogue based upon words. The experimenter's question was processed by the patient's left brain, which was unaware that the word *walk* appeared before left eye and the right brain—the corpus callosum had been cut, and signals could not traverse in a normal fashion. The left hemisphere of the brain had to make up a story to make sense of the right brain's actions.

To illustrate this further, let's review a second, classic experiment: images on a screen were presented in such a way that they would only be seen by the opposite visual area of the neocortex.[105] To understand this experiment, it is essential to recall that the brain swaps sides when visual images enter the brain (left cortex processes images on the right and vice versa) and that the opposite side of the brain commands the body (left brain commands the right arm and vice versa).

To help you follow the experiment outlined in this paragraph, refer to Figure 5.3 after reading each sentence. A chicken foot is displayed in such a way that it can only be seen by the right visual field and thus processed solely by the left cortex. The snow scene only appears in the left visual field; therefore, it is processed in the right visual cortex. The split-brain subject is asked to point with each hand to the card on the table that corresponds to the image he sees. The hemisphere that "saw" the image (left saw chicken foot, right saw snow scene) was able to command the arm that it controls to pick the correct corresponding image. That is to say, the left cortex, responding to the chicken foot commands the right hand to point to the image of the chicken and the right cortex commands the left hand to point to the shovel, relating it to the snow scene.

The remarkable nature of the split-brain patient shows up when the experimenter asks the subject why he pointed to each of the pictures. The subject notes the picture of the chicken (the language-enabled left hemisphere directs the right hand) and states that he pointed to the chicken because it relates to the chicken foot in his right visual field. This makes perfect sense; however, when asked why his left hand points to the shovel, there is a brief delay. His right hemisphere of the cortex does not contain language functions and, importantly, is not the location of the interpreter. After a short delay, the subject states that he pointed to the shovel to clean the chicken coop in which the chicken resides. In this experiment, the left hemisphere, which contains language and the interpreter, has to make up a story that matches the action of his right hemisphere and left hand. The incorrect (and concocted) response in this case is that he picked a shovel to clean out the chicken coop!

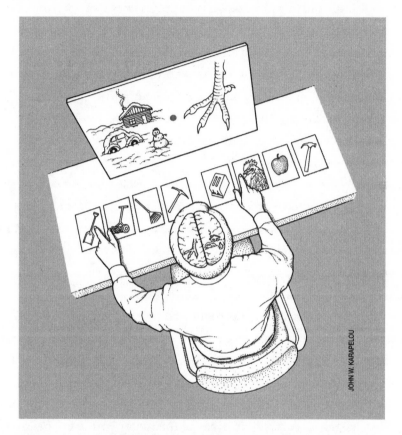

Figure 5.3 - Split-brain patients teach us about the interpreter

When reviewing this experiment, recall that sensory inputs (including vision) are processed by the contralateral hemisphere of the brain; the left brain processes our right visual field and the right brain processes our left visual field. Similarly, motor output (here control of the arm and hand) is controlled by the contralateral cortex. The left brain commands the right arm and vice versa. (Illustration © John W. Karapelou, CMI. Used with permission.)

Based upon this study and subsequent decades of additional research, Dr. Gazzaniga postulated that the left brain contains an interpreter, whose job it is to make sense of our actions and to create beliefs about the world around us. He points out that the interpreter does the best it can to decipher the environment around each individual—even when information it has at hand is faulty.

Studies from many other clinicians and researchers support this concept. Individuals with specific types of strokes may lose the ability to recognize parts of their body—a neurological condition called "anosognosia."[106, 107] When this happens, their brain's interpreter creates fantastical stories to make up for the lack of information. Patients with this condition often deny the limb or other body part is their own.

The implications of the interpreter are immense. First, this postulate supports other research suggesting language is deeply intertwined with consciousness. Second, it implies that the belief system we construct is to a large degree the product of our actions. Despite our convictions that we act in accordance with our beliefs, it may be the other way around. We believe things because we act a certain way. Said another way, the interpreter watches our actions and creates beliefs that fit past actions. Gazzaniga calls this concept "the post-facto world." Such a speculation has deep implications about whether or not we have free will.[108]

Gazzaniga's research is corroborated by Dr. Benjamin Libet, PhD, and his prescient studies from the 1980s. Libet observed electrical potentials in the motor cortex when a subject "decided" to act or not act.[109] He asked a participant to make a small movement while he measured the brain activity associated with the event. It had been previously known that certain areas of the motor cortex fire before the motor neurons that actually induce muscle movement. These neurons in the premotor cortex organize and prepare for movement, creating a "readiness potential." Libet compared the time when the subject became aware of the intention to move with the readiness potential and found that indeed that preparation for action preceded the conscious intention to move. This experiment posits that we take action before we "decide" what to do and questions whether or not we have free will or, at the very least, suggests that free will is constrained in some ways.

Libet's research brought about a tidal wave of heated discussion, valid criticism, and debate as to the proper interpretation of similar experiments. Nonetheless, we can conclude that everyone, including philosophers and neuroscientists cherish the belief that humans do indeed have free will but it is unclear how much we have and how it is expressed.

Using the construct of the interpreter, let us look at how we construct reality. The post-facto world hypothesis states that we react to events first and the brain subsequently interprets our responses. Our beliefs may or may not guide future actions, depending on how much free will we truly have. Shared beliefs create the rules of society. Such rules create a moral sense we are taught as children. The interpreter in the left hemisphere continually interprets events and creates stories that accommodate what we see and how we act. A perplexing moment occurs when the interpreter comes across information that does not fit the individual's actions. In such a case, the interpreter creates a belief that makes sense out of the new, ill-fitting data, at times discarding rational reality. This has significant implications about the disease of addiction that I will discuss next.

Consciousness and AddictBrain

Over the last few pages, I established that much of our brain's activity occurs outside the light of consciousness. More importantly, we explored the startling concept that the interpreter, a brain center posited by Dr. Gazzaniga, builds an ongoing narrative of our life. The interpreter creates a plausible story out of our actions under normal circumstances. In a reversal of cause and effect, the interpreter observes our behavior and posits intent based upon our actions, which in turn spins off life purpose and meaning. The stories we hold most dear are manufactured to make the most sense out of the data at hand. With all its elegance, the brain is subject to powerful misrepresentations of the external world.

How does this concept help us understand AddictBrain? It begins when addictive drug use triggers automatic learning—drug use shifts from a casual folly to a deep hunger. Priorities change, the importance of non-drug activities decrease; friends and family who stand in the way of continuing use become irritating impediments. Consciousness, the part of the brain that produces a continuous narrative about oneself, is twisted by powerful addiction-induced relearning and reprioritization. Working beneath conscious perception, AddictBrain creates situations and scenarios that are outside normal experience. The interpreter constructs the best reality it can, and in doing so, it manufactures stories that account for the facts but are nonetheless nonsense. A loved spouse who stands in the way of continued drinking becomes the enemy, and a fair but driven boss is seen as "out to get me." These subtle but pervasive twists of reality shift the blame away from addiction and toward external events and convenient scapegoats. Addiction literally reengineers the perceived reality of a person. The individual with alcohol or other drug use disorders is blinded to the self-destructive nature of his or her illness. Such a shift produces a grand denial of the real problem, the addiction itself.

Recently, the term "denial" has fallen out of favor in the addiction treatment world, presumably due to pejorative connotations that evolved out of overuse and misuse. In RecoveryMind Training I embrace this term rather than discard it. This is based upon one of the most important principles of conflict: the first step in defeating the enemy is to know it for what it really is. In RMT, the villain is named AddictBrain and its most important weapon, denial.

Chapter Five Notes

1. P. D. MacLean, *The Triune Brain in Evolution: Role in Paleocerebral Functions* (New York: Plenum Press, 1990).

2. We have carefully avoided calling this loosely coupled collection of nuclei the limbic system. The limbic area has many nuclei and nuclear clusters that are interconnected but often operate independently. They do have interconnections, share a close anatomical neighborhood, and emerged during the same general period of evolution.

3. This is especially true of more unusual species such as the monotremes (e.g. the Platypus) or the dodo (*Raphus cucullatus*).

4. Once we reached the complexity of the primate brain, many neuronal events appear to be completely disconnected from specific sensory stimuli and behavioral response. We will discuss this further in the section of this chapter titled The Default Mode Network.

5. D. Linden, *The Accidental Mind: How Brain Evolution Has Given Us Love, Memory, Dreams, and God* (Cambridge, MA: Belknap Press of Harvard University Press, 2007), 143.

6. Ibid.

7. A. Alcaro, R. Huber, and J. Panksepp, "Behavioral Functions of the Mesolimbic Dopaminergic System: An Affective Neuroethological Perspective," *Brain Res Rev* 56, no. 2 (2007): 283–321.

8. B. T. Chen, F. W. Hopf, and A. Bonci, "Synaptic Plasticity in the Mesolimbic System: Therapeutic Implications for Substance Abuse," *Ann N Y Acad Sci* 1187 (2010): 129–39.

9. J. LeDoux, *Synaptic Self: How Our Brains Become Who We Are* (New York: Penguin, 2003).

10. R. J. Davidson, K. R. Scherer, and H. H. Goldsmith, *Handbook of Affective Sciences, Series in Affective Science* (New York: Oxford University Press, 2009).

11. This is true up to a point. When an event is especially traumatic, our memory system can become swamped or overloaded. This may result in an intensely painful or traumatic memory being repressed. In such a case, lose the recollection of said event but keep its somatic correlates. This is one part of the post-traumatic stress disorder (PTSD) phenomenon.

12. J. B. Smaers, J. Steele, C. R. Case, A. Cowper, K. Amunts, and K. Zilles, "Primate Prefrontal Cortex Evolution: Human Brains Are the Extreme of a Lateralized Ape Trend," *Brain Behav Evol* 77, no. 2 (2011): 67–78.

13. S. J. Lynn, and K. Shindler, "The Role of Hypnotizability Assessment in Treatment," *Am J Clin Hypn* 44, no. 3–4 (2002): 185–97.

14. D. L. Schacter, *How the Mind Forgets and Remembers: The Seven Sins of Memory* (London: Souvenir, 2003).

15. L. R. Squire and D. L. Schacter, *Neuropsychology of Memory*, 3rd ed. (New York: Guilford Press, 2002), 97.

16. See above, n. 14.

17. E. Vermetten, M. J. Dorahy, D. Spiegel, and American Psychiatric Publishing, *Traumatic Dissociation: Neurobiology and Treatment*. 1st ed. (Washington, DC: American Psychiatric Pub., 2007).

18. J. E. Sherin and C. B. Nemeroff, "Post-Traumatic Stress Disorder: The Neurobiological Impact of Psychological Trauma," *Dialogues Clin Neurosci* 13, no. 3 (2011): 263–78.

19.   G. H. Seidler and F. E. Wagner, "Comparing the Efficacy of EMDR and Trauma-Focused Cognitive-Behavioral Therapy in the Treatment of PTSD: A Meta-Analytic Study," *Psychol Med* 36, no. 11 (2006): 1515–22.

20.   See above, n. 18.

21.   "CADTH Rapid Response Reports," in *Virtual Reality Exposure Therapy for Adults with Post-Traumatic Stress Disorder: A Review of the Clinical Effectiveness* (Ottawa, ON: Canadian Agency for Drugs and Technologies in Health, 2014).

22.   F. Shapiro, *Eye Movement Desensitization and Reprocessing (EMDR): Basic Principles, Protocols, and Procedures* (New York: The Guilford Press, 2001).

23.   A. Zeman, "What in the World Is Consciousness?" *Prog Brain Res* 150 (2005): 1–10.

24.   R. L. Buckner, J. R. Andrews-Hanna, and D. L. Schacter, "The Brain's Default Network: Anatomy, Function, and Relevance to Disease," *Ann N Y Acad Sci* 1124 (2008): 1–38.

25.   C. S. Soon, M. Brass, H. J. Heinze, and J. D. Haynes, "Unconscious Determinants of Free Decisions in the Human Brain," *Nat Neurosci* 11, no. 5 (2008): 543–45.

26.   T. C. Dalton and B. T. Baars, "Conciousness Regained: The Scientific Restoration of Mind and Brain," (2003).

27.   M. Jung-Beeman, E. M. Bowden, J. Haberman, J. L. Frymiare, S. Arambel-Liu, R. Greenblatt, P. J. Reber, and J. Kounios, "Neural Activity When People Solve Verbal Problems with Insight," *PLoS Biol* 2, no. 4 (2004): E97.

28.   J. Lehrer, "The Eureka Hunt," *The New Yorker*, July 2008.

29.   E. M. Dewan, "Consciousness as an Emergent Causal Agent in the Context of Control System Theory," in *Consciousness and the Brain*, eds. Gordon G. Globus, Grover Maxwell, and Irwin Savodnik (New York: Springer, 1976), 181–98.

30.   A. Combs, *Consciousness Explained Better: Towards an Integral Understanding of the Multifaceted Nature of Consciousness,* Omega Books, First ed. (St. Paul, MN: Paragon House, 2009).

31.   F. Crick, *The Astonishing Hypothesis: The Scientific Search for the Soul* (New York: Scribner, 1994).

32.   A. R. Damasio, *The Feeling of What Happens: Body and Emotion in the Making of Consciousness*, First ed. (New York/London: Harcourt Brace, 1999).

33.   *Looking for Spinoza: Joy, Sorrow, and the Feeling Brain*, First ed. (Orlando, FL: Harcourt, 2003).

34.   *Descartes' Error: Emotion, Reason and the Human Brain* (New York: Penguin Books, 2005).

35.   D. C. Dennett, *Consciousness Explained*, First ed. (Boston: Little, Brown, and Co., 1991).

36.   M. Donald, *Origins of the Modern Mind: Three Stages in the Evolution of Culture and Cognition* (Cambridge, MA: Harvard University Press, 1991).

37.   M. S. Gazzaniga, *The Mind's Past* (Berkeley, CA: University of California Press, 1998).

38.   *The Ethical Brain* (New York: Dana Press, 2005).

39.   E. Goldberg, *The Executive Brain: Frontal Lobes and the Civilized Mind* (New York: Oxford University Press, 2001).

40.   M. S. A. Graziano, *Consciousness and the Social Brain* (Oxford: Oxford University Press, USA, 2013).

41. J. E. LeDoux, *The Emotional Brain: The Mysterious Underpinnings of Emotional Life* (New York: Simon & Schuster, 1996).

42. R. Parasuraman, *The Attentive Brain* (Cambridge, MA: MIT Press, 1998).

43. S. Pinker, *The Stuff of Thought: Language as a Window into Human Nature* (New York: Viking, 2007).

44. J. R. Searle, *The Rediscovery of the Mind*. Representation and Mind. First MIT Press paperback ed. (Cambridge, MA: MIT Press, 1994).

45. A. Zeman, *Consciousness: A User's Guide* (New Haven, CT; London: Yale University Press, 2002).

46. S. J. Blakemore, *Conversations on Consciousness, What the Best Minds Think About the Brain, Free-Will and What It Means to Be Human* (Oxford University Press, 2006).

47. B. Baars, *In the Theater of Conciousness: The Workspace of the Mind* (New York: Oxford University Press, 1997).

48. M. L. Minsky, *The Society of Mind* (New York: Simon & Schuster, 1988).

49. M. Gazzaniga, *The Social Brain: Discovering the Networks of the Mind* (New York: Basic Books, 1987).

50. J. Jaynes, *The Origin of Conciousness in the Breakdown of the Bicameral Mind* (New York: Houghton Miffin, 1990).

51. See above, n. 31.

52. See above, n. 47.

53. R. Descartes, *Fourth Set of Replies, Ii, Sixth Meditation, Philosophical Writings of Descartes* (London: Cambridge University Press, 1637).

54. W. James, *The Principles of Psychology* (Cambridge, MA: Cambridge University Press, 1890).

55. See above, n. 47.

56. G. Makari, *Revolution in Mind: The Creation of Psychoanalysis* (New York: Harper Perennial, 2008).

57. J. A. Hobson, "REM Sleep and Dreaming: Towards a Theory of Protoconsciousness," *Nat Rev Neurosci* 10, no. 11 (2009): 803–13.

58. See above, n. 45.

59. J. E. Bogen, "On the Neurophysiology of Consciousness: I. An Overview," *Conscious Cogn* 4, no. 1 (1995): 52–62.

60. J. E. Bogen, "On the Neurophysiology of Consciousness: Part II. Constraining the Semantic Problem," *Conscious Cogn* 4, no. 2 (1995): 137–58.

61. G. M. Edelman, *Wider Than the Sky: The Phenomenal Gift of Consciousness* (New Haven, CT: Yale University Press, 2004).

62. G. M. Edelman, "Naturalizing Consciousness: A Theoretical Framework," *Proceedings of the National Academy of Sciences* 100, no. 9 (2003): 5520–24.

63. T. E. Feinberg and J. M. Mallatt, *The Ancient Origins of Consciousness How the Brain Created Experience* (Cambridge, MA: MIT Press, 2016).

64. G. Gallup, "Chimpanzes: Self-Recognition," *Science* 167 (1970): 86–87.

65. See above, n. 50.

66. H. Atmanspacher, "Quantum Approaches to Consciousness."

67. R. Bourtchouladze, *Memories Are Made of This* (London: Phoenix Press, 2002).

68. R. Hawkins, T. Abrams, T. Carew, and E. Kandel, "A Cellular Mechanism of Classical Conditioning in Aplysia: Activity-Dependent Amplification of Presynaptic Facilitation," *Science* 219, no. 4583 (1983): 400–05.

69. L. F. Haas, "Hans Berger (1873–1941), Richard Caton (1842–1926), and Electroencephalography," *Journal of Neurology, Neurosurgery & Psychiatry* 74, no. 1 (2003): 9.

70. D. H. Ingvar, "Hyperfrontal Distribution of the Cerebral Grey Matter Flow in Resting Wakefulness; on the Functional Anatomy of the Conscious State," *Acta Neurol Scand* 60, no. 1 (1979): 12–25.

71. E. Klinger, *Structure and Functions of Fantasy*, (Toronto, ON: John Wiley & Sons Canada, Limited, 1971).

72. R. L. Buckner, "The Serendipitous Discovery of the Brain's Default Network," *Neuroimage* 62, no. 2 (2012): 1137–45.

73. J. R. Andrews-Hanna, "The Brain's Default Network and Its Adaptive Role in Internal Mentation," *Neuroscientist* 18, no. 3 (2012): 251–70.

74. M. A. Killingsworth and D. T. Gilbert, "A Wandering Mind Is an Unhappy Mind," *Science* 330, no. 6006 (2010): 932.

75. R. L. Carhart-Harris and K. J. Friston, "The Default-Mode, Ego-Functions and Free-Energy: A Neurobiological Account of Freudian Ideas," *Brain* 133, no. Pt 4 (2010): 1265–83.

76. R. L. Buckner, J. R. Andrews-Hanna, and D. L. Schacter, "The Brain's Default Network," *Ann N Y Acad Sci* 1124, no. 1 (2008): 1–38.

77. D. T. Gilbert and T. D. Wilson, "Prospection: Experiencing the Future," *Science* 317, no. 5843 (2007): 1351–54.

78. R. N. Spreng, R. A. Mar, and A. S. N. Kim, "The Common Neural Basis of Autobiographical Memory, Prospection, Navigation, Theory of Mind, and the Default Mode: A Quantitative Meta-Analysis," *J Cogn Neurosci* 21, no. 3 (2008): 489–510.

79. R. L. Reniers, R. Corcoran, B. A. Vollm, A. Mashru, R. Howard, and P. F. Liddle, "Moral Decision-Making, TOM, Empathy and the Default Mode Network," *Biol Psychol* 90, no. 3 (2012): 202–10.

80. J. D. Greene, R. B. Sommerville, L. E. Nystrom, J. M. Darley, and J. D. Cohen, "An fMRI Investigation of Emotional Engagement in Moral Judgment," *Science* 293, no. 5537 (2001): 2105–08.

81. M. G. Berman, S. Peltier, D. E. Nee, E. Kross, P. J. Deldin, and J. Jonides, "Depression, Rumination and the Default Network," *Soc Cogn Affect Neurosci* 6, no. 5 (2011): 548–55.

82. See above, n. 24.

83. A. Anticevic, M. W. Cole, J. D. Murray, P. R. Corlett, X.-J. Wang, and J. H. Krystal, "The Role of Default Network Deactivation in Cognition and Disease," *Trends Cogn Sci* 16, no. 12 (2012): 584–92.

84. D. T. Gilbert, *Stumbling on Happiness*, First ed. (New York: A. A. Knopf, 2006).

85. See above, n. 77.

86. W. L. Dunlop and J. L. Tracy, "The Autobiography of Addiction: Autobiographical Reasoning and Psychological Adjustment in Abstinent Alcoholics," *Memory* 21, no. 1 (2013): 64–78.

87. J. Piaget, *The Construction of Reality in the Child* (New York: Basic Books, 1954).

88. A. R. Lindesmith, "The Drug Addict as a Psychopath," *American Sociological Review* 5, no. 6 (1940): 914–20.

89. See above, n. 48.

90. See above, n. 49.

91. M. L. Minsky, "Smart Machines," Chap. 8 in *Third Culture: Beyond the Scientific Revolution*, ed. John Brockman, 416: Touchstone, 1996.

92. P. S. Churchland, *Touching a Nerve: The Self as Brain*, First ed. (New York: W. W. Norton & Company, Inc., 2013).

93. Nature, *Neuropod Extra: Touching a Nerve*, podcast audio 16:072013, http://www.nature.com/neurosci/neuropod/index-2013-11-30.html.

94. See above, n. 27.

95. See above, n. 28.

96. U. Proske and S. Gandevia, "Proprioception: The Sense Within," *The New Scientist*, http://www.the-scientist.com/?articles.view/articleNo/46796/title/Proprioception--The-Sense-Within/.

97. J. T. Devlin, H. L. Jamison, L. M. Gonnerman, and P. M. Matthews, "The Role of the Posterior Fusiform Gyrus in Reading," *J Cogn Neurosci* 18, no. 6 (2006): 911–22.

98. See above, n. 49.

99. See above, n. 38.

100. See above, n. 37.

101. M. S. Gazzaniga, "The Science of Mind Constraining Matter," University of Edinburgh, http://www.ed.ac.uk/schools-departments/humanities-soc-sci/news-events/lectures/gifford-lectures/archive/archive-2009-2010/prof-gazzaniga.

102. M. S. Gazzaniga, "The Split Brain Revisited," *Sci Am* 279, no. 1 (1998): 50–55.

103. D. Wolman, "The Split Brain: A Tale of Two Halves," *Nature* 483, no. 7389 (2012): 260–63.

104. See above, n. 38.

105. In the brain's visual system, images from our right visual field travel to the left brain, and our right visual field information is interpreted by our left brain. This same type of neuronal crossover occurs in our sensory and motor systems.

106. K. M. Heilman, "Possible Mechanisms of Anosognosia of Hemiplegia," *Cortex* 61c (2014): 30–42.

107. A. Ananthaswamy, *The Man Who Wasn't There: Investigations into the Strange New Science of the Self* (New York: Dutton, 2015).

108. M. S. Gazzaniga, *Who's in Charge?: Free Will and the Science of the Brain*, Gifford Lectures, First ed. (New York: HarperCollins, 2011).

109. B. Libet, "Unconscious Cerebral Initiative and the Role of Conscious Will in Voluntary Action," Chap. 16 in *Neurophysiology of Consciousness: Contemporary Neuroscientists* (Boston, MA: Birkhäuser, 1993), 269–306.

Deeper into AddictBrain

Connecting personhood to biology is a ceaseless
source of awe and respect for anything human.
ANTONIO DAMASIO

In the previous chapter, I described how the brain is really a group of loosely interconnected structures that emerged sequentially in the evolution of the animal kingdom. Lower centers are more rigid and harder to turn off. Higher—and evolutionarily more recent—areas are capable of more complex and nuanced thought, but those thoughts are manipulated and overridden by the drives from the R-complex and emotional discharge in the limbic area. I also discussed the mind's problems with memory, even under normal circumstances, and how AddictBrain can exploit these problems to its own end. Finally, the baffling nature of consciousness was introduced and how it, too, may be enlisted in the service of AddictBrain.

In this chapter, I will look at the rapidly expanding body of addiction research and apply it to the AddictBrain concept. Over the history of addiction research, many models have been proposed, and many more will undoubtedly emerge over time. However, as of the writing of this text, three models predominate:

- The opponent process model[1, 2]

- The incentive salience model[3, 4]
- The aberrant learning model[5]

Decades of research have gone into these models. An excellent review of the research into the first two models is available.[6] They are not necessarily mutually exclusive. A recent review incorporates all three models into a heuristic system that delineates each phase of the addiction cycle.[7] RecoveryMind Training considers how each of the models contributes to different parts of the AddictBrain concept.

RecoveryMind Training contends the overall effect of AddictBrain is produced by changes in brain functioning that occur when someone progresses from casual use to the illness of addiction.[8-11] Four distinct brain-wide modifications, when combined together, comprise AddictBrain. The RecoveryMind Training model proposes that AddictBrain overwhelms an individual's conscious control, reorganizes life goals, and ensures its own survival in using these four mechanisms. The four components of AddictBrain are:

1. Shifting drug experience and drug wanting
2. Attention and prioritizing
3. Learning and memory
4. Cloaking

These components parturitate addiction's powerful grip on its victims. Each is part of the orchestrated whole of AddictBrain.

The first component of AddictBrain has two subparts—shifting drug experience (opponent process) and drug wanting (incentive salience). In shifting drug experience, the alcohol or drug user experiences changes as he or she shifts from casual to addictive use. Although pleasure and novelty drive initial drug consumption, desirable effects wane and are replaced over time by the negative consequences of continued use. The habitual opioid user, for example, experiences emotional pain and withdrawal when the drug is not available. Individuals who use alcohol, stimulants, and opioids develop anhedonia[12] and depression when use stops. These two opponent effects are paired, and each reinforces the other. In an effort to avoid the unpleasant aspects of withdrawal, the individual is driven by the hope of relief and pleasure. This opponent process studied by George Koob, PhD, and colleagues is now supported by decades of research[13, 14] and recent findings.[15-18]

The second subpart of the first component of AddictBrain is drug wanting. Robinson and Berridge have proposed a different and potentially complementary theory behind addictive drug use. According to this theory, reward induces wanting, which they defined with clarity using the term "incentive salience."[19] Drug, alcohol, or compulsive behaviors produce brain signals that earmark an event or situation as vital to an animal—be it human or otherwise. Wanting, i.e., incentive salience, impels the individual to repeat his or her initial drug experience.

Both subparts of the first component trigger changes in other brain circuits, which then kindle the remaining AddictBrain components. Once addiction is established, the afflicted individual develops a laser focus on effective drug or alcohol use. Even someone with severe attention deficit disorder who develops a drug use disorder can maintain focus on a series of complex interlinked tasks to procure and use his or her alcohol or drug. The addicted individual reprioritizes life goals, placing substance use at the top. These rearrangements in attention and priority comprise the second component of AddictBrain.

The third component of AddictBrain has to do with learning and memory. Component one induces drug wanting and a vicious cycle of use in the individual with addiction. Component two solidifies attention and changes priorities. Combined together, these first two components drive memory circuits to learn as much as possible about substance use. The individual becomes adept at procuring substances, memorizing phone numbers of suppliers, learning the route to and the hours of operation of a liquor store, or sneaking substances into treatment centers, jails, workplaces, and school. The brain earmarks substance use as a critical experience. The brain generates encyclopedic and hardwired memories about drug and alcohol use to ensure it continues in as efficient a manner as possible.

The fourth component of AddictBrain is the most perplexing. For the vast majority of individuals with the disease of addiction, a life focused on destructive substance use opposes their inborn and entrained value system. In order to sustain itself, AddictBrain builds a wall of deception and secrecy around itself. Self-awareness is hijacked. AddictBrain rearranges reality, preventing afflicted individuals from accurately recognizing the devastation wrought by their illness. Self-appraisal and self-correction centers go off-line. In perhaps its cruelest effect, AddictBrain shifts blame from itself to any other convenient target, often friends, work, or loved ones. "Reasons for using" may seem absurd or bizarre to others but fit perfectly in AddictBrain's handcrafted reality. This is cloaking, the fourth component of AddictBrain.

Table 6.1 identifies some of the brain areas that are instrumental in the development and continuation of addiction. Although it is not critical to know these brain areas, it may help you sort out the AddictBrain activities described in this chapter.

AddictBrain Component One: Shifting Drug Experience and Drug Wanting

Addiction research is a fast-evolving science with new discoveries emerging every day. Over the past several years, research has settled on three paradigms to describe the transition from casual drug use into addiction. They are the incentive salience, aberrant learning, and the opponent process theory. Each of the current paradigms is part of the AddictBrain concept. Two of the research models are relevant to AddictBrain Component One, the incentive salience and opponent process theories. Both of these theories are built on research from the latter part of the twentieth century. (Please refer to Chapter Three for

Table 6.1 - Brain Structures and AddictBrain

Brain System	Purpose	Benefit to *Homo sapiens*	Hijacked by AddictBrain
Mesolimbic Dopamine Circuit, primarily the Nucleus Accumbens and Ventral Tegmental Area	Alerts us to novel and important stimuli and triggers the brain to learn (neuroplasticity). Triggers the brain by generating curiosity, novelty seeking, and reward.	Ensures the procurement of food and water, procreation, child rearing, and potential living environments.	Changes dopamine firing produced by addicting substances reward use, triggering signal salience. Changing responsivity over time produces anhedonia, which negatively reinforces continued use.
Area of the Anterior Cingulate Gyrus	Once activated, focuses attention on important tasks (situations, places, and people who are defined by one or more of these terms: novel, significant, important, relevant, and fundamental).	Ability to attend to potentially harmful cues. Focuses human beings on attending to food and water supplies, procreation, learning, and life and species sustaining efforts.	Unintentional diversion from day-to-day activities to alcohol or drug procurement skills. Inappropriate attention to and focus on drug-related cues in the environment.
Striatum and Basal Ganglia, Limbic Area, Cerebellum	Complex and high priority procedural learning. Habit formation.	Ability to perform tasks without direct focus. Adaptation to changing environments helps species spread across the planet.	Creates habits that ensure continued use and promote relapse. In early recovery, using skills are more highly entrained than sobriety skills.
Neocortex	Thought, voluntary action, language, creation of a narrative, reasoning, and consciousness.	Complex socialization, culture, art, and inventions that improve survivability (and potential self-destruction).	Incorrect interpretation of historical information. AddictBrain rewrites reality, producing complex denial.

additional information.) The exact nature of the first component of AddictBrain has been well studied. It is best to consider this component as being built upon two theories: shifting drug experiences and drug wanting.

Shifting Drug Experiences: Opponent Process Theory

Dr. George Koob and colleagues have studied the addiction drive for decades, proposing that opponent process theory is the prime driver in addiction.[20] This theory argues that the rewarding effect of drugs promotes initial drug consumption. A novel and positive first experience makes an individual curious to repeat it. Negative consequences are minimal and transient at first. With each repeated use, the novelty and euphoria abate and post-use consequences increase. Chronic substance use induces a state of anhedonia that the individual with an alcohol or drug use disorder constantly tries to correct with additional substance use. Repeated use further exacerbates anhedonia and depression in a vicious cycle. The interaction between these two forces is the heart of opponent process theory. The individual with an incipient drug use disorder develops an aggravated sense that her alcohol or other drug consumption will repair her anhedonia and depression. This effectively releases the brakes on a runaway train. Chronic drug use is largely driven by abnormalities in the reward system, which accelerates the negative aspects of continued use.[21-29] Those struggling with alcohol and drug use disorders are driven in a downward spiral by this opponent process.

Drug Wanting: The Incentive Salience Theory

A second theory that makes up the first component of AddictBrain is "wanting." Neuroscientists define "wanting" as incentive salience. The concept of incentive salience evolved out of earlier research on the reward center in the brain. The reward center was discussed in Chapter Three; in this chapter I will bring that research up-to-date, highlighting the difference between reward and wanting prior to incorporating it into the AddictBrain model.

In the 1980s, research was reevaluating the actions of the ventral tegmental area, medial forebrain bundle, and the nucleus accumbens in the genesis and maintenance of addiction. When first discovered, this area was labeled the "pleasure center." Its moniker was changed to the "reward center" in the 1990s. When we think of reward, we naturally think of pleasure. As it turns out, the central effect of the reward center is not the production of pleasure but a drive to repeat the behavior or experience that triggered the event in the first place. Rewards incentivize us to continue life-sustaining behaviors, which include ingesting food and water, ensuring sexual responsiveness, maintaining safety, and child rearing.[30]

Our expanded understanding regarding the reward center comes from many research groups, notably the work of Kent C. Berridge and Terry E. Robinson.[31] Using carefully designed experiments, this group teased out critical differences between the pleasurable elements of drugs and food from the compulsive, highly motivated behaviors associated with the addictive drive. After ablating the core of the nucleus accumbens (part of the reward center) in rats, the animals were no longer motivated to seek out simple rewards, including food and sex and drugs. However, when food was supplied directly to the animal, without any effort on its part, it exhibited characteristic behavioral signs of pleasure. The destroyed neurons appeared to control incentive rather than pleasure. They concluded that the perception of pleasure is located in areas of the brain distinct from the nucleus accumbens.[32, 33] Their research suggests that the reward center be relabeled as the center for incentive salience.[34]

In this manner, wanting and pleasure are dissociated; that is, they do not necessarily occur together.[35] This is a common experience of individuals who develop addiction: once deep inside their addiction, wanting continues unabated, long after pleasure has gone. One of my patients with a drug use disorder described it this way:

> *In recent months, I knew with all my heart that using cocaine would be horrible. Instead of the intense euphoria I felt in the now-distant past, I would invariably become agitated and paranoid. I would hear voices, pace about the house incessantly, and wring my hands. Every time I started yet another binge, I recognized this truth. However, knowing this did not matter; I was mercilessly driven to use more and more.*

A similar experience occurs when one becomes tobacco dependent. As tobacco use has become more restricted in our society, smokers are better able to recognize the diminishing rewards from continuing their habit. After smoking for years, the pleasure from tobacco use diminishes. As a result, most smokers express a desire to quit. Attempts to quit fail, pleasure has decreased, but wanting continues unabated. Tobacco addiction combines increasingly elusive pleasures with unrelenting hunger.

Scientists and clinicians were both perplexed by these experiences in tobacco and cocaine dependent individuals prior to this work on incentive salience. Once elucidated, it became clear that midbrain dopamine systems are necessary for "wanting" incentives but not for "liking" them or for learning new "likes" and "dislikes."[36] The relationship between wanting, liking, and learning is schematized in Figure 6.1. Drug or alcohol use begins with low wanting, high liking, and little automatic learning. Over time, liking decreases and wanting increases. The likelihood and efficiency of continued use is ensured by continued activation of incentive salience by addictive drugs.[37]

The brain process referred to as "wanting" is complex, originating in drive centers more primal than conscious thoughts and urges. The center for incentive salience prioritizes and focuses the organism on continued drug procurement. In this manner, individuals with substance use disorders demote activities unrelated to drug use and consolidate efforts on the insatiable hunger of addiction.[39, 40] Drug use becomes the most desirable goal. Events leading up to procurement, setting up the environment, and the using event itself command attention and entrain future behaviors that ensure the process continues. Incentive salience shifts focus and rearranges a series of priorities, all beneath volitional control, i.e., at an unconscious level.

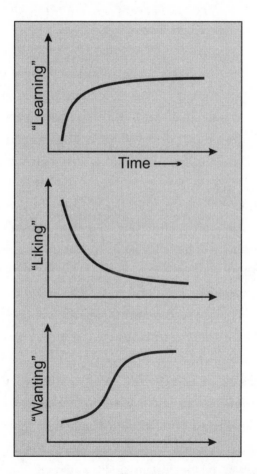

Figure 6.1 - Changes in wanting, liking, and learning over time (Adapted from Berridge and Kringelbach)[38]

Patients corroborate the concept of incentive salience. One patient described it this way:

I had tried opioids a couple of times, and it seemed to be no big deal. Then one day, I was sitting with my friends after taking a strong dose of oxycodone. Something magical happened. I felt ecstatic about where I was and whom I was with; the sights and sounds in that room were alive and wondrous. I have continued using opioids now for eleven years, each time trying to recreate that one incredible experience. It never comes close to that first experience, but that does not stop me from trying.

An apocryphal assertion is "Addicts take drugs to feel good." However, such folklore does not come close to describing the phenomenon of addiction. In fact, individuals with substance use disorders seek drugs knowing that little or no pleasure will result. Nagging craving recurs long after withdrawal has ceased, often with a seemingly random frequency and intensity.[41, 42]

The "wanting circuits" combined with the negative reinforcement that emerges when not consuming addictive substances lie at the center of the addictive drive. Pleasure is a common initial experience of addictive drugs; however, it is an epiphenomenon—and one that becomes increasingly elusive over time. Pleasure decreases, and the negative consequences of withdrawal increase. I often say to my patients, "If the desire for pleasure is truly the central motivating factor in your addiction, why are you having so little fun?"

It never ceases to amaze me how drug-induced wonderment is frequently attached to less than ideal circumstances or even horrid situations. I have heard patients wax eloquently about their friend's apartment only to find out it was nothing more than a drug-shooting hovel, or they recall the magical possibilities of their squalid crack house filled with poverty, sorrow, and sickness. Those with alcohol use disorder recall their favorite watering hole with a yearning, doleful look on their face. It often turns out the bar is a dull, dirty, and rancid hole-in-the-wall.

AddictBrain Component Two: Attention and Prioritizing

Through evolution, the mesolimbic dopamine circuit has served us well. Once activated, it shouts commands, such as "Wake up, pay attention, something important has happened!" and "Set aside other activities and focus your attention on this event. It is important for your survival!" The brain sets aside other activities and rivets attention on the situation that triggered the response. It activates learning circuits. Minute details are cataloged, and the body is poised for a next action. To ensure the signaling of the mesolimbic dopamine circuit is remembered, separate areas of the brain record its significance and pleasure. This sets up the organism to repeat the activity that promoted the response in the first place.

This brain circuit is important for the survival of our species. Food was scarce for *Homo sapiens* for the vast majority of his evolution. Imagine a hunter-gatherer as he happens upon a stand of fresh and nutritious berries growing in the wild. The pleasant surprise of finding the berries and their succulent sweetness triggers the mesolimbic reward (incentive salience) center to fire. Novelty increases the intensity of the response. The brain would record details, including images of the berry patch and the taste and texture as the sweet juice explodes in his mouth. The brain records how he happened upon this particular location, ensuring he would find it again. He would remember many details about his travel companions as they might also help him find this special location again. His brain would record the time of the year in order to find the berry patch at the peak of sweetness. The sweet prelude and tart aftertaste would be remembered as well. His brain would discern the color and texture of the ripest berries in the patch. His limbic system would assign a positive valence (positive feelings) to the experience. His traveling companions may be seen in a more positive light because, after all, it was they who helped find this sweet sustenance.

Drugs and alcohol (and presumably behavioral addiction) short-circuit this primitive response. Those with substance use disorders wax eloquently in exquisite detail about the first time they drank or used their drug of choice. They revel in the special—and novel—moment. For some, the first experience with such a substance becomes a life-changing event. Every aspect of the event can be brought up and played in three-dimensional Technicolor—often for the rest of one's life.

How does this experience translate into brain circuitry? When the various manifestations of addiction—drugs, alcohol, and certain behaviors—activate the mesolimbic dopamine circuit, the brain responds in stereotypical ways. As we can see from the previous example, this circuitry is thought to be responsible for transforming an event from the ordinary to one that is experienced as extraordinary. Firing in the nucleus accumbens—a central actor in the mesolimbic reward circuit—sends signals to other parts of the brain, first activating the attention and focusing systems. Addiction-related behaviors and chemical use are experienced as significant and crucial. Attention is concentrated on this important event, and the brain remains focused on everything surrounding the experience. The brain's learning mechanisms are activated. The individual's mind is primed to learn quickly and accurately. Each use of the drug retriggers the attention focusing centers in the brain as if the event is both novel and important, creating false meaning to the drugs and related rituals attached to substance use. Once recorded in memory, the limbic system tags the memory with the attributes of joy, surprise, happiness, and wonder.[43]

My patients often describe their chemical use as being more important than food, intimacy, and safety. The procurement of alcohol or other drugs, the continued access, and the time and place to use become paramount, occupying the same meaning as primitive instincts. Addiction "narrows the focus to drug seeking at the expense of natural rewards."[44] The reorganization of the reward system, in turn, demotes the importance of natural rewards. As individuals with drug use disorder mature into their use cycle, they fall into erratic and unhealthy food intake; poor hygiene and little attention to physical health; a loss of regard for personal safety; decreased interest in emotional connection and intimacy; abnormalities in sexual behavior; and diminished attention to childcare. Drug-induced incentive salience and its sequelae reorganize previous hardwired human priorities. Individuals set aside the most important tasks of being human, shifting their focus onto drug use behaviors.

Research has emphasized the concept of "attentional bias" in drug craving and subsequent relapse.[45, 46] Attentional bias, when applied to addiction, is the tendency for one's attention to focus preferentially on substances and their procurement, purchase, and subsequent use over other stimuli in the environment. When a drug cue occurs, the brain stops other activities and shifts its focus onto the drug cue.[47] Brain centers involved in this bias include a few areas of the frontal cortex, the amygdala, and the insula. The insula is located deep in the folds of the cerebral cortex. Goldstein et al. note that the insula correlates emotional states with the intensity of drug-related stimuli.[48] It is also generates internal awareness of the body, emotional states, and drug craving.[49] Clinical experience mirrors these findings; patients in early recovery are often unaware of intense craving until it is too late. For example, an individual with alcohol use disorder may say, "It does not bother me to watch other people drink; that never motivated me to imbibe." This statement might ring true to those with substance use disorders due to abnormalities in this interoceptive[50] system. Therapists, however, should avoid falling prey to this drug-induced delusion.

An article by Goldstein and colleagues discuss impairments in recognizing the severity of drug use and stress the importance of the anterior cingulate gyrus in cognitive control and generating responses to environmental cues.[51] Once drug or alcohol use is established, diminished activity in the anterior cingulate prevents the restraint of drug use and related behaviors. In contrast, higher levels of activation in the anterior cingulate cortex have also been shown to be predictive of successful treatment outcome.[52] As with many other aspects of AddictBrain, this impairment of inhibitory circuits emanates from brain centers that are below the level of conscious awareness. This information teaches us one simple relapse prevention technique: recovering individuals should decrease environmental cues (e.g., removing alcohol from the house) in the first years of recovery. This sidesteps impairments in the inhibition of actions that initiate the cascade of substance use. I will discuss this further in Chapter Fourteen, which focuses on relapse prevention.

Through thousands of interviews of patients over a period of thirty years, many common themes emerge. One of the cruelest AddictBrain tricks is how it imbues addiction-related events with profound, even spiritual qualities. I call this "deep meaning." Here is an example.

> *Jay had been a banker for many years. He worked hard in the corporate structure of nationwide banks for most of his life. He married Eleanor in his early thirties. The first few years of their marriage were strong and mutually supportive. In his late forties, he was approached by several investors who wanted to start a private bank in his community. It was the opportunity of a lifetime. He broke away from a secure job and dedicated all his energies to establishing a strong, local community bank. By his early fifties, his company was healthy and profitable. Jay secured a path to continued success.*
>
> *Oddly enough, this is when his drinking escalated. Jay lost interest in the day-to-day management of the bank and its employees. He spent his evenings at home, sitting in his favorite chair and drinking bourbon with his golden retriever at his side. Eleanor began to complain about his reclusive drinking. She became increasingly frustrated by his nightly inebriation. After several years of expressing her concern and with no response from Jay, Eleanor decided to move out of the house. Sitting in his chair through successive evenings, he found himself brooding about the meaning of his life. Eventually, his alcohol addiction took its toll: his health deteriorated, the bank board intervened, and he showed up at the doorstep of my treatment center.*
>
> *From information gathered during his intake interview, I recognized Jay as a thoughtful, reflective man*

who was open to the concept that he had developed an alcohol addiction; however, through a series of therapy sessions, I happened upon a major stumbling block. Over each succeeding month of his journey into the bottle, his evenings of sitting in his chair and looking out his back window with his dog at his side had become sacred. He could not imagine going through life without these moments. At times, he remembered ecstatic insights whose meaning seemed strangely elusive the following day. In therapy sessions he was flummoxed; he could not pull out why these moments were so important to him. Normally a reserved man, he walked out of one our sessions after standing and shouting, "You can't take those moments away from me!"

AddictBrain Component Three: Learning and Memory

AddictBrain affects how people with alcohol and drug use disorders learn and thus what is remembered. The human brain is a learning machine; we gather and process data whether or not we are consciously directing the process. We spend our waking hours gathering data and our slumber storing and cataloging the memories we collected throughout the previous day. Some of us focus our learning on books and extensive schooling while others learn through living. Everyone is constantly learning. Addiction is a learning process as well, and one that is prioritized in those who are destined to develop alcohol and/or drug use disorders.

Addiction and Learning

Addiction changes learning in the following ways:
- By improving learning skills related to drug and alcohol use. This includes finding and procuring substances, not getting caught, hiding one's use, obtaining money for continued use, and related talents.

- By inhibiting learning related to the negative consequences of drug and alcohol use.
- By decreasing the priority on the acquisition of other important life skills, crippling how those with addiction manage conflict, handle difficult emotions, etc.

Changes in learning are induced by dopamine signals from the mesolimbic dopamine system (the reward center). These signals activate the dorsal and ventral striatum, deep in the limbic area. Describing this process, Mary Torregrossa, PhD, states:

> Addictive substances create artificial learning signals that are of a greater magnitude and duration than what is observed neurophysiologically in response to natural events. Enhanced learning about a drug's positive effects results in an increased likelihood to use the drug again. This effect is magnified each time the drug is consumed. Drugs of abuse not only increase learning about the positive effects of the drug but they overshadow and diminish the impact of other features of the environment resulting in increased attention toward the drug and away from normal activities.[53]

Changes induced by aberrant learning also accelerate the formation of habits. Habits are stereotypical behaviors that, once acquired, are executed with little or no conscious awareness or control. When someone with alcohol use disorder calls his problem a "bad habit," he is at least partially correct. The acquisition of habits involves a shift from one set of brain structures to another; the ventral and medial striatum and dorsal prefrontal cortex (PFC) shift to a distinctly different habit executing brain circuit that involves the dorsal lateral striatum and ventral medial PFC.[54, 55] Once a behavior is entrained in this second brain circuit, it can, and will, execute without conscious control. Although habits are useful—most of us do not have to ponder whether we will brush our teeth when we walk in the bathroom in the morning—they are hardwired and difficult to unlearn. This progression has led Barry Everitt, PhD, and Trevor Robbins, PhD, to hypothesize that addiction is a process that moves from voluntary action (experimentation) to hardwired habits, ultimately leading to repetition compulsion.[56]

Those who know little about addiction are often stuck on the notion that alcohol or other drug use is a choice. When describing their position, such individuals bang their open hand sharply on the top of their desk, asserting, "Addiction is not a disease because you have to make a choice whether or not you use drugs or alcohol!" The central fallacy with this statement is exposed by the aforementioned transition from volition to compulsion. Before addiction takes hold, it is true that every individual makes a conscious choice whether or not to consume addicting chemicals during early experimentation. For some individuals, the ability to choose slips away in a matter of months. Others seem to use addictive substances under volitional control for an extended period, only to later discover that it has silently slipped away. In either case, once addiction takes hold, choice has long left.

Looking at the behavior from the outside, it does appear that choice is still occurring. The person with alcohol use disorder, despite promises to his wife, drives to the liquor store on the way home. He decided to turn the wheel and drive into the liquor store parking lot, didn't he? The best response from a neurophysiological perspective is to point out the four elements of AddictBrain discussed so far: wanting, attentional bias and reprioritization, learning, and memory. Together they drive continued use that may appear to the casual observer as being willful action. Nora Volkow, MD, and her colleagues elegantly describe how this loss of choice occurs.

> The dysfunctions reflect (a) decreased sensitivity of reward circuits, (b) enhanced sensitivity of memory circuits to conditioned expectations to drugs and drug cues, stress reactivity, and (c) negative mood, and a weakened control circuit. Although initial experimentation with a drug of

abuse is largely a voluntary behavior, continued drug use can eventually impair neuronal circuits in the brain that are involved in free will, turning drug use into an automatic compulsive behavior. The ability of addictive drugs to co-opt neurotransmitter signals between neurons (including dopamine, glutamate and GABA) modifies the function of different neuronal circuits, which begin to falter at different stages of an addiction trajectory. Upon exposure to the drug, drug cues or stress this results in unrestrained hyperactivation of the motivation/drive circuit that results in the compulsive drug intake that characterizes addiction.[57]

To summarize, the use of addicting substances activates the attentional and prioritizing areas of the frontal cortex; this pressures the learning centers to acquire the knowledge that ensures continued access to addictive chemicals or behaviors. Much of this learning is automatic, well below the level of conscious intent and volitional control. The repeated use of chemicals or enactment of other addictive behaviors entrains the mind to further habitual use.[58] Previous activation of the mesolimbic dopamine circuit produces wanting, which, in turn, focuses attention and realigns the brain's priorities. These two elements commit the brain's immense learning resources to change and adapt; to learn more efficient ways of obtaining alcohol or other drugs; to protect and hide the supply of drugs; to eliminate extraneous people and situations; and, ultimately, to live a life filled with finely honed AddictBrain behaviors.

When the brain is flooded by the chemical response produced by addiction, other areas of learning and growth move to a secondary position—they do not seem as important as the drug use. The addicted individual is less motivated by normal concerns, learning how to get along with others, managing conflict, and deepening meaning through interpersonal relationships and other fundamental human pursuits. When the individual with a drug use disorder enters treatment, her socially normative human skills have withered. In the case of an individual who began drug or alcohol use early, such skills are most likely never learned in the first place.

Addiction and Memory

Learning and memory are deeply intertwined processes. In the previous chapter, I discussed how normal distortions of memory cause problems in everyday life and how this may also affect how a patient may understand his disease. I also discussed how certain addiction-related events create extreme stress, which, in turn, builds intrusive memories similar to post-traumatic stress disorder (PTSD).

Addiction is, to a large extent, a disease of memory.[59, 60] Ann E. Kelley, PhD, states, "The process of addiction shares striking similarities with neural plasticity associated with natural reward learning and memory."[61] This concept is illustrated by the following vignette from a patient with alcohol use disorder.

> *David has long known that liquor stores in his state close at 11:00 P.M. on Saturday night and do not reopen until Monday morning. Sitting in a therapy session, he described his usual drinking bouts that extended late into Saturday night while sitting home alone. He became animated as he described the events of one particular evening.*
>
> *On this particular Saturday evening, he drank until his supply of vodka was exhausted. He shuffled off to bed at 10:30 P.M. At the moment of falling asleep, he described bolting upright in bed. He proceeded to get out of bed, put on his clothes, search for his keys, and walk out the door, all before he realized where he was going. As he put his key in the car's ignition, it suddenly dawned on him that he'd run out of vodka. Recounting this episode, he remembered saying to himself, "It's a good thing I'm going to the store. I've run out of vodka!"*

This clinical vignette describes a fascinating aspect of memory in the addicted individual. The brain undergoes a number of unconscious motivations and reorganizations in priority once the illness of addiction is active. In this case, my patient had an alarm clock in his head that would go off whenever he needed to restock his alcohol supply. His actions and behaviors were unconscious for quite some time. It was as if his conscious mind had to catch up with hardwired, deeper neural circuits programmed by his alcoholism to ensure a continued supply.

Another memory perturbation is the tendency to "go vague" about details of past use and use consequences. Part of this can be attributed to the "Seven Sins of Memory" described in Chapter Five. However, the pervasive and repeatable problems in remembering substances used, frequencies, amounts, and consequences of that use are way out of proportion to minor problems of recall. Memory is blocked by the psychological defenses of repression and suppression. Treatment should counteract these lapses using a thorough written and verbal "use history." Once completed and disclosed to others, the shame that occurs during disclosure is replaced by a quiet, centering calm. The truth is finally out. Individuals say, "I no longer have to hide." This process decreases addiction's wholesale distortions of reality. Such distortions are not a product of faulty or misguided recall or caused by psychological repression. Rather, they are part of a deeper reconstruction of past reality called "cloaking."

AddictBrain Component Four: Cloaking

This last effect of AddictBrain is especially devious, hiding the negative consequences of the disease from its victim. The purpose of this fourth function is to conceal AddictBrain's true intent and destructive nature. Brain circuits that suppress and sidestep self-understanding are pulled into play as the illness progresses. Most of us have observed baffled and befuddled patients, clients, family, or friends say, "I don't understand what is happening to me!" This, I believe, is an accurate portrayal of the disease.

In Chapter Five, I discussed Gazzaniga's interpreter and other misattributions that occur in the human mind. Gazzaniga's studies show that significant judgment errors related to cause and effect arise after the corpus callosum has been severed. Yet individuals who have had this surgery seem quite normal and lead typical everyday lives. Individuals who have suffered strokes limited to the motor and left parietal areas of the cortex suffer from a condition called anosognosia[62] (or better named asomatognosia). They are unable to reconcile that their limb is not moving and wind up with rationalizations that are strangely reminiscent of a patient in denial of a substance problem. They report that the limb "is not mine" or "I do not feel like moving it now" or have other patently incorrect interpretations of their condition.

But are we leaping to the conclusion that the disease of addiction imparts structural damage similar to brain surgery or stroke? The short answer is "no." After decades of research, Gazzaniga describes the vast power of the interpreter in our everyday lives by stating the following:

> Any time our left brain is confronted with information that does not jibe with our self-image, knowledge, or conceptual framework, our left-hemisphere interpreter creates a belief to enable all incoming information to make sense and mesh with our ongoing idea of ourself. The interpreter seeks patterns, order, and causal relationships.[63]

He highlights situations when the interpreter generates the most havoc, stating, "The interpreter tells us the lies we need to believe in order to remain in control."[64] Although he was not addressing addiction per se, Gazzaniga captures important qualities of addiction denial when he writes, "The left-hemisphere interpreter is not only a master of belief creation, but it will stick to its belief system no matter what."[65]

How would this work in addiction? Addiction overwhelms the interpretive circuits and causes a response in susceptible individuals that is outside the scope of normal events. The reward response of certain substances is beyond normal experience because it is exogenously induced and has no blueprint in evolution. Learning circuits reinforce related environmental cues (e.g., "I must have had such a great time because of the people I was with and the interesting new music I heard"). Extraordinary echoes are set up in the brain, caused by previous riveted attention and detailed learning. The interpreter does its best to understand this initial event. Subsequent use fails to live up to the initial hype. The individual with alcohol and drug use disorder develops rebound dysphoria, which is projected onto family, work, or any available scapegoat. The central actor—addiction—has no context; as a result, the interpreter projects its rationalizations onto the external environment. Denial of the problem arises when the brain is unable to create contextual understanding for the intense reward, compulsion, attention, prioritization, and learning built up through chronic drug use. Anything and everything else seems to be the cause of life problems.

Therapists who do not understand addiction are often swept up into the witch hunt. They carefully walk the individual with addiction through the plusses and minuses of her home life or current job without ever recognizing that fixing an unhappy relationship or employment is a red herring, skillfully fabricated by AddictBrain. It continuously knocks the patient and her therapist off track, subverting interventions to arrest addiction and preventing her from establishing Recovery Skills.

Summary

Addiction affects many brain mechanisms; the sum of these is labeled AddictBrain. AddictBrain has four prongs of attack that work together to create a formidable foe, one that has flummoxed treatment for the past 100 years. In the 1960s, many types of cancer were thought to be incurable. Somehow, the National Cancer Institute, organized medicine, and basic research worked together to study all available techniques, assembling them in different combinations in a concerted effort to improve long-term survivability. Surprisingly, new medications were not the central component of the initial success. Research determined which methodologies worked in select types of cancer and certain patients; such exhaustive studies sparked a revolution in cancer survival.

We are "in the 1960s" with addiction care. We have a hodgepodge of treatment efforts that are seemingly unconnected. We know very little about how and what to combine together to create the best long-term outcome. RecoveryMind Training, described in Section Two of this text, is my humble framework for a quantifiable and systematic approach to addiction care. Other addiction specialists will propose additional treatment frameworks. When various treatment combinations are studied, research will determine which approaches work for which people with the myriad addiction variations. Effective treatment for addiction will be the eventual result, ensuring a sustainable recovery for all who suffer from the most complex disease of humankind.

Chapter Six Notes

1. G. F. Koob, L. Stinus, M. Le Moal, and F. E. Bloom, "Opponent process theory of motivation: neurobiological evidence from studies of opiate dependence," *Neurosci Biobehav Rev* 13, no. 2–3 (Summer-Fall 1989): 135–40.

2. R. L. Solomon, "The opponent-process theory of acquired motivation: the costs of pleasure and the benefits of pain," *American Psychologist* 35, no. 8 (1980): 691.

3. K. C. Berridge and T. E. Robinson, "What is the role of dopamine in reward: hedonic impact, reward learning, or incentive salience?" *Brain Res Brain Res Rev* 28, no. 3 (Dec 1998): 309–69.

4. K. C. Berridge and M. L. Kringelbach, "Affective neuroscience of pleasure: reward in humans and animals," *Psychopharmacology (Berl)* 199, no. 3 (Aug 2008): 457–80.

5. M. M. Torregrossa, P. R. Corlett, and J. R. Taylor, "Aberrant learning and memory in addiction," *Neurobiol Learn Mem* 96, no. 4 (Nov 2011): 609–23.

6. G. F. Koob and N. D. Volkow, "Neurocircuitry of addiction," *Neuropsychopharmacology* 35, no. 1 (Jan 2010): 217–38.

7. G. F. Koob and N. D. Volkow, "Neurobiology of addiction: a neurocircuitry analysis," *The Lancet Psychiatry* 3, no. 8 (2016): 760–73.

8. N. D. Volkow, G. F. Koob, and A. T. McLellan, "Neurobiologic Advances from the Brain Disease Model of Addiction," *New England Journal of Medicine* 374, no. 4 (2016): 363–71.

9. B. Adinoff, "Neurobiologic Processes in Drug Reward and Addiction," *Harv Rev Psychiatry* 12, no. 6 (2004): 305–20.

10. R. Z. Goldstein, A. D. Craig, A. Bechara, H. Garavan, A. R. Childress, M. P. Paulus, and N. D. Volkow, "The neurocircuitry of impaired insight in drug addiction," *Trends Cogn Sci* 13, no. 9 (Sep 2009): 372–80.

11. N. D. Volkow, J. S. Fowler, and G. J. Wang, "The addicted human brain viewed in the light of imaging studies: brain circuits and treatment strategies," *Neuropharmacology* 47 Suppl 1 (2004): 3–13.

12. Anhedonia is defined as the inability to experience pleasure from activities usually found enjoyable (e.g., exercise, hobbies, music, sexual activities, or social interactions).

13. G. F. Koob, "Neurocircuitry of alcohol addiction: synthesis from animal models," *Handb Clin Neurol* 125 (2014): 33–54.

14. G. F. Koob, C. L. Buck, A. Cohen, S. Edwards, P. E. Park, J. E. Schlosburg, B. Schmeichel, *et al*, "Addiction as a stress surfeit disorder," *Neuropharmacology* 76 Pt B (Jan 2014): 370–82.

15. See above, n. 7.

16. See above, n. 8.

17. I. Willuhn, L. M. Burgeno, P. A. Groblewski, and P. E. Phillips, "Excessive cocaine use results from decreased phasic dopamine signaling in the striatum," *Nat Neurosci* 17, no. 5 (May 2014): 704–9.

18. D. Caprioli, D. Calu, and Y. Shaham, "Loss of phasic dopamine: a new addiction marker?" *Nat Neurosci* 17, no. 5 (Apr 25 2014): 644–6.

19. T. E. Robinson and K. C. Berridge, "The neural basis of drug craving: an incentive-sensitization theory of addiction," *Brain Res Brain Res Rev* 18, no. 3 (Sep–Dec 1993): 247–91.

20. G. F. Koob and M. Le Moal, "Plasticity of reward neurocircuitry and the 'dark side' of drug addiction," *Nat Neurosci* 8, no. 11 (Nov 2005): 1442–4.

21. See above, n. 1.

22. See above, n. 13.

23. See above, n. 20.

24. G. F. Koob and E. J. Nestler, "The neurobiology of drug addiction," *J Neuropsychiatry Clin Neurosci* 9, no. 3 (Summer 1997): 482–97.

25. A. Kelley, "Memory and Addiction: Shared Neural Circuitry and Molecular Mechanisms," *Neuron* 44, no. 1 (2004): 161–79.

26. A. E. Kelley and K. C. Berridge, "The neuroscience of natural rewards: relevance to addictive drugs," *J Neurosci* 22, no. 9 (May 1 2002): 3306–11.

27. G. F. Koob and M. Le Moal, "Neurobiological mechanisms for opponent motivational processes in addiction," *Philosophical Transactions of the Royal Society B: Biological Sciences* 363, no. 1507 (07/24 2008): 3113–23.

28. G. F. Koob, "Neurobiology of addiction. Toward the development of new therapies," *Ann N Y Acad Sci* 909 (2000): 170–85.

29. G. F. Koob, and E. J. Simon, "The Neurobiology of Addiction: Where We Have Been and Where We Are Going," *J Drug Issues* 39, no. 1 (Jan 2009): 115–32.

30. K. C. Berridge, T. E. Robinson, and J. W. Aldridge, "Dissecting components of reward: 'liking', 'wanting', and learning," *Curr Opin Pharmacol* 9, no. 1 (Feb 2009): 65–73.

31. See above, n. 19.

32. See above, n. 30.

33. K. C. Berridge and T. E. Robinson, "Parsing reward," *Trends Neurosci* 26, no. 9 (Sep 2003): 507–13.

34. K. C. Berridge, "The debate over dopamine's role in reward: the case for incentive salience," *Psychopharmacology (Berl)* 191, no. 3 (Apr 2007): 391–431.

35. See above, n. 9.

36. See above, n. 3.

37. J. J. Day and R. M. Carelli, "The nucleus accumbens and Pavlovian reward learning," *Neuroscientist* 13, no. 2 (Apr 2007): 148–59.

38. K. C. Berridge and M. L. Kringelbach, "Building a neuroscience of pleasure and well-being," *Psychology of well-being* 1, no. 1 (2011): 1–3.

40. R. A. Wise and M. A. Bozarth, "A psychomotor stimulant theory of addiction," *Psychol Rev* 94, no. 4 (Oct 1987): 469–92.

41. See above, n. 19.

42. See above, n. 40.

43. J. E. LeDoux, *The Emotional Brain: The Mysterious Underpinnings of Emotional Life* (New York: Simon & Schuster, 1996).

44. See above, n. 6.

45. See above, n. 30.

46. See above, n. 33.

47. P. W. Kalivas and N. D. Volkow, "The neural basis of addiction: a pathology of motivation and choice," *American Journal of Psychiatry* (2014).

48. See above, n. 10.

49.   See above, n. 10.

50.   A. D. Craig, "Interoception: the sense of the physiological condition of the body," *Curr Opin Neurobiol* 13, no. 4 (Aug 2003): 500–5.

51.   See above, n. 10.

52.   S. M. Grusser, J. Wrase, S. Klein, D. Hermann, M. N. Smolka, M. Ruf, W. Weber-Fahr, *et al*, "Cue-induced activation of the striatum and medial prefrontal cortex is associated with subsequent relapse in abstinent alcoholics," *Psychopharmacology (Berl)* 175, no. 3 (Sep 2004): 296–302.

53.   See above, n. 5.

54.   S. Killcross and E. Coutureau, "Coordination of actions and habits in the medial prefrontal cortex of rats," *Cereb Cortex* 13, no. 4 (Apr 2003): 400–8.

55.   A. Nelson and S. Killcross, "Amphetamine exposure enhances habit formation," *J Neurosci* 26, no. 14 (Apr 2006): 3805–12.

56.   B. J. Everitt and T. W. Robbins, "Neural systems of reinforcement for drug addiction: from actions to habits to compulsion," *Nat Neurosci* 8, no. 11 (Nov 2005): 1481–9.

57.   N. D. Volkow, G. J. Wang, J. S. Fowler, D. Tomasi, F. Telang, and R. Baler, "Addiction: decreased reward sensitivity and increased expectation sensitivity conspire to overwhelm the brain's control circuit," *Bioessays* 32, no. 9 (Sep 2010): 748–55.

58.   S. E. Hyman, R. C. Malenka, and E. J. Nestler, "Neural Mechanisms of Addiction: The Role of Reward-Related Learning and Memory," *Annu Rev Neurosci* 29, no. 1 (2006): 565–98.

59.   Ibid.

60.   S. E. Hyman, "Addiction: a disease of learning and memory," *Am J Psychiatry* 162, no. 8 (Aug 2005): 1414–22.

61.   See above, n. 25.

62.   E. Bisiach, G. Vallar, D. Perani, C. Papagno, and A. Berti, "Unawareness of disease following lesions of the right hemisphere: Anosognosia for hemiplegia and anosognosia for hemianopia," *Neuropsychologia* 24, no. 4 (1986): 471–82.

63.   M. S. Gazzaniga, *The Ethical Brain* (New York: Dana Press, 2005), 151.

64.   M. S. Gazzaniga, *The Mind's Past* (Berkeley, CA: University of California Press, 1998), 138.

65.   See above, n. 63, p. 149.

SECTION TWO

CHAPTER SEVEN

An Overview of RecoveryMind Training

The greatest revolution of our generation is the discovery
that human beings, by changing the inner attitudes of
their minds, can change the outer aspects of their lives.

WILLIAM JAMES

In Section One, I introduced you to AddictBrain, a complex covert brain learning response that occurs in patients who develop addiction. I discussed the depth and breadth of its action on its unsuspecting host. As drug or alcohol use transitions from casual to compulsive, a baffling malady results. Now that we recognize the progenitor of the disease—AddictBrain—and understand how it works within the brain, our task is to build a treatment solution that dismantles its control systems and constructs a platform for systematic recovery. This chapter is an overview of that solution.

Addiction treatment has taken it on the chin over the past twenty-five years. Our division of medical and psychological care is berated for any number of problems, many of which are unfortunately true. The popular press displays the treatment failures of celebrities, highlighting that treatment does not work by showing them returning again and again to short-term rehabilitation centers. Treatment centers have been the subject of investigative reports; they overcharge for many alternative therapies and fail to provide systematized care. Individuals who fall into the public limelight are criticized when they profess they are cured and subsequently go down in flames from spectacular publicized relapses.

This type of controversy always occurs in the years or decades before proven approaches to a medical illness are available. In the 1970s, cancer patients flocked to Laetrile (amygdalin) as a cancer cure without scientific evidence. Even when it was shown to be ineffective and potentially dangerous, cancer victims made pilgrimage to Laetrile clinics, hoping for a magical cure. Over the ensuing forty years, medicine developed systematized and proven cancer treatments, and we rarely hear about Laetrile today. In the addiction world, we are still in the "Laetrile stage," lacking research-backed treatment and searching for snake oil. Unfortunately, addiction treatment has been in this place for over 150 years.[1]

To date, research shows that any singular addiction treatment technique is ineffective when studied over a sufficiently long period.[2] However, combining multiple methodical interventions over extended time frames does provide hope.[3] This is analogous to cancer treatment, where multiple drugs and multiple modalities, when put together in the right combination, are the most effective in inducing remission. I think this same approach will prove most effective for addiction treatment; that is, a specific combination of modalities tailored to the individual and consistently applied will prove the most effective route to long-term remission. Research into which techniques and combinations of techniques prove most effective will take decades to complete and wind up costing hundreds of millions of dollars.

According to the Center on Addiction and Substance Abuse at Columbia University (CASA Columbia), the United States spends $500 billion on the consequences of addiction, but prevention, treatment, and research accounts for only 3 percent of those dollars.[4] If we had done the same thing for cancer, we would all be searching for Laetrile clinics instead of going to oncologists who can give us clear survival rates for almost every type of cancer, long remissions for many cancers, and cures for some. If we spend no money on addiction treatment research, we will never realize effective treatment.

In 1997, Alan Leshner, PhD, then the head of the National Institute on Drug Abuse (NIDA), published a position paper that shifted the scientific community. The paper was "Addiction Is a Brain Disease, and It Matters."[5] Research into the neurophysiology of addiction intensified, and remarkable findings have followed. Unfortunately, the treatment field has experienced no commensurate uptick in clinical research to determine what really works. The vast majority of addiction care in the United States "treats a chronic disease with an acute care model."[6] So today, we have mounting evidence that addiction causes wholesale and diffuse changes in the brain that leads to the ferocity and recalcitrant nature of the addiction illness; however, our care tools remain poorly crafted and hardly studied.

What Is Recovery?

To study addiction treatment, it seems intuitively obvious that we need to know what constitutes a success. RMT defines recovery as its desired outcome. Individuals who overcome addiction often say they are "in recovery." But what does this mean? In an effort to better define this state of being, many groups have developed consensus documents that define the state of recovery.[7, 8, 9] More recently, the Alcohol Research Group, a part of the Oakland-based Public Health Institute led by Lee Ann Kaskutas, DrPH, conducted an online survey that was completed by 9,341 people from different pathways to recovery.[10, 11] The researchers distilled the survey responses and published their results in 2014.[12] Central themes about recovery arose from this work and were grouped into five areas: abstinence in recovery, essentials of recovery, enriched recovery, spirituality of recovery and uncommon elements of recovery. By serendipity, these groupings turned out to be quite similar to the care domains of RecoveryMind Training, which will be introduced in Chapter Eight (i.e., Containment, Recovery Basics, Emotional Awareness and

Resilience, Healthy Internal Narrative, Connectedness and Spirituality, and Relapse Prevention). Therefore, the definition of recovery provided by Dr. Kaskutas' empirical research most closely fits the framework and philosophy of RecoveryMind Training.

The struggle to define our desired treatment outcome underscores a glaring problem in the field of addiction medicine: We ask our patients to work toward a goal that we cannot even universally define! Even if we accept that we cannot clearly define the end point (recovery), we disagree vociferously how to get there. In short, we are asking our patients to work toward an ambiguous goal with methods to which no one agrees.

Despite all this confusion, most trained specialists agree that recovery is intuitively recognizable. Indeed, many lay people sense something fundamentally different in their friends and loved ones once they enter into true recovery. Spouses, parents, and peers tell me, "Something feels different this time; Keisha seems different." When family members of a patient tell me this, it is highly predictive of a good long-term prognosis. Human beings seem to be able to detect multiple clues that point to pervasive change in others, such as the transformation of recovery. Unfortunately, science has not yet been able to define such states with objective, measurable criteria.

Most individuals who attain a solid recovery see the world through "a new set of glasses."[13] It almost always involves seeing others in a different light and changes internal self-perspective. Many people begin to explore a broader spiritual view of themselves as well. This change is called recovery.[14, 15] But how does one get there? Unfortunately, the exact path can be elusive and often shrouded in mysticism. RecoveryMind Training makes the bold claim that practicing a specific set of skills will induce this ineffable recovery, even though the exact definition of the end goal remains murky to this very day.

Standardized Treatment

Although RecoveryMind Training is a cohesive model, I make no claims that the system as a whole has undergone rigorous scientific examination. It is borne out of three decades of work with many colleagues and has shown to be effective through clinical experience. Each module of treatment has been systematized with definable goals.[16] The RMT model was built for clinical clarity and to be studied; its treatment goals are defined and measureable. If a particular component has no discernable effect on outcome, it can simply be discarded when the time comes. Certain components appear to be synergistic on first principles, but time will tell.

RMT's standardization arises naturally from its structure. Patients or clients are taught that recovery comes when you learn, internalize, and practice a set of defined skills. These skills are organized into "buckets" called domains. In general, a patient begins with the mission-critical skills first. From there, he or she moves on to work on skills that interrupt AddictBrain thinking and build an emotionally resilient life. Simply enough, these skills are called Recovery Skills.

The biggest single challenge in addiction treatment is ensuring every patient acquires primary, critical skills while at the same time avoiding the same cookie cutter approach with all patients who arrive at the door. RecoveryMind Training accomplishes this by offering many services in many areas of behavioral healthcare. Some patients will spend more time in one domain than another, depending on need, and most patients will touch on each of the six domains over the course of their treatment.

Even with all this, RMT does not cover the entire gambit of ancillary support services that are essential to specific populations. Specifically, family therapy needs are not directly defined. Other concomitant psychiatric or medical disorders or the need for legal, social, and financial counseling is not described. Specific populations have different and critically important needs. For brevity, I have not addressed them here, but that does not mean that addressing co-occurring conditions is not central to addiction care. For example, studies show that, in the addicted and homeless population, addiction care is but one aspect of comprehensive and effective care for this vulnerable population and must be accompanied by housing assistance and other recovery support services.[17, 18] My focus is on the nucleus of addiction treatment while at the same time recognizing that distinct but highly correlated life problems need be addressed in every patient.

Part of the standardized RMT system is regular patient and staff assessments. Patients complete evaluation forms for the particular domain(s) they are addressing. Once the patient completes his or her assessment, the staff does the same. Differences in treatment status are discussed. Patients and staff reset goals and expectations as to treatment progress and length of stay, using this assessment process. Several sample assessment forms from the companion workbook appear at the end of this volume.

The Qualities of RecoveryMind Training

RecoveryMind Training uses components of each of the following therapeutic techniques:

- Cognitive Behavioral Therapy (CBT) specific to addiction[19-22]
- Addiction-treatment contingency management[23]
- Motivational Interviewing[24-26]
- Understanding addiction as a biopsychosocial illness[27-29]
- Twelve-step facilitation[30-35]
- Drug screening technology[36]
- A healthy examination of addiction denial[37, 38]
- Attachment theory,[39] especially as it relates to addiction[40]
- The complexity of therapist and patient self-disclosure in addiction treatment[41]
- Spiritual principles in addiction treatment[42-44]
- The ASAM Criteria, especially regarding Levels and Dimensions of Care[45]
- Viewing addiction as a chronic disease[46, 47]

Other techniques were involved in the actual treatment process, including:

- Understanding the difference between problem-solving and process-oriented, emotions-based group therapy[48]
- Reflective listening[49]
- The use of paradox[50]
- Family Systems Theory[51]
- Understanding of character and temperament[52-54]
- Mindfulness meditation[55-62]

RecoveryMind and Twelve-Step Treatment Models

Because RecoveryMind Training uses twelve-step concepts and the support provided by Alcoholics Anonymous, readers may have a tendency to say, "Oh, this is just a twelve-step program." My response to this is mostly "no" but at times "yes." If you travel to addiction programs across the United States—and to a more limited degree outside of the US—many programs incorporate AA into their care model. Yet, if you examined their day-to-day schedule, you will see a plethora of other care models and philosophies. Addiction treatment is a disparate and idiosyncratic industry.

RecoveryMind Training implements twelve-step principles and techniques because they are practical, effective, and often result in a persistent change or even transformation. Recovering individuals need a lot of support. Twelve-step meetings are readily available and very inexpensive. Twelve-step meetings, when used alone, have low potency in helping individuals transition from chemical use to abstinence but are quite effective in sustaining recovery (see Chapter Ten for further discussion of the research in this regard). Many patients who use AA and its sister organizations complain at first but undergo an ineffable process of transformation over time. Despite all this, I do not insist that patients who are treated using RecoveryMind Training must remain in twelve-step meetings. I hope they will do so; insisting that this be the case often sets up oppositional or defiant behavior in certain patients. Involvement with twelve-step meetings and step work is a low cost, readily available transformational system. Why not use all the tools at hand to combat the disease?

RecoveryMind Training has minor disagreements with some interpretations of the twelve-step philosophy. Many treatment providers portray addiction as an indecipherable malady, and they feel trying to understand addiction is dangerous. This comes from three words in the AA's Big Book: "cunning, baffling, powerful."[63] RMT states that AddictBrain has a clear purpose and intelligence. Although we cannot yet fully understand its mechanisms or attempt to outfox it,[64] we can understand AddictBrain's motive (continued use) and eventual outcome (self-annihilation). Addiction is indeed powerful, but RMT trains patients and caregivers to use alternative life responses that thwart AddictBrain and hold the disease in remission.

RecoveryMind Training also questions another notion that seems to be popular today. We hear, "I am not only powerless over my addiction, I am powerless over everything." This, I believe, is a distortion of the original twelve-step philosophy.[65] Those with substance use disorders are certainly powerless over their addiction when in the throes of AddictBrain's control. However, an informed recovery provides tools that, when practiced, can keep the illness at bay. These tools are effective at changing individuals' lives, and recovery empowers them to do so. The notion of powerlessness is, at its core, an elegant mental jiu-jitsu, one that throws off the opponent, AddictBrain.

This notion of powerlessness is anathema to many. Disenfranchised populations—those subject to discrimination, sexism, and victims of abuse—have justifiable difficulties with the concept of powerlessness. RMT uses the concept carefully and applies it in a well-circumscribed context: we are powerless over alcohol (or drugs), but not everything.

A Chronic Disease

RecoveryMind Training looks at the treatment of addiction as a long-term process, stretching out over years. Most individuals begin their treatment with an initial burst of high intensity care. Good treatment follows this up with support group attendance, disease management through contingency contracting, psychotherapy, and relapse prevention training. The initial treatment dose may run for weeks or months. The entire course of treatment should continue for years.

Because addiction is a lifelong illness, it requires lifelong care. This does not mean intensive treatment has to occupy many hours in each day for the rest of one's life. Most patients have to establish recovery as their number one priority for the first year of abstinence. During that time, patients practice a set of proven Recovery Skills, which soon become an automatic response to life's stressors. Recovery becomes a part of one's day, integrated to the point that it is indistinguishable from the rhythm of everyday life.

The change of recovery is similar to other chronic illnesses. Imagine Ashley, a preteen who is newly diagnosed with Type 1 diabetes mellitus (insulin dependent). Soon after diagnosis, counting carbohydrates, checking blood glucose, and preparing and administering insulin several times per day seems daunting. She feels overwhelmed and becomes frustrated. "Do I really have to do this every day for the rest of my life?" she cries. Ashley's mood alternates between depressed compliance and defiance, with occasional moments of acceptance. She attends a diabetes camp during her first post-diagnosis summer. She meets others who have the same illness and finds comfort and camaraderie with them. She gradually learns to count her "carbs" automatically. She carries her insulin in a small, insulated pouch and gracefully retreats to the restroom when at her friend's house to inject insulin before meals. Her diabetes stabilizes and she becomes a candidate for an insulin pump. Although she looks longingly at candy and desserts, she learns how to control her food choices carefully. Her recovery responses become automatic and life goes on.

Ashley's stages of change in accepting her diabetes apply just as well to addiction. Addiction recovery requires acceptance and ingrained responses to external stressors. Accepting the illness is difficult, and patients are emotionally labile and alternate between acceptance and denial at first. Failure to adhere to the treatment can cause life-threatening consequences. Spending time with others who have the same illness decreases shame and provides hope and companionship in the common journey. This chronic illness is held in remission by defining and practicing Recovery Skills. RecoveryMind Training strives to delineate these skills (in diabetes: accept the diagnosis, count carbs, calculate activity level, check glucose, and take insulin) with as much clarity as possible (in addiction: accept the diagnosis, prevent access, adjust attitude, disclose addictive thinking and craving, and seek support).

The first task in treatment is containing the behavioral aspects of the illness. In RMT, this work occurs in Domain A: Addiction Containment. Some patients need to be locked in an inpatient facility to interrupt destructive use. Other patients can come to an addiction therapist once a week and contract with them not to use in between sessions (more discussion on this in Chapter Nine). Too much or too little treatment is counterproductive.[66] The intensity of treatment should taper organically over time. Different patients need differing intensity to establish initial abstinence and the length of that higher intensity varies from individual to individual.

Too often, third-party payers insist that a patient should be stepped down to a less intensive (i.e., less expensive) level of care once they show any signs of independent functioning. They are not suicidal and are no longer hypertensive and delusional from alcohol withdrawal. Such edicts are based upon co-morbid medical illness and imminent lethality.

Treatment providers, on the other hand, insist that every patient needs to stay as long as the average patient remains in treatment at their particular facility. Too often providers set the length of treatment based upon their particular treatment model or program. The determinants of either of these stakeholders fail to consider the illness as the determining factor that should define the length of stay at a given level.

RecoveryMind Training has simple, patient-centered ways of determining if a patient remains at the current level of care. These simple guidelines suggest that a patient should remain at a current level of care if

- Medical management, detoxification, and the observation of withdrawal risk can only safely be performed at the current level of care;
- The patient has co-occurring psychiatric or psychological conditions that demand this level of care;
- The current level of care is needed to protect him or her from imminent relapse into substance use or unhealthy/maladaptive behaviors;
- The current level of care is needed to provide the intensity of support required to motivate the patient to accomplish recovery management skills;
- The patient needs accountability and staff encouragement at a level that cannot be obtained at a lower level of care; or
- The patient has treatment tasks that necessitate involvement in the current milieu due to staff expertise or interpersonal dynamics with his or her fellow patients. A transfer to a different milieu would be counterproductive at the current time.

While in RMT treatment, both the patient and staff track progress with defined Recovery Skills. Once a series of skills are met and the above criteria do not preclude decreasing the intensity of treatment, transfer should occur, if an appropriate lower level of care is available to that patient.[67]

RecoveryMind Training uses the infrastructure of the ASAM Criteria,[68] developed by David Mee-Lee, MD, and colleagues. The ASAM Criteria define levels of care clearly and concisely.[69] These guidelines encourage treatment along a continuum and define six areas of treatment, called Dimensions, matching them to a given patient's needs. RMT is not a replacement for or a subset of the ASAM Criteria. Instead, RMT delineates the details of the addiction-focused elements of comprehensive patient care. The ASAM Criteria are more global, canvassing the entire physical, medical, psychiatric, and social network of the patient, and RMT provides a granular description of the addiction components of a larger comprehensive treatment. The ASAM Criteria and RMT are synergistic and should be used together for best results.

We must help our patients accept that they have a lifelong disease and, at the same time, comfort them that the rest of their life will not be solely focused on wrestling the hunger to relapse. From the outset, patients or clients need to hear a consistent model that reflects chronic disease management. Many physicians use metaphors from the medical world—diabetes, hypertension, rheumatoid arthritis, and chronic gastrointestinal diseases. It often helps if the patient has a family member with a chronic medical condition. I usually say, "If I had to pick one chronic illness, it would be addiction. It is the only disease that, after you obtain proper treatment, you are healthier than you were before the illness started."

RecoveryMind Nomenclature

RecoveryMind Training strives for clarity at all times. Patients arrive in treatment confused and befuddled by their illness. As addiction treatment professionals, we should always use clear terminology to help them overcome confusion. RecoveryMind Training uses consistent terms to help patients and providers describe the course of care. During any given day, the strife and emotional upheaval of our patients' lives induce confusion in everyone within the treatment arena. RecoveryMind

Training keeps a steady path to recovery by using clear and consistent terms. I will define the main terms in the next section.

Recovery Skills

When trying to describe the qualities and state of recovery, I often use Potter Stewart's phrase "It is very difficult to describe, but I know it when I see it."[70] Despite problems with definition, RMT asserts that recovery emerges by developing and practicing a set of proficiencies called **Recovery Skills**. Recovery Skills are wide-ranging and include changing behavior, responding to a cue in a new fashion, rethinking self-concept, and learning how to experience but not react to destructive emotions.

Recovery Skills are a comprehensive, defined set of responses. Once learned and practiced with diligence, they establish an alternative way of living. Recovery Skills suppress AddictBrain and promote RecoveryMind. Please note that practicing RMT Recovery Skills does not completely eliminate AddictBrain thinking. When you talk to individuals with many years of abstinence and recovery from alcohol or other drugs, most of them report they still have residual past addictive thinking, i.e., AddictBrain. A better way of thinking about RecoveryMind Training is that the Recovery Skills lay down a second track or path alongside AddictBrain. Over time, it becomes easier for the recovering individual to hop off the AddictBrain track and onto the RecoveryMind track. Patients are introduced to Recovery Skills through written assignments and discussion—most often in a group setting called Assignment Group which is described later in this chapter). Most are practiced and internalized in a second group therapy called Skills Group (also defined later). Staff members encourage patients to continue newly learned skills throughout treatment.

Domains

RecoveryMind Training is built upon a long list of Recovery Skills. These skills are divided into six domains (see Chapter Eight). The domains contain logical groupings of these skills. This creates cohesion and structure to the RMT treatment process.

Worksheet

Self-exploration is an important component of addiction treatment. The process of self-exploration often begins when patients complete worksheets. When work in a domain is indicated, a staff member assigns one or more worksheets in that domain. The patient completes the worksheet during scheduled work periods in ASAM Level 2.5, 3, and 4 programs and outside normal treatment hours in ASAM Level 1 and 2.1. Patients often refer to their worksheets as "homework." The patient then hands the worksheet to a staff member who reviews it. If the work is incomplete or a patient misunderstands the assignment, the staff member provides clarification and motivation to complete the assignment. Once a worksheet is complete, the patient is instructed to bring it to assignment group for further discussion.

Types of Group Therapy

Many of the components of RecoveryMind Training can by implemented by a sole practitioner in a therapy office. Most experts believe, however, that addiction care is most effective in organized settings. RecoveryMind Training focuses on group therapy, similar to most addiction treatment centers today. In either case, RMT is very careful about clear language. Therefore, RMT uses three different types of group therapy; announces the type of group; and explains at the beginning the procedure, actions, and expected outcome of each of the three group modalities. Too often, therapists launch into a group where many of the participants have no idea of group norms and expectations. Such patients spend weeks trying to understand the unspoken rules of engagement in group therapy. Their energy is spent on learning unspoken rules; as a result, they miss the real purpose of the group in which they sit.

Assignment Group

In assignment group, worksheets are read aloud and discussed. At the beginning of assignment group, the staff leader reviews group tasks in order to properly pace that day's therapy. A patient slowly and clearly reviews the assignment and her worksheet entries. It is helpful to provide clarity as to the purpose of a given worksheet multiple times during the patient's recitation. Once read, other patients and staff provide feedback. The feedback helps the patient better understand her answers, consider other alternatives, and deepen her appreciation of the worksheet task.

At times, assignment group might slide into interactions that are more akin to process group (description in forthcoming section). When this occurs, the group leader may choose to allow process work to proceed but limit its scope. If such process work is too extensive (or the therapist senses it will become too extensive), the therapist might gently encourage participants to hold onto such discussion and revisit it during the time allotted to process group.

Skills Group

Skills group is a staff-led therapy where all participants are introduced to a recovery skill. The leader introduces the skill, e.g., "Today, we will learn drug refusal skills," and goes on to describe what the skill is and how it fits into a comprehensive recovery program. The leader then invites one participant to walk through the skill with him. A volunteer (or leader conscripted "volunteer") is chosen. It is helpful to decrease performance anxiety with a statement such as "Great, Jenny, let's walk slowly through this together." At this point, the group often stands and sets up a "stage"[71] to begin the role-play. The skill is demonstrated, and the leader stops and starts the process along the way, asking for feedback and discussion by the group.

Once the demonstration is complete, group participants discuss the process again, to deepen understanding. Additional patients are brought in to be the protagonist, repeating the skill sequence. Group members are enrolled into the experience (e.g., a using friend who shows up at the house or who calls on the phone, a waiter or waitress asking for drink orders, or a drug dealer who shows up unannounced). Feedback from the audience, enrolled "auxiliaries," and the "protagonist" occurs at the end of each role-play. Discussion is brief and pointed, asking questions such as "What worked?"; "What did not?"; and "What feelings came up while practicing the skill?" A playful, "let's try that too" mood helps the group experiment in alternative approaches to the skill. A talented leader learns as much as the patient participants.

Process Group

During all stages of treatment, patients report one of the most valuable experiences is process group. Process group is a here-and-now, emotions-based group therapy. Patients should be discouraged from giving advice, engaging in long soliloquy, extensive storytelling, and attempts at caretaking the feelings of other members. The vast majority of times, process group does not directly address specific treatment assignments. Patients are encouraged to bring emotional conflict, interpersonal issues, and events from their past life into process group. The central goal of process group is healthy interpersonal connection and shared empathy.

Staff members will often need to retrain process group participants. In a high functioning process group, members often police themselves to avoid advice giving, speak from personal experience, use "I" statements, and express emotions about the current group experience. In addiction treatment, group participants come from all levels of sophistication and experience. Therefore, the group leader often finds himself training and retraining group members to ensure a productive experience for all.

Progress Assessment

As patients move through treatment in a RecoveryMind Training program, they complete worksheets, become familiar with Recovery Skills through assignments and skills groups, and practice newly learned behaviors throughout the day. Each of these techniques is focused on acquiring the Recovery Skills that build a solid recovery. The Progress Assessment rounds out the RecoveryMind Training treatment process. With this tool, patients routinely review their progress in the domain(s) where they are currently working. The progress assessment form describes each of the Recovery Skills within that domain and asks patients to rate themselves as to their progress. A simple three-point scale is used (has **B**egun, is **I**ntermediate, or has **C**ompleted the skill). Once a patient completes the self-assessment, he or she hands it to his or her therapist or case manager who also evaluates progress using the same three-point evaluation scale. Next, one or more staff members meet with the patient to review the progress assessment form. Using this process, a patient always comprehends the work that has been completed or needs to be completed for an effective outcome in the given domain.

Where Are All These Worksheets and Forms?

This text provides an overview of RecoveryMind Training. The forms and worksheets involved in RecoveryMind training are available in upcoming companion book titled, *RecoveryMind Training: A Guide to Implementation.* Two worksheet examples appear in the Appendix.

Treatment Flow

RecoveryMind Training states the goal of treatment is recovery. Further, it asserts that one learns how to recover by studying, understanding, and practicing specific skills, which are called Recovery Skills. Treatment, then, becomes a place where individuals learn skills. But exactly how does this occur? What does treatment with RMT look like?

To provide a sense of treatment flow, let's follow James, an alcohol-dependent patient through a snippet of his longer care in a RecoveryMind Training program.

> *James is a forty-five-year-old, unmarried man with twenty years of sustained alcohol use. He arrives in treatment at the behest of his attorney, who urged him to enter treatment after his third DUI/DWI arrest. James lives alone and has a steady job with an insurance agency. His career has stalled, mostly because of his increasingly problematic drinking.*
>
> *James goes to his family physician who directs him to a local treatment center with multiple levels of care and community outreach. James arrives at his initial appointment late and with ambivalent feelings about addressing his drinking. After a lengthy initial assessment, James reluctantly agrees to enter an evening intensive outpatient program (IOP, ASAM Level 2.1). He is detoxified from alcohol using an ambulatory detoxification profile (ASAM Level 2.1-WM) with frequent medical and nursing checks. A comprehensive psychosocial assessment is completed. His primary care provider is a physician familiar with addiction recovery who supplies a recent history, a physical, and lab work that validate he is medically appropriate for this level of care.*
>
> *James enters ASAM Level 2.1 treatment that meets Monday through Friday from 6:30 p.m. to 9:30 p.m. On his first day, Carolyn is assigned as James's case manager. She reviews the RecoveryMind Training model used at the center and provides a patient manual describing the important elements of care. During the first few hours of his treatment, Carolyn asks James to read the manual while she leaves to run a skills group. After she returns, she answers his questions. At the end of his first day, James is familiar with the treatment model and understands the clear goals he needs to accomplish during his time*

at the center. He finishes his first day by sitting in on an assignment group. As he leaves, Carolyn asks James to read information about Domain A in the patient manual.

On his second day, Carolyn meets with James briefly to answer any questions. James has never been in treatment and is affronted by having to provide urine drug screens. Carolyn explains how abstinence provides safety for all patients. She asks James to complete two assignments in Domain A over the next two days. James enters the flow of group sessions through the ensuing several days. Carolyn and other staff members make sure James understands the purpose of each exercise. James has many questions about the skills being taught. Brief individual sessions combined with education from peers who are further along in treatment buttress group training. The combination ensures that James understands each step of his care.

Once James completes his first assignments in Domain A, he submits them to Carolyn who reviews them for completeness. She asks him to bring the first two worksheets in Domain A to assignment group. James does so and reads the assignments, which examine James's feelings about addiction containment). Peer feedback in assignment group helps everyone understand that James has had difficulties controlling his drinking in the past. Reluctantly, he accepts the need for disease containment. He states, "I'll go along with this, at least for right now." Smiling, the group leader says, "That's great. No one likes to give drug screens or to be told what to do. We'll look at your feelings about this over the next few days."

Soon, James becomes more comfortable with his peers. Although he is quiet and has kept to himself most of his life, he begins participating in skills group, much to his surprise. He participates in a Domain B skill building exercise where he is introduced to the concept of AddictBrain. In a role-

play, James plays the part of the protagonist's AddictBrain. When instructed, he whispers "You could have just one!" to the protagonist in the role-play. During feedback, James reports that he enjoyed the role, but the experience was spooky. "I knew exactly what to say because I've been hearing that voice in my head for years." Through his participation role-play, he begins to understand his own internal AddictBrain. Unexpectedly, he begins to enjoy treatment, if just a little bit.

Through the ensuing weeks, James completes all assigned worksheets, reviewing them in assignment group. He participates in role-plays and skill building in Domains A and B. After weeks one and two, Carolyn asks James to complete a progress assessment form for Domain A. James does so. Carolyn reviews it with him. Surprisingly, James underestimates his progress, and Carolyn uses this opportunity to help him recognize all the work he has done to date. By the end of the second week, all assignments and work in Domain A are complete. James shows up for assigned urine drug screens with an occasional grumbling comment.

At the end of the time in his initial phase of treatment, Carolyn encourages James to continue in a step down, ASAM Level 1 program. This program meets weekly and continues assignments in Domains C, D, E, and F. This weekly group spends quite a bit of time working on relapse prevention topics contained within Domain F. James remains in this level of care for six months. Despite his isolated past, he develops a strong relationship with his peers in treatment. Much to his surprise, the experience of bonding with his peers increases his interest in support groups. At first, he attends twelve-step meetings with other members of his treatment group. At the encouragement of others, he seeks out a sponsor and begins working

> *the Twelve Steps. He is well on his way to a durable and*
> *healthy recovery.*

As you can see, the combination of worksheet assignments, review in assignment group, building Recovery Skills in skills group, and progress review using progress assessment forms create a fluid and coherent whole. If the stay in an ASAM Level 2.1 program is short, most patients will only be able to complete assignments in Domains A and B. If more time is available, additional assignments in Domains C through F can be addressed at this level of care.

Chapter Seven Notes

1. W. L. White, *Slaying the Dragon: The History of Addiction Treatment and Recovery in America* (Bloomington, IL: Chestnut Health Systems/Lighthouse Institute), 1998.

2. The single most effective treatment, when studied over the short term, is opioid replacement therapy. Treatment of opioid dependence with buprenorphine or methadone is effective at reducing the harmful consequences of opioid dependence. However, two problems that need to be resolved. Both medications are difficult to discontinue if a client wishes to do so, and relapse often occurs when their use is interrupted. Should they therefore be prescribed forever? The second problem is more philosophical: Are there psychological and psycho-spiritual consequences that come from chronic administration of these medications? If there are, should we take a pragmatic approach, trading off the more minor psychological traps—the individual has to continue to take the medication to ward off painful withdrawal—for the greater good—they are no longer addicted to illicit or ill-gained opioid medications? In addiction medicine at present, vociferous arguments about these questions occupy center stage.

3. M. Adler, K. B. Brady, G. Brigham, K. Carroll, R. Clayton, L. Cottler, D. Friedman, *et al,* "Principles of Drug Addiction Treatment: A Research-Based Guide," edited by NIH Publication No. 12–4180: NIDA, 2012.

4. CASA, "State spending on Addiction and Risky Use," CASA, http://www.casacolumbia. org/addiction/state-spending-addiction-risk-use.

5. A. I. Leshner, "Addiction Is a Brain Disease, and It Matters," *Science* 278, no. 5335 (October 3, 1997 1997): 45–47.

6. This quote is attributed in many forms to A. Thomas McLellan, PhD.

7. W. L. White, "What is recovery? A working definition from the Betty Ford Institute," *J Subst Abuse Treat* 33, no. 3 (Oct 2007): 221–28.

8. United States Substance Abuse and Mental Health Services Administration, "SAMHSA's Working Definition of Recovery Updated," SAMHSA, http://blog.samhsa. gov/2012/03/23/defintion-of-recovery-updated/.

9. American Society of Addiction Medicine, "The State of Recovery," http://www.asam.org/ docs/default-source/public-policy-statements/1state-of-recovery-2-82.pdf?sfvrsn=0.

10. L. A. Kaskutas, "What is Recovery?" http://www.asam.org/magazine/read/ article/2015/04/10/what-is-recovery.

11. L. A. Kaskutas and L. A. Ritter, "Consistency Between Beliefs and Behavior Regarding Use of Substances in Recovery," *SAGE Open* 5, no. 1 (2015).

12. L. A. Kaskutas, T. J. Borkman, A. Laudet, L. A. Ritter, J. Witbrodt, M. S. Subbaraman, A. Stunz, and J. Bond, "Elements That Define Recovery: The Experiential Perspective," *J Stud Alcohol Drugs* 75, no. 6 (2014): 999–1010.

13. This is a reference to a classic book from the twelve-step literature by Chuck C. called *A New Pair of Glasses.*

14. See above, n. 7.

15. W. L. White, "Addiction recovery: its definition and conceptual boundaries," *J Subst Abuse Treat* 33, no. 3 (Oct 2007): 229–41.

16. A "first pass" at a clinical training manual that describes how to conduct each of the Domains of care is complete. Several treatment programs are using this model, and refinements will be necessary along the way. Definitive research as to the effectiveness of this treatment model has not been done, and I make no claims that it has been properly studied at the time of publication of this text.

17. S. Tsemberis, D. Kent, and C. Respress, "Housing Stability and Recovery Among Chronically Homeless Persons With Co-Occuring Disorders in Washington, DC," *Am J Public Health* 102, no. 1 (2012/01/01 2011): 13–16.

18. A. P. Sun, "Helping homeless individuals with co-occurring disorders: the four components," *Soc Work* 57, no. 1 (Jan 2012): 23–37.

19. See above, n. 3.

20. P. C. Ouimette, J. W. Finney, and R. H. Moos, "Twelve-step and cognitive-behavioral treatment for substance abuse: a comparison of treatment effectiveness," *J Consult Clin Psychol* 65, no. 2 (Apr 1997): 230–40.

21. R. Kadden, K. Carroll, D. Donovan, N. Cooney, P. Monti, D. Abrams, M. Litt, and R. Hester, *Cognitive-Behavioral Coping Skills Therapy Manual: A Clinical Research Guide for Therapists Treating Individuals With Alcohol Abuse and Dependence* (Rockville, MD: National Institute on Alcohol Abuse and Alcoholism, 2003).

22. S. A. Brown, S. V. Glasner-Edwards, S. R. Tate, J. R. McQuaid, J. Chalekian, and E. Granholm, "Integrated Cognitive Behavioral Therapy Versus Twelve-Step Facilitation Therapy for Substance-Dependent Adults with Depressive Disorders," *J Psychoactive Drugs* 38, no. 4 (2006): 449–60.

23. N. M. Petry, "A comprehensive guide to the application of contingency management procedures in clinical settings," *Drug Alcohol Depend* 58, no. 1–2 (Feb 2000): 9–25.

24. W. Miller and S. Rollnick, *Motivational Interviewing: Preparing People for Change*, Second ed. (New York: Guilford Press, 2002).

25. W. Miller and S. Rollnick, "Ten things that motivational interviewing is not," *Behav Cogn Psychother* 37, no. 2 (Mar 2009): 129–40.

26. W. Miller, A. Zweben, C. C. DiClemente, and R. Rychtarik, *Motivational Enhancement Therapy Manual: A Clinical Research Guide for Therapists Treating Individuals with Alcohol Abuse and Dependence* (Rockville, MD, 1999).

27. British Columbia Ministry for Children and Families, "The Biopsychosocial Theory: A Comprehensive Descriptive Perspective on Addiction," ed. British Columbia Ministry for Children and Families, 12. Vancouver, B.C., 1996.

28. D. H. Angres and K. Bettinardi-Angres, "The disease of addiction: Origins, treatment, and recovery," *Disease-a-Month* 54, no. 10 (2008): 696–721.

29. W. L. White, M. Boyle, and D. Loveland, "Alcoholism/Addiction as a Chronic Disease," *Alcoholism Treatment Quarterly* 20, no. 3–4 (Jul 2002): 107–29.

30. J. Nowinski, S. Baker, and K. Carroll, *Twelve Step Facilitation Therapy Manual* (Rockville, Maryland: U.S. Department of Health and Human Services, 1995).

31. Narcotics Anonymous, *Narcotics Anonymous Basic Text*, Sixth ed. (Chatsworth, CA: Narcotics Anonymous World Services, Inc., 2008).

32. Alcoholics Anonymous, *Alcoholics Anonymous*, Fourth ed. (New York: A.A. World Services, Inc., 1976).

33. L. A. Kaskutas, M. S. Subbaraman, J. Witbrodt, and S. E. Zemore, "Effectiveness of Making Alcoholics Anonymous Easier: A group format 12-step facilitation approach," *J Subst Abuse Treat* 37, no. 3 (2009): 228–39.

34. AA World Services, *Twelve Steps and Twelve Traditions* (New York: AA World Services, Inc., 2002).

35. J. N. Chappel and R. L. DuPont, "Twelve-Step and Mutual-Help Programs for Addictive Disorders," *Psychiatric Clinics of North America* 22, no. 2 (6/1/1999): 425–46.

36. American Society of Addiction Medicine, "Drug Testing: A White Paper of the American Society of Addiction Medicine (ASAM)," Chevy Chase, MD: ASAM, 2013.

37. R. J. Goldsmith and B. L. Green, "A rating scale for alcoholic denial," *J Nerv Ment Dis* 176, no. 10 (1988): 614–20.

38. P. Dare, and L. Derigne, "Denial in alcohol and other drug use disorders: A critique of theory," *Addiction Research & Theory* 18, no. 2 (2010): 181–93.

39. M. S. Ainsworth and J. Bowlby, "An ethological approach to personality development," *American Psychologist* 46, no. 4 (1991): 333–41.

40. P. J. Flores, *Addiction as an Attachment Disorder* (Oxford: Jason Aronson, Inc., 2004).

41. G. G. Forrest, *Self-disclosure in Psychotherapy and Recovery* (Oxford: Jason Aronson, Inc., 2010).

42. M. Galanter, "Spirituality, evidence-based medicine, and alcoholics anonymous," *Am J Psychiatry* 165, no. 12 (2008): 1514–17.

43. J. M. White, R. S. Wampler, and J. L. Fischer, "Indicators of Spiritual Development in Recovery from Alcohol and Other Drug Problems," *Alcoholism Treatment Quarterly* 19, no. 1 (Jan 2001): 19–35.

44. W. R. Miller and M. P. Bogenschutz, "Spirituality and Addiction," *South Med J* 100, no. 4 (2007): 433–36, 10.1097/SMJ.0b013e3180316fbf.

45. ASAM, *The ASAM Criteria: Treatment Criteria for Addictive, Substance-related and Co-occuring Disorders*, Third ed., ed. David Mee-Lee (Carson City, Nevada: The Change Companies, 2013).

46. See above, n. 29.

47. A. T. McLellan, J. R. McKay, R. Forman, J. Cacciola, and J. Kemp, "Reconsidering the evaluation of addiction treatment: from retrospective follow-up to concurrent recovery monitoring," *Addiction* 100, no. 4 (2005): 447–58.

48. I. Yalom and M. Leszcz, *Theory and Practice of Group Psychotherapy*, Fifth ed. (New York: Basic Books, 2005).

49. N. Katz and K. McNulty, "Reflective Listening," ed. Maxwell School of Citizenship and Public Affairs, 1994.

50. D. M. Foreman, "The ethical use of paradoxical interventions in psychotherapy," *J Med Ethics* 16, no. 4 (Dec 1990): 200–5.

51. M. J. Cox and B. Paley, "Families as Systems," *Annu Rev Psychol* 48, no. 1 (1997): 243–67.

52. C. R. Cloninger, D. M. Svrakic, and T. R. Przybeck, "A psychobiological model of temperament and character," *Arch Gen Psychiatry* 50, no. 12 (Dec 1993): 975–90.

53. D. Angres, S. Bologeorges, and J. Chou, "A two year longitudinal outcome study of addicted health care professionals: an investigation of the role of personality variables," *Subst Abuse* 7 (2013): 49–60.

54.   D. H. Angres, "The Temperament and Character Inventory in Addiction Treatment," *FOCUS: The Journal of Lifelong Learning in Psychiatry* 8, no. 2 (2010): 187–98.

55.   T. N. Hanh, *The Miracle of Mindfulness: An Introduction to the Practice of Meditation* (Boston: Beacon Press, 1976).

56.   G. A. Marlatt and N. Chawla, "Meditation and Alcohol Use," *South Med J* 100, no. 4 (2007): 451–53.

57.   B. E. Carlson and H. Larkin, "Meditation as a Coping Intervention for Treatment of Addiction," *Journal of Religion & Spirituality in Social Work: Social Thought* 28, no. 4 (2009): 379–92.

58.   J. Kornfield, *Meditation for Beginners* (New York: Bantam Books, 2005).

59.   A. Zgierska, D. Rabago, M. Zuelsdorff, C. Coe, M. Miller, and M. Fleming, "Mindfulness Meditation for Alcohol Relapse Prevention: A Feasibility Pilot Study," *J Addict Med* 2, no. 3 (2008): 165–73.

60.   K. Witkiewitz, G. A. Marlatt, and D. Walker, "Mindfulness-Based Relapse Prevention for Alcohol and Substance Use Disorders," *Journal of Cognitive Psychotherapy* 19, no. 3 (2005): 211–28.

61.   D. Lama, *Stages of Meditation*, (Boulder, CO: Snow Lion Publications, 2001).

62.   J. Forem, *Transcendental Meditation: The Essential Teachings of Maharishi Mahesh Yogi* (Carlsbad, CA: Hay House, 2012).

63.   See above, n. 32, pp. 58–59.

64.   After all, it is hard-wired deep in our brain. Think of the childhood game "Don't think about an elephant."

65.   The word "powerless" occurs seven times in the *Alcoholics Anonymous* text and the step book, *Twelve Steps and Twelve Traditions*. Each time, it refers to alcohol. It never states "we are powerless over everything."

66.   M. Stallvik and D. R. Gastfriend, "Predictive and convergent validity of the ASAM criteria software in Norway," *Addiction Research & Theory* 22, no. 6 (2014): 515–23.

67.   See above, n. 45.

68.   Formerly known as the *ASAM Patient Placement Criteria, Second Edition, Revised (PPC-2R)*.

69.   See above, n. 45.

70.   This is a phrase that came into the popular lexicon following a United States Supreme Court decision regarding a pornography case. The phrase came from a concurring opinion by Justice Potter Stewart. The case centered on Louis Malle's movie *The Lovers*. The film was judged not to be hard-core pornography by this Supreme Court ruling.

71.   Skills group uses techniques and nomenclature from psychodrama. As a therapeutic technique, role-play is powerful. Therefore, the role-play in these trainings should not expand into a full-blown psychodrama experience. If not trained in psychodrama or psychomotor, staff should stick with specific assignments. Undertrained therapists can inadvertently fall into a situation they are ill-equipped to manage if they revisit unaddressed childhood wounds, for example. However, RMT therapists should be encouraged to obtain additional training in experiential therapy.

Domains and Techniques

The synopsis provided in this chapter lays the groundwork for the remainder of the text, where each domain is discussed in depth in its own chapter (Chapters Nine through Fourteen). I will also discuss the theory behind and practice of three techniques used in RMT that differentiate it from traditional treatment methods.

Domains

RecoveryMind's Recovery Skills are divided into six domains. Domains provide logical groupings of these skills and help patients and therapists conceptualize the overall goals of this treatment process. They include the following:

- Domain A: Containment
- Domain B: Recovery Basics
- Domain C: Emotional Awareness and Resilience
- Domain D: Healthy Internal Narrative
- Domain E: Connectedness and Spirituality
- Domain F: Relapse Prevention Skills

Within each domain, multiple skills collectively form the core aptitudes of that domain. Any given patient will not master *every*

Recovery Skill in *every* domain while in treatment. The Recovery Skills in Domains A and B tend to be the most critical in the short run, and those in Domains C though F, when internalized, prove important for long-term recovery.

RecoveryMind Training breaks down the acquisition of a particular skill or competency into discrete steps. RMT believes skills are best learned by doing. Specific groups train Recovery Skills. In such a group, a Recovery Skill is described using a brief lecture (less than ten minutes), which is followed by group learning and practice. This cycle of describing the skill, watching a demonstration of that skill, and following this up with practice entrains the brain at both a conscious and habitual level. For example, training in drug refusal skills might begin by having the leader describe the process of drug refusal. He describes the intent of learning the skill, times when it should be executed, and its importance in maintaining recovery then provides examples of that skill to the entire group. The group then watches the leader as he works with one patient who walks through that skill, actively managing this high-risk situation.

Several other patients then practice this skill using a context that fits their own history and future risks. If the training occurs in a smaller group, the leader moves from patient to patient until every participant practices the skill. The focus of the group is on one patient at a time. At the end of each patient interaction, brief feedback and discussion occurs. This draws the entire group into the learning process and produces interdependent learning. In a larger group, patients may pair off; multiple staff members may need to be present, coaching several pairs or groups in learning the skill. Experiential groups entrain automatic learning—in contrast to factual learning. Automatic responses are essential to maintaining sobriety/recovery. Important skills may be revisited multiple times, if need be. Patients are encouraged to practice these skills throughout their treatment.

To improve procedural learning, staff members must move from the traditional lecture format (talking *at* patients) to a collaborative learning paradigm (interacting *with* patients). For some staff members this can be quite a stretch. In a program that has fully embraced RMT, there are few "lecture hours" on the schedule. I also encourage RMT-based programs to limit the times when chairs are arranged in rows, lecture style. Staff members should arrive at each training module prepared with brief descriptions of the skill, which may contain examples for demonstration. At times, it may be helpful to stop the interaction before the session has elapsed, asking patients to fill out feedback forms for quality improvement. The forms encourage self-reflection to help patients internalize what they learned during that specific training period.

RMT domains are described briefly in the following sections.

Domain A: Containment

To begin the recovery journey, a patient must be abstinent. Stopping addictive chemicals for the individual with alcohol and drug use disorders, discontinuing compulsive betting for those suffering with gambling addiction, interrupting compulsive sexual behaviors for individuals struggling with sex addiction, and stopping compulsive food behaviors for those addicted to food is recovery's *sine qua non*. Maintenance medications—especially for opioid dependence—do not compromise abstinence if they are not abused. Very few individuals with substance use disorders have the initial resolve to interrupt their addictive use of chemicals without outside help. The same can be said for other addiction disorders. Early in the recovery process, we cannot expect our patients to be able to stop using and/or remain abstinent using willpower. If it has failed in the past, it is time for a different plan.

In Domain A, RecoveryMind Training catalogues external constraints that assist in efforts at abstinence and guides the patient, helping construct her containment system and take the first step of her journey. The patient must look outside herself, using whatever it takes to stop the destructive cycle of use. Occasionally a patient or client might be able to use a contractual containment procedure, such as a commitment to a spouse or therapist. This is one type of containment. In most cases, the containment needs to be stronger. Entering an outpatient program, a residential treatment program, or a detoxification facility provides increasingly intense levels of initial containment. A small number of people with prolonged substance use disorders who have failed less aggressive treatment may need to be "locked up" for a period to ensure disease containment.

It is important to remember that applying external containment upon one's addiction disorder is not the same thing as recovery. One uses containment to begin recovery; it is not recovery itself. When describing containment to patients, you should clearly differentiate containment from recovery.

Over time, the need for containment will decrease. Three years into recovery, someone with an alcohol use disorder might only need the gentle reminders that come from attending AA meetings. However, should that person fall into a place of increased stress or loss, he would benefit from a temporary increase in his external containment to ensure continued abstinence. Data from many sources supports the hypothesis that the longer one is abstinent, the longer that person will remain abstinent.[1] Containment can be physical, social, contractual, and biological.

Domain B: Recovery Basics

Once a patient has the temporary protection provided by disease containment, he or she is ready to learn recovery basics: the essential elements of a recovery program. Recovery basics combine some of the principles of Alcoholics Anonymous with elements of self-care. One of these elements is mindfulness meditation. Meditation is powerful medicine; it quiets the mind and prepares it to consider new options. Domain B also teaches self-reflection and organizational skills. A structured daily written reflection helps plan each day and prioritize recovery activities.

In Domain B, the patient undertakes a thorough examination of how substance use has taken over her life. Assignments gently lead the patient to an in-depth examination of how her addiction has created wholesale damage to herself and her family. By completing worksheets and reviewing them in assignment group, she pierces the fog of unknowing that enshrouds her substance use and its consequences. Past behaviors are compared with her values, recalibrating and placing her on a recovery path aligned to her deeper core values.

In Domain B, patients are trained to use Recovery Reflection, a tool that helps them plan the day, reflect upon their feelings, attitudes, and progress, excavate addiction denial, and establish healthy recovery goals. Once learned, the patient completes the Recovery Reflection worksheet once or twice per day, depending on treatment intensity.

Patients also learn simple meditation techniques in a Domain B skills group. A patient's initial meditation practice may be only a few minutes in length. It slowly increases in length and benefit as treatment progresses and into the first year of recovery. Mindfulness meditation has been shown to decrease emotional lability[2] and impulsiveness, decrease the probability of relapse,[3] and improve connectedness with others.[4] Individuals who find they cannot meditate after repeated diligent attempts can be taught a substitute skill, most commonly, auditory brain entrainment.[5]

Domain C: Emotional Awareness and Resilience

Addiction, by its very nature, befuddles the brain, creating intense confusion and conflict. AddictBrain whips up emotional cacophony as part of its plan for survival. Even if an individual enjoyed a modicum of emotional stability prior to the onset of his addiction, chaos soon rules. The patient who is younger or lacks maturity—and as a result is not facile in sitting with feeling states and reacting in a healthy manner—or the individual who has preexisting emotional distress is fertile soil in which addiction grows. AddictBrain exacerbates emotional problems, using the resultant chaos for self-preservation.

The first step to emotional balance is awareness of one's feeling states. Some individuals are all too aware of their feelings. Others seem to register negative emotions but remain unaware or misjudge mirth, happiness, and joy. A third group seems partly or completely out of touch with any emotional experience inside themselves or in others; they report facts not feelings. The first competency in Domain C for each of these groups is emotional awareness.

A healthy recovery can only emerge when those with substance use disorders develop emotional balance. Emotional balance is not emotional flatness. Individuals in solid recovery enjoy a wide range of emotions, living life at its fullest. In RecoveryMind Training, the term for this state is emotional resilience.

The skills learned in Domain C, emotional awareness and resilience, increase emotional balance and simultaneously decrease the probability of relapse. Using techniques borrowed from Emotional Intelligence[6] (EI) and Dialectical Behavioral Therapy (DBT),[7] RecoveryMind Training builds skills in the recovering patient that allow him or her to experience a full emotional life; use these skills to connect with others in a healthy manner; and, at the same time, prevent overwhelm caused by counterproductive, runaway emotional states.

Patients who have concurrent mood disorders or other psychiatric diseases require assessment for medication management as well. Most modern psychiatric medications do not derail recovery and can, therefore, be used judiciously. At the same time, using psychiatric medications to chase ephemeral symptoms and emotional states that invariably pop up in early recovery is strongly contraindicated. Medication management is an additional Domain C intervention. All individuals who have simultaneous mood and substance use disorders should spend time discussing the interaction between the two conditions. Staff members need to be clear that these two conditions are deeply interactive but should never be considered to be causative of the other. Junior staff members or those who have more extensive training in either camp will have a tendency to fall into this trap. Statements such as the following are dangerous and happen far too often: "I know your depression dragged you down and eventually you began drinking excessively just to cope," or "Everyone who uses drugs gets depressed, it will go away once you are clean for a while." While common, these statements are downright dangerous. When a staff member or patient makes such an error of causation, it should be gently but swiftly corrected.

Domain D: Healthy Internal Narrative

In Domain D, patients are taught about the many maladaptive internal thoughts (referred here in as voices) that accompany addiction. At first, the strongest is that of denial. Denial is resilient, recurrent, and pervasive. It also shows up using a patient's previously perfected defense mechanisms.[8, 9] For example, a patient who has used blaming defenses since childhood—perfecting them along the way—will have a denial complex loaded with blame: "My boss drives me to drink." But the internal narrative contains more than just the voice of denial. The internal narrative in many addicts contains elements of inevitable doom: "I may be doing well in treatment but I always eventually relapse." Addicted individuals often have a litany of "negative self-talk." In Domain D, each patient catalogs his or her own unique narrative and builds corrective responses that protect recovery.

Repairing a self-destructive internal narrative is a three-step process. The first step is identifying the laundry list of voices specific to each particular patient. When building such a list, the patient is surprised by the number of voices in his narrative, yet, at the same time, he is reassured that the number is finite. This jump-starts the patient on the process of reengineering his internal narrative. The second step is to create a corrective narrative for each voice. And finally, the third step is practicing the corrective narration over and over. One cannot glibly make negative internal narration go away by "thinking nice thoughts." Laying down a parallel track of realistic truths will, however, temper the impact over time.

Domain E: Connectedness and Spirituality

Addiction is a disease of isolation and loneliness. Even if someone with addiction was highly social or his or her use began in a social setting, isolation eventually wins out. As addiction matures, most people with addiction disorders fall into painful solitude. Treatment is, in its very essence, a resocializing and reconnecting experience. An often-heard truism is "We get sick alone but we recover with others." Interpersonal support is critical in reducing denial, creating hope, and building a network that establishes healthy norms.

Some experts in attachment theory assert that addiction is driven by failures in healthy attachment.[10] Substance use is a way of assuaging the hunger produced by this failure. In the pragmatic arena of addiction treatment, it matters not whether unhealthy attachment is the cause or effect of addiction—the treatment remains the same. The exercises in Domain E teach and strive to repair deficits in healthy connection. The result of this work improves the patient's ability to use support group networks; learn and relate to others and hopefully to one's sponsor; and repair addiction-induced family dysfunction.

The second area of skill building in Domain E is spirituality. The goal of the spirituality exercises in this domain is to expand a patient's willingness to explore spiritual principles and practice in one's daily life. They do not mandate any religious beliefs. Spirituality exercises encourage patients to parlay their gains in interpersonal connection onto a higher plane. Some patients may return to their previous religious practices or seek out a new faith; however, treatment should never imply this is mandatory.

Domain F: Relapse Prevention Skills

In Domain F, we return to a pragmatic set of Recovery Skills, i.e., relapse prevention. More than any work in other domains, these skills must be learned experientially. Patients will develop a personalized list of high-risk situations, role play them, and explore and practice responses that subvert relapse. In relapse prevention training, every response needs to be practiced until procedural learning occurs.[11] The reason for this is simple. By the time an individual arrives in treatment, AddictBrain has already preprogrammed explicit responses to environmental stimuli, feelings, and even specific thought patterns. To overcome AddictBrain-induced procedural memory, the recovering individual needs to practice explicit RecoveryMind responses to these same triggers.

In RecoveryMind Training, patients also learn to recognize and acknowledge cravings, recognize conditioned cues in their environment, and program other important behaviors. RMT relapse prevention training uses a specific set of terms. Patients should be conversant in these terms and be able to use them in constructing a practiced response to the many dangers they will face in recovery.

RecoveryMind Training Techniques

I will highlight three of the many techniques used in RecoveryMind Training in this section: clarity of language, procedural learning, and role-playing. This information should be used as a guide to understanding how some of the RMT concepts are implemented. It is by no means exhaustive. Education and training in these techniques as well as the many other aspects of RecoveryMind Training is essential to properly implement this care model.[12]

Clarity of Language

While sitting with a group of patients nearing the completion of their initial phase of treatment many years ago, it hit me how muddled addiction treatment really is. In this meeting, patients reflected back on their eight- to twelve-week treatment course. Every member of that group vociferously agreed when two of the group members stated, "It took me three weeks just to figure out what I was supposed to be doing. I never did understand why I was assigned certain tasks!" I recognized the panoply of terms, definitions, and often-conflicting concepts that exist in the addiction treatment industry only serves to obfuscate. What happens when one treatment provider discusses a patient's progress to another provider in an attempt to communicate a comprehensive understanding of the patient's condition? Not surprisingly, there is much hand waving, interruptions, and conversational retracements. I set out to fix this muddle.

When building RecoveryMind Training, I recognized that clear language should be one of the foundational elements of the treatment system. Clarity was created on multiple levels. The first is in clearly defining the problem: the destructive brain circuits that combine to produce AddictBrain. The problem, AddictBrain, has a reparative alter, RecoveryMind. Addiction creates AddictBrain; RecoveryMind induces recovery. Clarity is increased by defining clear goals, subdivided into logical units (i.e., Recovery Skills grouped into domains).

Clear language will come easiest to the student of RecoveryMind Training who has not yet been burdened by years of previous treatment jargon. By itself, treatment jargon is bad. Over time, however, treatment terms have become inconsistent, vary from therapist to therapist, and are not fully explained to patients. When John, who was trained at treatment center "A," begins working at treatment center "B," he brings with him a whole different set of concepts and words to describe treatment. Most centers have a hodgepodge of staff members, trained at different universities and facilities, who use different language when working with patients. If we add the illness of addiction to this mix, which creates its own chaos, then we have the perfect formula for a failed treatment, regardless of staff dedication.

Many more terms will be introduced in this book. I urge you to discard past terms when implementing RecoveryMind Training. Hold each other accountable for clarity of language so you can build a clear path to recovery for your clients or patients.

Language and the Perception Reality

The content and syntax of language alters our perception of the world around us, yet the extent and qualities of reality that are altered as a result of language remains a hotly contested topic in linguistics. However, linguists agree that language "provides a medium for describing the contents of our conscious experience."[13] Language also provides a handle to grab onto when considering complex subjects. For example, studies on the efficacy of medications in the treatment of mood disorders enjoyed a great leap forward when research scientists and clinicians were able to agree on the definition and qualities that define depression or bipolar illness. Discussion was ignited by the publication of the APA's first *Diagnostic and Statistical Manual: Mental Disorders* (*DSM-I*) in 1952.[14] Despite the controversy that still seems to swirl around it and worries about the accuracy of this empirically derived manual, the *DSM* has improved communication and increased meaningful debate about psychiatric diseases throughout the world.

The *DSM-5* defines substance use disorders by specific criteria. I believe the treatment of addiction needs clear terminology as well. In RecoveryMind Training, this starts with the definition of AddictBrain (the sum of all brain changes that occur when addiction is established, including those that lock in continued addictive urges, thoughts, actions, and behaviors) and RecoveryMind (the sum of all changes in thinking, behavior, self-concept, and action that are needed to induce a remission of the addictive disorder). Clearly defining the culprit and providing a system that contains elements of its treatment help clinicians and staff members agree upon the problem and focus on tasks that restore health. Clear definitions of the goals in treatment remove the sense that recovery is an elusive state.

Procedural Learning

AddictBrain rewires neural circuitry in the brain. To recover, one needs to rewire the brain in a similar manner. Fortunately, the brain is doing this all the time. The depth to which the brain's control centers are rewired gives addiction its power. You can't recover by changing your mind; you have to practice new behaviors. Psychotherapy works at many levels; changing your thinking occurs first, then emotional changes are next. Hardwired behaviors are the most resistant to change. Recovery can only occur after changes occur at every one of these levels.

Most treatment centers offer lectures to patients. I have noted over the years that, at the time of discharge, patients only vaguely remember the content of such lectures. They report which staff member gave an inspiring or amusing talk but frequently cannot describe, execute, or even remember the skills taught in those lectures. RecoveryMind Training avoids using lectures as a sole means of communicating a concept or skill. Rather, it imparts complex skills through acquisition and practice. Attaining skills and rehearsing them through body movement is called procedural learning.

To understand procedural learning, we need to investigate how the brain learns and stores memories. I will address this in the following sections.

Types of Learning and Memory

The human brain does not store memories in a singular location or by using one process. There are many types of memories and storage locations; some memories are even stored outside of the brain. A simple diagram of the different types of human memory appears in Figure 8.1.

Sensory memory (①) is the first type of memory. It holds raw data briefly before sending it on for further processing. The remainder of our memories is divided into short-term (②) and long-term (③) memory. Short-term memories are gathered and held in the hippocampus and related structures. We hold on to short-term memories for minutes, and repetition helps us retain such information. One good example of short-term memory occurs when we repeat someone's phone number to ourselves as we enter it into an address book or contact list.

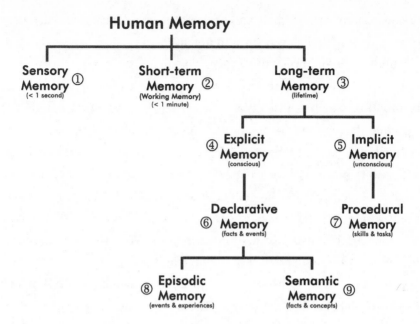

Figure 8.1 - Types of Memory[15] (Courtesy of
Luke Mastin. Used with permission.)

Long-term memory is measured in days, months, or years. We
collect short-term memories as we go through our day. We may recall
this information off and on throughout the day, and as we do so, this
information is placed into context. During sleep, additional processing
occurs, and information is transferred from short-term to long-term
memory where further associations, context, and meaning occur. Long-
term memory is divided into explicit (④) and implicit (⑤) memory.
Explicit memory is conscious; it is also called declarative memory (⑥). Our
explicit, declarative memory is divided into two separate buckets: episodic
(⑧) and semantic (⑨) memory. Episodic memory contains information
about past events or experiences and has rich associations. You may recall
receiving an award several years ago, remembering the location, time of
day, and the people with which you shared this experience. This is episodic
memory. Episodic memory is not fixed. Each time we recall a past event,
the brain alters it, adding new meaning and even new information to a
past event. We also have a fickle explicit memory system, called semantic

memory. Here we store facts and concepts, such as our friend's birthdate or the names of each part of an automobile engine.

Implicit memory is the other type of long-term memory. It is unconscious. We have several forms of implicit memory;[16] the most common of which is procedural memory (⑦). Procedural memory is stored in deeper areas of the brain: the stratum and basal ganglia, the cerebellum, and the limbic area. Procedural memory is often associated with habits but can be very complex. Anyone who has learned to drive a car or ride a bicycle has experienced procedural learning. During the learning process, a task is practiced over and over. At first it may seem incomprehensible and strains the brain. With repeated practice, however, very complex skills are acquired and mastered.

When a skill is internalized through procedural learning, our response becomes automatic; it shifts from difficult to effortless. When we first learned to drive an automobile, coordinating the multiple tasks and operating in a smooth and efficient manner seemed nearly impossible. Our trip behind the wheel in traffic was exhausting. Over time, driving becomes second nature. We zip down the expressway humming our favorite tune while deftly and automatically avoiding another driver who zooms into our lane.

RecoveryMind Training posits that procedural learning is a central part of a solid recovery. Those with addiction cannot overcome the unconscious procedural learning entrained by AddictBrain using happy thoughts or good intentions. They have to *practice* recovery.

To witness AddictBrain-induced procedural memory, one simply has to observe a smoker who is deep in thought, completing his college term paper. Unbeknownst to him, his non-dominant hand wanders across the desk, fumbles for his pack of cigarettes, removes a single cigarette with a practiced motion, and places it in his mouth. He unconsciously reaches for the lighter and lights up the cigarette. Only after taking his first puff and removing the cigarette from his mouth, he is conscious that he is smoking. The shift of his stream of thought away from his writing comes from the bolus of nicotine that reaches the mesolimbic reward center.

For a moment, he gazes in contemplation at the shaft of the cigarette with familiar appreciation for the gratifying effect of nicotine.

In RecoveryMind Training, procedural learning occurs in skills groups and should be practiced throughout the course of one's treatment. For example, AddictBrain hides cravings and thoughts about substance use. Addiction-driven learning is partially or completely unconscious, automatic, and stereotypical. The RecoveryMind antidote is to practice frequent disclosure of craving episodes and random desires to use. In RMT, I like to say, "Action defeats action." Said another way, the only way of overcoming AddictBrain's procedural memory is to engage in the procedural learning inherent in RecoveryMind Training.

Role-playing and Experiential Therapy

I have repeatedly made the point that acquiring and practicing Recovery Skills is at the core of the RecoveryMind Training treatment process. So how is this actually implemented? Such learning occurs through the use of practicing new behaviors and learning new behaviors through role-play. Role-play relies upon the natural ability human beings have for simulation. In Chapter Five, I discussed the Default Mode Network and described one of its functions, future simulation. When at rest, we think about the future. In doing so, we enact future situations and interactions with others. For example, someone struggling with alcohol use disorder may plan out her response when faced with an old friend asking if she would like an alcoholic beverage. Although this is a powerful modeling tool, it cannot override procedural memory. AddictBrain continues to drive her to drink. Thinking through possible responses to abort a relapse has little power over AddictBrain's procedural memory where procuring and consuming alcohol has become as effortless as riding a bike.

Instead, she needs to act out her responses to such situations. Procedural learning occurs when an individual plans out and physically executes a specific task. Repeated task enactment builds procedural memory or habit. This process must be a central component of a

RecoveryMind Training-based treatment program. Human beings have a natural capacity for storytelling and simulation. Role-playing uses our ability to simulate potential future events to entrain Recovery Skills. Continuing with the previous example, someone role-plays the "old friend" who asks the woman if she would like an alcoholic beverage. The patient then walks through several responses, finding and practicing the ones that are most effective and natural in preventing relapse.

Examples of skills that are part of RecoveryMind Training and practiced in treatment include accepting addiction containment, becoming comfortable with support groups, and drug refusal skills. Role-playing is also used to concretize important RMT concepts. One of the most important of these is helping patients have a visceral understanding of AddictBrain. The following is an example of one role-play based upon a clinical scenario. In this skills group, a person with drug use disorder experiences AddictBrain firsthand.

> *Malik is a thirty-two-year-old male who enters treatment for his opioid use disorder. He first used opioids after a significant work-related musculoskeletal injury. His injury was caused by a construction accident and a subsequent fall. Thanks to his generally good health and excellent orthopedic treatment, Malik has returned to being close to fully functional. His treatment required multiple surgeries scattered across several months. During the course of those treatments, he was introduced to two opioid painkillers, oxycodone and hydrocodone. Malik's orthopedic physician continued him on these medications for almost eight months to ensure he was pain-free and mobile during the recovery process. At that point, he transferred him to a rehabilitative medicine physician and physical therapy.*
>
> *Malik noticed his alcohol intake decreased during the course of his rehabilitation. He grew up with a father who drank heavily; this resulted in a deep commitment that he would never drink like his father. He was quite pleased*

with himself about his decreased alcohol intake, unaware that his problematic alcohol use was quietly switching to something much more problematic, opioid dependence.

Malik's rehabilitation physician immediately began tapering the narcotics. Malik complained that his pain still made it difficult to function. His physician, in an effort to return Malik to full functionality, insisted on a consistent taper, discontinuing the hydrocodone and oxycodone in a matter of weeks. Malik felt worse. His sessions with the rehabilitation physician became increasingly contentious. Although he understood he needed to discontinue the pills at some point, Malik was not convinced that this was the right time. Nonetheless, he cooperated with a slow consistent taper and eventually discontinued all opioids.

One day, Malik experienced a minor re-injury. The pain was intense, so he decided to go to an urgent care clinic. The physician at the center examined the injury, telling Malik that part of the pain came from an exacerbation of his past physical trauma. He prescribed large doses of oxycodone with multiple refills. As he was leaving the urgent care clinic, Malik felt strangely like a little boy at Christmas.

Upon arriving home, Malik immediately started taking the oxycodone with a ferocious appetite. His daily use escalated quickly. He felt surprisingly well. During his physical therapy sessions and visits with the rehabilitative medicine physician, he did not disclose his return to opioid use. His rehabilitation physician confused Malik's drug-induced improvement with genuine improvement and announced that his course of rehabilitation was complete.

This was when his oxycodone use got out of hand. Malik started going from physician to physician, describing his injuries to obtain additional drugs. As this became too costly and time-consuming, he soon began purchasing oxycodone and hydrocodone from "friends." Malik's wife and family grew increasingly concerned about his behavior. He avoided work, was moody, and disappeared for hours at a time. His wife discovered Malik's stash of pills and confronted him late one afternoon. Surprisingly, he admitted that his "pill problem" was out of hand. After discussing his situation with his family, Malik decided to enter a treatment program.

Early in his treatment, Malik made the connection between his father's drinking, the change in his alcohol consumption, and his use of opioid pain pills. He was wary of the staff and other patients at first but soon found the treatment unburdened his dishonesty and secrets.

One day in skills group, the group leader, Linda, asked Malik if he would like to role-play his AddictBrain. Malik had watched others in skills group and understood the basics of role-playing. He had never been the protagonist in such a role-play; however, Linda, smiling widely while standing in the center of the circle, invited Malik to join her. He walked into the circle and looked around. At the moment he entered the circle, he felt awkward and a little scared.

Linda started by saying, "It's time we introduce you to your AddictBrain. Think of a time in your past use where you were fighting the urge to get more pills but at the same time had misgivings about this being the right thing to do." Malik immediately recalled the second time he went to a "Doc in a Box," hoping to get hydrocodone or oxycodone. Linda sequentially enrolls two auxiliaries: the physician and nurse at the urgent care clinic. The scene is played out briefly. Linda asks Malik, "What was going on in your head?" Malik replies that he really wanted the physician to prescribe the drug, but he felt somewhat guilty. Linda enrolls group members as these two voices in Malik's head, labeling one AddictBrain and the other "the voice of caution." Malik then instructs these voices to verbalize the thoughts he had at that moment. The actors repeat back Malik's words exactly. Linda may coach the actors to change emphasis or tone to clarify Malik's experience. In hearing the voices repeat his words, Malik's shoulders fall, his head bows, and a look of resignation moves across his face. "Yeah, that was what it was like," he sighs.

Linda follows Malik's lead, expanding the enrolled voices. She may carry those voices to different points in time, asking Malik to describe how they changed as his illness progressed. After twenty minutes of this work, Linda checks in with Malik, ensures he is okay, and instructs the characters in the scene and the voices in Malik's head to disenroll from their assignment. The other group participants relate to the experience and discuss what they felt watching Malik's work in this group. All members of the group deepen their understanding of AddictBrain in this manner.

When exercises like this occur at the right time in treatment, most patients transition from verbal understanding to visceral appreciation. When they review their treatment experience at a later date, I often hear, "That was when I *got* it."

Although such role-plays are not full-blown experiential psychotherapy sessions, RMT staff members who run skills group should obtain some training in action-oriented psychotherapy. Several schools of training exist, including psychodrama,[17] Pesso Boyden System Psychomotor,[18, 19, 20] social therapy,[21] and others. Each of these schools has their own techniques and emphasis; however, all of them involve action and interaction with others as a method of learning and change. RMT agrees the body has to move (stand, walk, touch, push, fall, and other actions) to overcome the powerful behavioral training that AddictBrain has already produced. Using this type of exercise and subsequent practice of skills, patients are well prepared to engage with the outside world.

Chapter Eight Notes

1. M. L. Dennis, M. A. Foss, and C. K. Scott, "An Eight-Year Perspective on the Relationship Between the Duration of Abstinence and Other Aspects of Recovery," *Eval Rev* 31, no. 6 (Dec 2007): 585–612.

2. C. L. M. Hill and J. A. Updegraff, "Mindfulness and its relationship to emotional regulation," *Emotion* 12, no. 1 (2012): 81–90.

3. K. Witkiewitz, G. A. Marlatt, and D. Walker, "Mindfulness-Based Relapse Prevention for Alcohol and Substance Use Disorders," *Journal of Cognitive Psychotherapy* 19, no. 3 (2005): 211–28.

4. C. A. Hutcherson, E. M. Seppala, and J. J. Gross, "Loving-kindness meditation increases social connectedness," *Emotion* 8, no. 5 (2008): 720–24.

5. G. Oster, "Auditory Beats in the Brain," *Sci Am* 229, no. 4 (1973): 94–102.

6. J. D. Mayer, P. Salovey, D. R. Caruso, and G. Sitarenios, "Emotional intelligence as a standard intelligence," *Emotion* 1, no. 3 (2001): 232–42.

7. M. M. Linehan, *Skills Training Manual for Treating Borderline Personality Disorder*, First ed. (New York: The Guilford Press, 1993).

8. J. Wallace, *John Wallace: Writings - The Alcoholism Papers* (Newport, RI: Edgehill Publications, 1989).

9. J. Wallace, "Working with the Preferred Defense Structure of the Recovering Alcoholic," in *Practical Approaches to Alcoholism Psychotherapy*, eds. S. Zimberg, J. Wallace, and S. B Blume (New York: Springer, 1985), 432.

10. P. J. Flores, *Addiction as an Attachment Disorder*, (Oxford: Jason Aronson, Inc., 2004).

11. W. T. Maddox and F. G. Ashby, "Dissociating explicit and procedural-learning based systems of perceptual category learning," *Behav Processes* 66, no. 3 (2004): 309–32.

12. Look online at RecoveryMind.com.

13. N. Klemfuss, W. Prinzmetal, and R. B. Ivry, "How Does Language Change Perception: A Cautionary Note," *Front Psychol* 3 (2012): 78.

14. American Psychiatric Association, "DSM: History of the Manual," APA, http://www.psychiatry.org/practice/dsm/dsm-history-of-the-manual.

15. L. Mastin, "Types of Memory," http://www.human-memory.net/types.html.

16. Non-declarative or implicit memory also includes priming, emotional responses, and muscle memory.

17. T. Dayton, *The Drama Within: Psychodrama and Experiential Therapy* (Deerfield Beach, FL: Health Communications, Inc., 1994).

18. A. Pesso and J. Crandell, *Moving Psychotherapy: Theory and Application of Pesso System/Psychomotor Therapy* (Cambridge, MA: Brookline Books, 1991).

19. A. Pesso and J. Crandell, *Moving Psychotherapy: Theory and Application of Pesso System/Psychomotor* (Cambridge, MA: Brookline Books, 1991).

20. G. Slaninová and P. Pidimová, "Pesso Boyden System Psychomotor as a Method of Work with Battered Victims," *Procedia - Social and Behavioral Sciences* 112 (2014): 387–94.

21. L. Holtzman and R. Mendez, *Psychological Investigations: A Clinician's Guide to Social Therapy* (New York: Routledge, 2003).

CHAPTER NINE

Domain A: Addiction Containment

Even though the monkey is off your back, it
doesn't mean the circus has left town.
ANONYMOUS

Overview

The primary goal of Domain A in RecoveryMind Training is containing the addictive use of substances or addiction-related behaviors. RMT uses the concept of locus of control to help understand the concepts in Domain A. The construct of locus of control was developed by one of the preeminent psychologists of the twentieth century, Julian Rotter.[1] Rotter defined locus of control as "the degree to which persons expect that . . . an outcome of their behavior is contingent on their own behavior or personal characteristics versus the degree to which persons expect that the outcome is a function of chance, luck, or fate, is under the control of powerful others, or is simply unpredictable."[2] At the extremes, individuals could see themselves as having an internal locus of control (everything is self-determined) or an external locus of control (everything is determined by others, fate, the whim of the gods, or bad luck). Most of us lie somewhere in between these extremes.

How does the concept of locus of control provide clarity about addiction containment? Prior to a period of abstinence and treatment, individuals with alcohol and drug use disorders lack control over their alcohol or other drug use. This is a defining characteristic of the illness. They have a focal loss of insight; they believe their locus of control is internal when it is not. In the midst of continual use, they mistakenly believe they can stop anytime. As they examine their illness under the watchful eye of a competent therapist or treatment team, they begin to accept their drug or alcohol use is out of control. Their locus of control shifts from internal to external (i.e., they shift from the false belief their use is under control to accepting they have little power over it). Paradoxically, the patient gains a bit of power over the addiction by seeing the problem for what it really is. This is a subtlety that those who oppose twelve-step philosophy frequently miss when they dismiss the powerful, yet paradoxical, concept of Step One (admitting one is powerless over addiction).

The AddictBrain concept brings clarity to this confusion. The patient or client is encouraged to visualize her core self as distinct from AddictBrain. Exploration of this duopoly helps a patient recognize how, over the course of her illness, the locus of control has shifted away from self and toward AddictBrain. By the time she falls into treatment, control over her life is external. AddictBrain is in charge. To gain control over this beast, it must be constrained first. When we use the word "containment" in RMT, we are talking about containing AddictBrain, not the patient or client.

Other patients arrive in treatment after multiple failed attempts at recovery. Many such individuals feel helpless; their lives are spinning completely out of control. Addiction has run rip shod through their world, destroying health, family, work, and self-esteem. They fully admit their disease has captured their locus of control. These patients benefit from the AddictBrain concept as well, and therapy helps them realize that AddictBrain is the holder of their locus of control. Caregivers can help them construct containment sufficient to hold the illness at bay while they collect tools and gain needed strength for recovery. Over time, the locus of control moves inward, partly propelled by differentiating self from illness.

Addiction containment occurs when a patient or client and his or her recovery team constrain AddictBrain behaviors (chemical use in substance use or addiction behaviors in process addictions). At first, individuals with alcohol and drug use disorders have a tendency to conceptualize containment as coming from others. It feels as if their caregivers are doing something *to* them. Despite the fact they have long since given control to AddictBrain, many patients have a natural tendency to rebel against containment, even if they participated in its construction. Patients and staff alike should approach addiction containment as a collaborative process. Patients discuss potential containment procedures and, when possible, participate in selecting the containment procedures that are both effective and acceptable. As a patient accepts the need for help and practices his or her new containment skills, it feels less onerous, even freeing. Over time, the depth and breadth of containment decreases, and external control and protective barriers drop away. The individual internalizes the core competencies of Domain A and begins his or her recovery journey.

Is Containment a Form of Contingency Contracting?

Contingency contracting, also known as contingency management (CM), is a research-based treatment technique where a treatment system—or a patient and his or her caregiver—develop a verbal or written contract that outlines positive contingencies for a limited set of desired behaviors and/or negative contingencies for undesired behaviors. Contingency management is based upon operant conditioning. Well-designed studies confirm the efficacy of this intervention.[3-10] CM can be used to shape any number of behaviors, such as showing up for therapy, completing assignments, maintaining personal hygiene, and completing chores in the treatment community. CM tends to use positive reinforcement (e.g., vouchers, prizes, or increased privileges) more than negative reinforcement (e.g., loss of privileges or work detail).

Much of the initial research in contingency management occurred in settings where drug use continued at varying frequencies; the contracting is designed to shape and decrease drug use. The theoretical construct behind this research is that one can override the biological drives of addiction using operant conditioning. Like all interventions in addiction treatment, contingency contracting is not 100 percent effective—about 55 percent of patients change their using patterns incorporating these protocols. What is striking, however, is how effective it is for an illness characterized by hardwired biological drives and rigid learning. Simple operant techniques work to override primal brain circuits that subtend the addictive use of chemicals. In several special populations, such as physicians,[11] it has been shown to be highly effective in maintaining abstinence once the physician-patient has received an initial strong dose of treatment including a period of abstinence.

Addiction containment uses elements of contingency contracting but is distinct in many ways. Containment focuses on gaining initial control over substance use—the first goal in addiction care once basic medical and self-care needs are met. If there is a containment breech, some previously agreed upon action is executed. Well-defined contingent actions occur if any substance use arises; it is partially based upon operant conditioning as well. However, containment does have significant differences from contingency management.

First and foremost, addiction containment encapsulates additional modalities such as the norming and transforming effect of a social milieu and containing the illness though biological intervention (e.g., disulfiram for alcohol dependence). In addition, addiction containment tapers over time but should never stop. For example, a patient with five years of recovery might contract with his or her sponsor to disclose thoughts or cravings the moment they first appear. Speaking these thoughts and urges aloud to a trusted support person decreases their power and thus decreases the tendency to relapse. The chronic, tapering nature of addiction containment addresses one concern about contingency management: it is an effective treatment tool, but effectiveness drops when contingencies are discontinued.[12] Addiction containment is closely tied to a patient's understanding of his or her addiction, more so than for contingency management. On the other hand, addiction containment can lack the immediacy of CM. In contingency management, a patient receives positive reinforcement as close in time to the shaped behavior as possible. Containment can also be seen as focusing more on negative reinforcement: "You will have to come into the recovery residence if we cannot contain your addiction in the intensive outpatient program." Nonetheless, I have witnessed patients transform what starts out feeling like jail to a path of freedom. Tying containment to the concept of AddictBrain produces an empowering indignation. The patient or client cries, "I am not going to let you (AddictBrain) keep doing this to me!"

Contingency management alters behavior and treatment compliance by shaping behaviors that are prerequisite to RecoveryMind. It does not directly improve emotional resilience (Domain C), internal narrative (Domain D), connectedness and spirituality (Domain E), or teach relapse prevention skills (Domain F). Contingency management can be used alongside RMT when based upon two separate precepts: the contingency is swift and sure, and the contingent response is graded according to the degree to which addiction has reemerged (as reflected in the contracts or rules that have been violated).[13] For example, a patient who fails to show up in time for a urine drug screen and is late for several groups later in the day may not be eligible for extended family visitation that same night.

Implementing Addiction Containment

Once a patient has entered the action stage in the Transtheoretical Stages of Change Model,[14] she is ready to begin RecoveryMind Training. Domain A, disease containment, is the first goal of RMT. An Alcoholics Anonymous slogan says, "First things first." Recovery cannot begin until the disease is contained because brain circuits activated by substance use would continue to cloud judgment and subvert insight until substance use is halted. This may seem like a self-evident truth, but even seasoned therapists are blinded by AddictBrain, especially when dealing with complex patients. To replace AddictBrain thinking, an individual must use techniques that appear to arise from outside the self. At first, a patient may experience containment as being done to her rather than a necessary barrier that thwarts self-destruction. The concepts of RMT make the recovery struggle tangible and the enemy clear. As the patient deepens her understanding of AddictBrain and its rampant destruction, containment feels more and more acceptable. Control of AddictBrain behaviors begins a slow methodical transition from external to internal control; this occurs over years but is never complete.

In the early days of addiction treatment, providers would talk about the need of those with alcohol use disorder to "hit bottom." Patients who fell into a deep well of despair do appear to be more compliant as they enter treatment. A part of this ease comes from the fact that such individuals "have surrendered," their denial has been shattered, and they acknowledge they are unable to control their substance use. On the other hand, such patients are prone to helplessness and readily accept any level of containment, knowing they cannot do it on their own. Many more patients arrive in a therapist's office or treatment center before they have hit such a bottom. RMT provides a respectful road to recovery for those who have not fully accepted the gravity of their situation. It helps those who have difficulties with trust, reducing reflexive oppositional patient responses in those who are blinded by AddictBrain thinking.

Containment has both a short- and long-term horizon. In the short term, containment must be intense and multifocal to interrupt the destructive use of substances early in the battle. Control feels distinctly external ("I'm stuck in this treatment center, aren't I?"). Even patients who vociferously profess a desire to recover require moderate to strong containment at the very start; the desire to stop use rarely correlates with an ability to put out the all-consuming addiction fire. Alcohol or drug withdrawal, intense cravings, and an active AddictBrain require a strong firewall between patients and their substance use. The treatment program staff or therapist carefully reviews past attempts to quit, looking for containment methods that did or did not help. This type of survey often reveals inadequate containment and/or a too rapid containment taper are the cause of previous treatment failures early on in the course of treatment.

Looking over the longer term, the numbers and intensity of containment techniques decrease, and control of the patient's life internalizes. Recovering individuals learn their stability waxes and wanes; they respond by increasing containment during high-risk periods.

> *Jerry enjoyed a successful recovery from his opioid dependence disorder for fifteen months. In fact, he was surprised by how successful he was in treatment. He continued with a relapse prevention specialist and support meetings in Narcotics Anonymous (NA) and Alcoholics Anonymous (AA). For the first time in decades, he was free from the gnawing desire for pain pills. He talked frequently with his therapist about his difficult childhood. Jerry grew up in a violent household. While in treatment, Jerry acknowledged that both his father and mother struggled with alcohol dependence for most of their lives. When Jerry was between the ages of seven and thirteen, his father's illness was at its worst; he would be emotionally and physically violent toward both Jerry and his mother.*
>
> *Jerry arrived at his fifteen-month mark in early December. Late one evening, his mother called to tell Jerry that his father had been diagnosed with lung cancer. Despite all that happened, Jerry was a dutiful and loving son. He loved his parents with all their faults. In his therapy and step work, he had begun the long process of forgiveness. Despite all he had done in recovery, the call from his mother set him back. Jerry knew he had to go home. He also knew that his past was waiting for him.*

By now, he had accepted the close relationship between his earlier trauma and his tendency to relapse. Jerry recognized that returning to his childhood home, his mother's worries, his mixed feelings about his father, and the strong emotions that always seem to emerge at Christmas would combine to create a high-risk situation. At fifteen months, Jerry's recovery had become dear to him, and he did not want to lose it.

After discussing the situation with his friends from the treatment center, his newfound friends in AA, his therapist, and his sponsor, Jerry knew he needed to be well prepared for this trip. Jerry recalled the odd protection he felt when he was housed in treatment (addiction containment). He could not go back there; besides, he did not need to go back there. Therefore, he needed a temporary increase in containment. After discussing his upcoming trip with just about everyone, Jerry came up with the following plan: 1) he would call his sponsor every day while at home; 2) he would find support group meetings in his hometown before he left on the trip and committed to his sponsor that he would attend meetings daily; 3) he set up a phone session with his therapist midway through the sad holiday visit; 4) he would go back on oral naltrexone for two weeks before he left, during his entire visit home, and for two months after returning.

As you can imagine, with all this containment in place, Jerry did well; however, surviving this painful time required a concerted effort. Importantly, the construction and execution of a solid plan of protection from AddictBrain strengthened his recovery moving forward as well. He learned how to protect himself from relapse and, with the help of his support system, increased his addiction containment during his time of incredible stress.

The need for containment never completely disappears. Individuals with multiple decades of stable recovery will say, "I have to frequently remind myself that the disease of addiction has not disappeared . . . sometimes as often as once a day." Nothing speaks to the chronic nature of the addiction illness more than this concept. This is no different from the diabetic who, when faced with a highly caloric dessert, has to tell himself "that will wreak havoc with my diabetes; it is not worth the trouble." Over many decades, I have treated patients with alcohol or drug dependence who relapse after ten to twenty years of good recovery. They arrive in treatment, grievous and crestfallen, saying," I just forgot I have an illness that never completely goes away" or "I thought one drink wouldn't be a problem after all this time."

Psychotherapists who pride themselves on being client-centered often struggle with the concept of addiction containment. They attend my seminars with a heartfelt belief that every client should find his or her own internal strength—addiction containment feels contrary to their belief system. They want their clients to function from an internal locus of control, and I could not agree more. The problem with addiction is that the individual with alcohol and drug use disorders who is in the first several years of recovery often cannot distinguish his true internal guidance voice from that of AddictBrain. It takes many years for an individual to pull himself out from under the sly thoughts and beliefs carefully constructed by AddictBrain. AddictBrain serves up its "good ideas" in droves, each time reminding its victim that the idea du jour is his and his alone.

As the previous story shows, most recovering individuals soon find relief in the containment techniques of Domain A. As they experience that relief, containment shifts from an external to internal locus of control. Such individuals may say something similar to the following:

> *I used to hate calling my sponsor every day, I thought she was meddling in my life, and it irked me to no end. Over time, something strange happened. I saw that she really cared. She saw things in me I could not see in myself. Now*

> *I look forward to calling her, although I no longer need to*
> *talk every day. The ritual of calling helps me remember that*
> *I have support and guidance. I feel stronger inside because*
> *of what I have learned from her. I can accept outside*
> *suggestions without bristling in defiance, as I did in the past.*

The long-term goal of the Recovery Skills in Domain A is to learn, accept, and find relief from internal and external constraints that contain AddictBrain and prevent relapse. Work in Domain A helps the patient choose containment techniques that match the severity of his or her illness and, at the same time, respect patient preferences.

Patient Responses

Some patients reflexively rebel from the external control inherent in containment. A number of patients are hounded by deep-seated dynamics that reject any type of help that hints at a smidgen of external control. In the vast majority of cases, a patient's ability to stop or even limit substance use has long since failed by the time he arrives in a therapy office or treatment center. His life is already under external control by AddictBrain. The peculiar blindness to this obvious fact obscures this simple but vital truth. Patients who have an aggressive disease and have yet to comprehend its severity will say, "Why can't you just trust me? I really want to recover!" The confusion comes from the misunderstanding of "me." Early in the process of healing, the organism is in the throes of a battle for control. AddictBrain is constantly pushing its victim to give in to the insatiable drive to use. It bamboozles the unwitting patient into thinking his caregivers are the enemy when, in truth, AddictBrain is his real nemesis.

Once a methodical and least restrictive containment system is formalized, many patients find relief from AddictBrain's incessant hounding. Drug or alcohol hunger lifts, and containment feels protective. Containment helps patients when they literally are not in control of themselves. The intensity of containment and the type of containment is best matched to the patient's current needs, although in multi-patient treatment settings, this may prove to be difficult.

I should mention a particularly vexing patient presentation. This is the patient who states, "I love to drink (or use other drugs); it is what I like best about life!" This statement is often uttered by an individual with a prolonged history of substance abuse who is in the end-stages of his illness. Libertarians might assert that such an individual has a right to continue his self-destructive chemical use to the bitter end. When you spend time in a careful inquiry into his beliefs, in the vast majority of cases, such an individual is also holding onto a fantasy that he can continue his use without lethal consequences. This individual has rarely accepted the gruesome conclusion of his current trajectory. A good response is to suggest that a healthy examination of his decision to continue or stop substance use necessitates a clear mind. Of course, a clear mind requires detoxification followed by a period of complete abstinence from addicting chemicals. After a genuine recovery trial lasting six months or a year, he can decide then whether or not to return to his past life.

Patients with oppositional characteristics tend to push against containment and respond best to a cognitive approach. Explain the goals of containment and reiterate that no one likes to be told what to do. Some patients may need additional therapy that explores the origins of their oppositional stance. Individuals with childhood trauma require a consistent and empathetic approach. With a compassionate but firm hand, the therapist points out how addiction has become yet another abusive actor in their life. In such cases, AddictBrain takes on the attributes of past abusers, be it seductive or a cruel taskmaster. Implementing addiction containment brings up dynamic issues that are then lightly explored after such a patient completes the Recovery Skills in Domain A.

Addiction Containment: Types and Details

Each type of addiction containment has benefits and snags. Patients benefit most from a containment plan that balances efficacy with acceptability. Treatment providers should fill their toolbox with every containment tool available. The tools used in a given case will depend on addiction type, severity, and their acceptability by the patient or client. One tool I believe to be the most universally effective is the drug screen. The aforementioned variability of containment is constrained when the patient and his or her counselors are housed in an organized treatment system. This is for a good reason; it is impractical and counterproductive, for example, to have some patients in an organized treatment program be subject to drug screens while others are not.

Physical, social, contractual, and biological measures produce containment. Please note that effective treatment uses a combination of these elements with varying degrees of intensity. Physical containment tapers first; the others taper and are internalized along the road to a healthy recovery. For example, the most common scenario in residential settings is a combination of Physical Containment (housed in the building), Social Containment (accountability with peers in treatment), Contractual Containment (community rules that are a prerequisite for continuing at the current level of care), and Biological Containment (e.g., observed ingestion of disulfiram, buprenorphine, or naltrexone).

Physical Containment

Physical containment is, to a large degree, a remnant from centuries old alcoholism care. In the nineteenth and early twentieth centuries, the only way to separate alcohol dependent individuals from their substance was to lock them away in an inebriate asylum. Many early treatment centers were physically isolated, and one or two even had their own police forces that barred access to alcohol and prevented patients from escaping.[15] As treatment increased in sophistication over the past thirty years, physical containment has become less necessary.

Social, contractual, and biological containment are more cost effective and humane. However, when battling the most aggressive addiction cases, physical containment saves lives. It should be considered when less intense methodologies fail.

When AddictBrain has complete control of an individual, some patients may literally need to be locked up in order to interrupt a drug use cycle. Once the illness has progressed to a certain point, the individual with alcohol and drug use disorders is unable to stop use during a binge, for example. Locked doors in an inpatient hospital or sequestering him or her without transportation in a rural center can save lives.

Note that containment is not synonymous with the need for physician-managed detoxification. Third party payers and managed-care companies may only permit an inpatient stay when life-threatening withdrawal is present. Detoxification may occur alongside containment, but RMT asserts that physical barriers, including locked doors, are clinically indicated when less aggressive containment has heretofore failed or has a high probability of failure in the given circumstance. Hopefully, third party payers will one day recognize this simple truth.

Physical containment should be tapered as soon as possible. It is humane and cost effective to move a patient from a locked psychiatric or detoxification unit when he or she becomes medically and psychiatrically stable and able to remain safe using less restrictive containment. Most patients who require a locked door for their initial containment do poorly if physical containment is not continued—albeit at a lower level—immediately after discharge from an inpatient stay. The most common transfer is to a treatment program with strong barriers that prevent access to drugs and alcohol. Some treatment centers are located in remote areas; they achieve physical containment by their isolated location. Others limit access to car keys or transportation. Removing or limiting access to cell phones and the Internet are also part of physical containment.

Social Containment

Social containment uses social pressure and group norming to prevent substance use. The most effective form of social containment occurs in a community whose central purpose is addiction recovery. Such a community stands between the addicted individual and his or her illness. At the same time, social containment shifts the addicted individual from hedonistic, self-focused pleasure to the nurturing effect of a caring community that strives toward recovery.

All addicted individuals experience ambivalence about or outright rebellion against treatment from time to time. Attitudes wax and wane for months on end. The norming of a social environment supports patients during periods of ambivalence, acknowledging and accepting their defiance during periods of rebellion. The individual who openly professes thoughts of "going back out" is pressured by the other community members to not make hasty decisions and consider the benefits of staying. The urge to abort treatment passes, and soon that individual is helping to prevent someone else from jumping ship. Experiencing both sides of this process helps reinforce the internal decision to stay. It also helps a patient understand the drive to return to substance use is often covert and can come and go—learning to "surf the urge"[16] rather than acting on every impulse to use alcohol or drugs.

Social containment also uses the power of the milieu to identify how AddictBrain controls the individual. When a patient experiences an urge to return to substance use, the community accepts these natural events with a knowing equanimity. When one patient brings his reasons for leaving to the community, other patients calmly describe how they have experienced something similar in the past. Group discussion ensues; patients who have suffered the most with toxic ambivalence become the most strident participants in such a discussion. If shepherded properly by staff, everyone in the community learns from the experience, and a recommitment to abstinence and recovery occurs. The community confirms that toxic ambivalence is part of the journey through early recovery. Importantly, years of work in residential programs have taught me that social containment is never created by a staff alone. A staff provides the framework for a healthy milieu, which in turn creates the interpersonal environment that produces a healthy community that contains itself.[17]

Not every treatment setting has the needed critical number of patients or a sufficient intensity of interpersonal interaction to produce a community of recovery. Social containment works best in a residential setting when patients are living together twenty-four hours per day. However, even an intensive outpatient program (IOP, ASAM Level 2.1)[18] where patients interact for at least three hours per day and five days per week has a modicum of social containment. Social containment is fostered by clear, carefully crafted rules of interaction that promote a healthy treatment community. Centers that have "alumni" or former patients who return to the center for support or group meetings help foster community development. One crucial mistake IOP treatment providers are prone to make occurs when they drop their attention from the treatment milieu itself. Naïve or misinformed managed care providers, working in any level of care, may miss the importance of social containment if training and supervision are not provided by supervisory staff.

Lower levels of care also provide social containment. Outpatient group therapy and support group meetings provide meaningful social containment. The individual who fails to come to a group session or AA meeting might receive a call from concerned friends to check on her. The social containment here comes from a long-term but low intensity milieu. Longer-term groups, such as an AA home group an individual attends for years, may occur only once a week but make up for the decreased frequency with a deep caring for the missing member. This model of caring, practiced in AA groups for decades, has saved thousands of individuals from certain demise.

Social containment is a crucial element of treatment that is difficult to accomplish in a solo practitioner's office. Several solutions to this dilemma have been proposed. Marc Galanter, MD, describes

Network Therapy as one answer.[19] Outpatient practitioners may offer group therapy to a group of addiction patients; such groups hold its participants accountable to the group as a whole. The participants may interact outside the formal therapies using a variety of social media networks. Many outpatient therapists direct their patients to support groups. Regardless of the type of outside group a therapist uses, he or she invokes social containment by tracking patients' attendance and exploring their responses to that support network. RecoveryMind Training encourages attendance at Alcoholics Anonymous and/or its sister organizations as the best-studied support system.[20] It is far and away the most available support system no matter where the patient lives, works, and travels. A good addiction therapist discusses his or her patient's reaction to being in the group, resistance to attending, commitment to a sponsor, and asks for a list of attended meetings at each session until social containment is fully engaged.

Several themes are present in all levels and intensities of social containment. These elements include the following:

- A critical mass of individuals focused on overcoming a common malady.
- Sufficient time together, interacting in a manner that induces interpersonal connection.
- Therapists who provide support that reinforces healthy attachment in many, but not all, types of milieux.
- Rules that define the milieu and interactions within it.
- Boundaries that ensure the safety of all members.

Social containment grows in intensity with the degree of identification and the strength of commitment to a given social structure. A therapist can reinforce the level of containment by exploring a patient's conflicts and what he appreciates about group participation.

Difficulties with attachment have been postulated to be generative in the development of addiction.[21] Patients who have anxious, avoidant, disorganized, or other maladaptive attachment styles will struggle with the healing and structure that typically comes from a group. John Wallace, PhD, noted that assimilative projection was part of normal treatment binding, and this temporary mild distortion helps to promote social containment.[22]

Contractual Containment

Once a patient has emerged from the most intense period of craving, he or she can be managed adding contractual containment to the social containment part of organized treatment. RMT defines contractual containment as any interaction with the patient that is structured by a verbal, rules-based, or written agreement that defines and limits all addiction behaviors up to and including chemical relapse. Contractual containment often includes contingencies and is closest to contingency management in its theory and implementation. The positive and negative reinforcement paradigms vary widely from one treatment setting to another. Positive reinforcement rewards small behaviors that reinforce abstinence. Although negative reinforcement is thought to be less desirable, it is part of contractual containment and ranges from loss of minor privileges to jail time. Contractual containment describes a larger sphere of influence than contingency contracting, as it includes larger treatment rules (some of which are held in place by social containment) and drug screen monitoring (which overlaps with biological containment).

A well-designed treatment system should be explicit about a wide variety of behaviors contained within that milieu. Some behaviors may seem unrelated to addiction recovery when seen by the casual observer. For example, addicted individuals live behind a complex web of deceit. Simple rules that encourage rigorous honesty may prove difficult for the patient at first, but they are critical in helping the patient shift from compulsive dishonesty to honest self-disclosure and self-appraisal. Please note, each rule should be carefully crafted and anchored in the principles of RMT rather than staff convenience.

Once a rule is developed, the reason behind each rule should be clearly described in patient literature and reviewed frequently in sessions because most patients arrive in treatment under a mental fog of past chemical use. Providers hand a sheaf of rules to a patient whose brain has been scrambled by toxic substances. Some individuals have survived up to that point in their life though subtle or flagrant violation of rules. Is it any wonder why it is difficult to get such patients to abide by a center's list of common-sense guidelines? Using RMT, all contractual containment statements are paired with a recovery principle. This transforms a seemingly capricious dictum into a value system that a patient can slowly incorporate into his recovery. Similarly, when a contractual violation has occurred, the patient is given a brief assignment to describe why the rule should or should not apply to him based on past behaviors. I have repeatedly watched centers improve patient adoption and alignment after they add seemingly obvious recovery principles to each community rule. When the elements of contractual containment are more coherent, the path to recovery will be clearer.

Separate from center rules, a treatment program may apply specific contractual obligations to individuals with special needs or to families who have had difficulties with their addicted family member. Consider a young adult patient with a history of bringing illicit drugs into the home. Staff members may sit with the family to develop a set of safety goals that must be accomplished both prior and subsequent to the patient returning to the family domicile. This sets healthy expectations for the entire family system. The earlier this is accomplished in treatment, the more time a patient has to gain acceptance of his or her situation. Treatment centers should have a prepared library of common contracts that can be modified for a patient's specific condition.

Drug Screening Is Contractual Containment

The single most effective form of contractual containment comes from frequent analysis of body fluids and other material for drug screen analysis. At first glance, it may seem more appropriate to place this type of containment with the Biological Containment section of this chapter. However, I think the most important element of screening is the contractual relationship between the caregiver and the patient. The medical technique to determine abstinence is much less important than the contract for abstinence. Drug screens should always be used during initial treatment of substance dependence. Best practice is to continue screens during the first several years of recovery.

I have used the term "body material analysis" to describe drug screening because in the twenty-first century, many body materials and fluids can be used to analyze for drugs of abuse. At present, urine is the most common material. Many other materials are effectively used for analysis, including blood, hair, fingernails, saliva, and sweat. Each of these materials has its positives and negatives for drug analysis. Hair and nail testing, for example, can often detect drugs of abuse during the past several months post consumption. Such screens evaluate the veracity of statements, such as "I haven't used oxycodone for years." The type of material, the type of screens, and the timing of screens are part of a complicated process that requires a fair amount of expertise for proper interpretation. A certified Medical Review Officer should be employed in all centers to ensure appropriate test selection and results analysis.[23, 24] A comprehensive introduction to the science and application of screening can be found in the recently published ASAM white paper on drug testing.[25]

For purposes of this text, I will review the logistical and therapeutic uses of drug screening as a contractual containment system, as well as several of the important elements of an effective drug screening system and how it is best implemented within the larger subject of addiction containment. Two terms are important for every caregiver to know. In toxicology, a *false positive* test states substance use occurred when it did not, and a *false negative* report claims no drug use when in fact it did occur.

If a treatment center, individual therapist, or physician has decided to use body material analysis to determine a patient's recovery state, the single most important ingredient is drug screen accuracy. Staff members must have complete faith in screen results despite the attestation of the patient or client. Difficulties with accuracy arise in three separate areas: false positives, false negatives, and natural (but misleading) attempts to interpret screens as strictly binary. We desire screens to be unequivocally positive (a substance was used) or negative (a substance was not used). Science dictates that at times this will not be the case.

The first accuracy concern is that of the false positive test. A false positive occurs when the screening technology reports a drug is present when it is not. Done properly, screens for alcohol and other drug use are extremely accurate; remarkably few tests show a false positive. Quality drug screens are not inexpensive, but attempts to use less expensive screening produces the worst kind of error: a false accusation that the patient is using when indeed he or she is not.[26] Most inexpensive "rapid test cup" screens have *few* false positives—those few are, however, important. Any presumptive positive screen should be followed up with definitive confirmation using GC/MS[27, 28] or LC/MS[29] technology. Caregivers do not need to know everything about the science of toxicology, but addiction physicians and therapists should recognize that laboratory testing is fallible and know when to ask for interpretive help.

The second accuracy concern arises when staff members believe they are testing for all substances a patient might use, but their drug testing system is limited in its scope. Test cups and one size fits all drug-testing panels often miss the one or two abusable substances they really need for testing. This leads to false negative results—a drug was consumed but does not show up in testing. Although it is less likely, it is also possible to have a false negative screen simply because the drug screening system fails to detect a particular substance in certain situations.

False negatives are seen most frequently in adolescents, young adults, individuals in criminal justice systems, and healthcare professionals. Today, synthetic cannabinoids and other designer drugs are readily available, and naïve drug experimenters and younger at-risk individuals frequently use such substances. Healthcare professionals use drugs to which the public has low access, thus they may not be included on standard panels. People in criminal justice systems learn about current screen protocols and teach each other how to beat the screening system. When such a patient is known to be consuming abusable substances and the tests return negative, the therapist or treatment center staff should seek experts in toxicology to reevaluate their current screen protocols. One solution is to have multiple panels available, matching test panels to the population at risk. Expert consultation ensures drug screen protocols are clinically appropriate. Making the decision about drug screening based upon finances alone is courting disaster.

The third type of error arises when a physician, therapist, or treatment center staff begins to view drug screens as simple yes/ no (positive/negative) decisions. This is especially vexing when screening for ethyl alcohol (ethanol). Addiction treatment has several newer biological markers for alcohol consumption, including ethyl glucuronide[30, 31] (EtG), ethyl sulfate[32] (EtS), and phosphatidylethanol[33] (PEth). Due to their sensitivity, screens with these markers often come back as an initial presumptive positive, suggesting alcohol use. This is due in large part to the use of ethanol in many cosmetics, pharmaceuticals, and even cleaning agents in the home and at work.

Individuals who are in solid recovery may show up with a screen that is positive for these newer markers due to incidental exposure in the environment. Conversely, a relapse might be heralded by a low-level positive in any alcohol marker, but it is all too often written off to incidental environmental exposure. Thus, all drug screens, especially those for ethyl alcohol, have to be interpreted within a clinical context. Consider healthcare workers who sanitize their hands between each patient. The active ingredient in most hand sanitizers is ethyl alcohol (although several isopropyl alcohol sanitizers are just as effective[34] and readily available). If a recovering individual has had clear instruction to avoid ethanol-based hand sanitizers and shows up with a low-level positive ethanol marker, he or she may indeed have ingested alcohol. On the other hand, if a screen reports a low-level positive EtG from a healthcare worker with no previous training in avoiding ethanol-based hand sanitizers, no definitive conclusion about past alcohol use can be reached.

Finally, I cannot emphasize enough the importance of having a skilled and experienced toxicologist or physician review and interpret drug screens as part of treatment. The reviewer should be familiar with the patient populations being treated and the day-to-day patient care. It may not be possible for every individual addiction therapist to have a toxicologist or physician on hand to help them decipher drug screens on their patients or clients. However, many third-party services are available to assist in the drug screening process, including timing of screens, helping patients get to a screening site, and interpreting the results for you. Whenever drug screens are used, proper review by a Medical Review Officer (MRO) is a must.[35] A MRO is a physician trained in the interpretation of toxicology/drug screen results. Good MROs are also familiar with addiction treatment procedures and work with treatment staff to ensure firm, compassionate care.

How does one determine the screening frequency? No statistical analysis of drug screen frequency is available at this writing.[36] It may be tempting to obtain screens often enough to ensure that no substances are used (e.g., testing for methamphetamine every two to four days because it can be detected in urine two to four days after use). This proves expensive and impractical for many reasons. Instead, the best protocol is to test an individual for a wide variety of substances at decreasing frequency over many years. The testing frequency is randomized within a given time frame and varies as to the substances tested. Randomization keeps costs lower. Random, lower frequency testing does not guarantee zero substance use, but the random nature prevents a patient from "counting days" since the last screen. The best testing systems use computer-based (i.e., true) randomization rather than staff-generated (pseudorandom) test dates. Such protocols have proved to be effective with safety-sensitive workers, such as physicians, airline pilots, and attorneys who return to work and at the same time ensure public safety. When a patient says, "I will just tell you when I use, and that way we can avoid all this drug screening," the RMT response by the therapist is "Both of us are trying to get a handle on AddictBrain, the drug screen process will help us do that." This approach avoids conversations about lying that always promulgate shame and threaten the therapeutic alliance.

Alcohol detection requires special attention. Patients who are subject to alcohol screens need education to prevent environmental exposure. Gregory Skipper, MD, Bruce Merkin, MD, and I have published a medication guide to assist in this training.[37] In the initial phase of outpatient treatment for alcohol dependence (ASAM Level 1 or 2.1), it is often best to randomly screen weekly or more often, if needed. Decrease as the patient responds to other containment techniques and cravings abate. The random and reasonably frequent nature of screens improves accuracy despite the fact that an EtG may only detect alcohol for two to four days following use. Centers that add a finger stick for blood PEth to this protocol will gain a high degree of confidence regarding their patients' alcohol recovery status.[38]

During assessment and initial treatment, high-frequency screening validates a patient's illness status when he or she is most vulnerable to relapse. Screening frequency also varies according to the intensity of other types of containment. A patient in a day hospital program combined with a recovery residence (ASAM Level 2.5 plus 3.1) will need fewer screens compared to a patient in an evening intensive outpatient program (ASAM Level 2.1), for example. In the first case, near continuous observation combined with a high level of social containment provide sufficient supervision thus less frequent screening. Screening is combined with other forms of containment; together they have a high probability of preventing and discovering substance use should it occur. Screen frequency may be tapered at varying rates but should always be random. The frequency of screens during a taper should vary according to the patient's history, compliance in other areas, and work- or home-related issues. Addiction is a chronic disease and varies widely in its severity, thus no single tapering protocol works in all cases. Based upon research in several different cohorts,[39, 40–42] the best outcomes occur when drug screening tapers over many months or years.

Screens should not be limited to substances previously used. Once one door closes, AddictBrain will try to sneak through another. The benzodiazepine-dependent individual may fully recognize that using benzodiazepines caused significant problems. AddictBrain will begin whispering in her ear, "Hey, a glass of wine might help with anxiety." When varied as to substances studied, drugs will intermittently cover substances other than a given patient's past use pattern.

Biological Containment

Biological containment is a technique that blocks the effect or alters the body's response to an abusable substance. As of this writing, there are three available medications that provide biological containment; hopefully, others will appear over time. At least one addiction vaccine has been under development for some time.[43] Biological containment is one of the most promising areas of research and addiction treatment today.

The first medication used for biological containment was disulfiram (Antabuse). Disulfiram, when consistently consumed and continuously present in the blood stream, is quite effective in preventing the use of ethyl alcohol. For most individuals, consuming any alcohol while taking disulfiram produces a violent allergic and gastrointestinal reaction. In this manner, an alcohol dependent individual has a wall of containment that separates him or her from a drink. However, the biggest single problem with disulfiram is getting the alcohol dependent individual to take it.

Patients who are in the earlier stages of change are commonly ambivalent or consciously or unconsciously opposed to abstinence. In such cases, when a healthcare practitioner prescribes disulfiram, the person with alcohol use disorder simply stops taking it. Even patients who are in the action stage of change will suffer from periods of waning commitment. The first sign of a drop in commitment is often an unconscious "forgetting" to take disulfiram. In such cases, disulfiram is of limited use. When practitioners prescribe it during these phases, they often sabotage its effective use later on in the treatment cycle. Patients who have violent swings in motivation or severe cravings are most problematic. During high commitment, such individuals regularly take the disulfiram. Unfortunately, motivation falls rapidly, followed by urges to drink; they consume alcohol on top of the disulfiram, often resulting in painful results and emergency room visits.

Disulfiram is most effective with patients with moderately high and consistent motivation to change. If a therapist, physician, or treatment center wants to use disulfiram, it must be combined with additional contract items that ensure its efficacy and safety. Every patient with an alcohol use disorder has heard of disulfiram, and many have been prescribed it in the past. When the caregiver brings up disulfiram, the first response is often, "I have tried that and it did not work." For disulfiram treatment to work, the caregiver must first find a way to ensure that it is consumed every single day. It is helpful to have a family member consistently observe its consumption. Also I have found it helpful to crush the tablets and place them in water so their consumption can be confirmed; cheating a dose is prevented. If a patient "forgets a dose," then it is recorded and immediately discussed in a psychotherapeutic setting. If the family member who is charged with observing disulfiram consumption forgets to witness a dose, the therapist carefully explores his or her ambivalence as well.

Disulfiram proves its worth in one more specific situation for an individual in recovery from alcohol addiction with a strong acceptance of his alcohol dependence and a commitment to sobriety. Disulfiram is quite helpful when he is preparing to enter a high-risk situation or a period of high stress. For example, such a patient may have to travel to a series of business meetings in another city where he will be repeatedly exposed to alcohol. Start disulfiram several weeks in advance to ensure the patient becomes acclimated to the medication. Upon returning home, the drug is maintained for a period to prevent a "success relief relapse."

The second currently available biological medication is naltrexone. Naltrexone is available as an oral tablet, an extended release injection, and extended release subcutaneous pellets. The pellets, available through a few physician practices, are placed under the skin and disperse the medication over several months. Naltrexone is a potent blocker of all opioids. If an individual consumes opioids while on naltrexone, nothing happens. This experience is different from the aversion therapy that is provided by disulfiram. Like disulfiram, naltrexone only works if it is present in the blood stream. Those with opioid dependence who are prescribed oral naltrexone commonly discontinue their use of the drug when their commitment to recovery is subverted by AddictBrain. Patient compliance is a significant problem with oral naltrexone because every individual with opioid dependence suffers from early recovery ambivalence.[44] They may "forget" or delay taking oral naltrexone for one day, leaving them vulnerable.

This compliance problem has led to extended release formulations of naltrexone. If a patient is given extended-release naltrexone, he or she only has to make the decision not to use once a month (or less often in the case of subcutaneous naltrexone pellets). This dampens or eliminates the constant chatter that often fills the head in early recovery.

Naltrexone is not just an agent of biological containment. It also decreases cravings for both opioids[45] and alcohol.[46] It also ameliorates the pleasure perceived from alcohol use in many patients.[47] The exact neurophysiological mechanism is unknown at this time, and part of it may simply be the loss of "perceived availability"[48] similar to what happens when opioid dependent individuals are incarcerated, away from drug access. Neural circuits respond to naltrexone below the level of conscious awareness as well; its effects are, therefore, partly unrelated to perceived availability. Everyone who has treated opioid dependent individuals is struck by the persistent, unpredictable, and recurrent nature of opioid cravings. This alone might be considered sufficient reason to use this drug. However, two other reasons for naltrexone emerge. The first is that naltrexone, as a biological containment vehicle, builds time in abstinence. During time on naltrexone, the individual may discuss strongly triggering emotions or encounter high-risk situations.

When these events remit without inducing relapse, fatalistic internal self-talk begins to fade. While in a cycle of use, a craving of sufficient magnitude inevitably leads to use. When contained by naltrexone, cravings continue to occur; however, the patient's prediction of inevitable relapse does not come to pass. The importance of decoupling craving from relapse cannot be overstated. In some patients, it may be the difference between recovery success and failure. Previously defenseless against an episode of drug craving, individuals with addiction learn that cravings come and go and will do so without using.

The third group of medications that provide biological containment are opioid agonists (e.g., methadone) and mixed agonist/antagonists (e.g., buprenorphine). Buprenorphine and methadone are extremely effective at tapering drug hunger.[49] Methadone requires special licensing, but buprenorphine can be prescribed in office-based practices.[50] At present, the terminology for describing the use of these medications is undergoing change. Previously, these drugs were called "replacement therapy." In an effort to destigmatize the use of these drugs, several newer terms have been proposed. In this text, I will use the term promoted in the ASAM Criteria, Opioid Treatment Services (OTS).[51] The OTS moniker refers to the use of these medications in treatment past the point of detoxification.

The use of OTS in the treatment of addiction has had a complex past. Proponents and opponents to the use of agonists and mixed agonist/ antagonist medication line up on both sides of the debate. Proponents state that opioid treatment services are a humane and research-proven way of handling a lethal disease. OTS provides a steady state of medication to the mesolimbic dopaminergic system, quelling drug hunger and preventing withdrawal. OTS decreases addiction-related antisocial behaviors and helps the person with opioid use disorder disconnect from the drug culture and other social situations where drug use is common. Data confirm that OTS saves lives and helps individuals reenter society.

Opponents express concerns about starting patients on a medication that at least partially activates the μ-opioid system in a manner similar to an opioid user's drug of choice. They express concern about difficulties discontinuing this medication if a patient chooses to do so in the future.

RMT takes no sides in this debate except to emphasize that a comprehensive treatment process is imperative when fighting addiction. In the balance, the benefits of the mixed agonist/antagonist medication buprenorphine strongly override concerns. However, using a medication by itself, without teaching Recovery Skills is folly. Addiction is a complex disease of brain rewiring. Transformative recovery in the vast majority of cases necessitates a reciprocal repair that untangles and reworks brain changes produced by AddictBrain. This involves psychiatric, psychological, social, and spiritual training that medication alone cannot provide. However, OTS combined with well thought out treatment, such as RecoveryMind Training, are synergistic. Buprenorphine, similar to naltrexone, is effective biological containment. Lastly, OTS with methadone and buprenorphine should be considered in every case but never used reflexively. Instead, they should be administered to opioid dependent patients after a thorough evaluation and consideration of other treatment options.

Biological containment addresses one or, at most, two drug types. Consider the individual who is dependent on alcohol but has used benzodiazepines in the past. He is placed on disulfiram, and AddictBrain silently shifts its focus away from the alcohol—containment has closed the door to alcohol. Cravings for benzodiazepines may stealthily increase. Or, if an individual is dependent upon both opioids and cocaine and his access to opioids is blocked by buprenorphine, AddictBrain begins whispering in his ear about the joys of his past cocaine use. Therefore, biological blocking agents and replacement therapies are best used in patients with a singular drug of abuse or who have one substance that is overwhelmingly problematic.

When looking over longer-term horizons, I have watched many patients stop using one drug only to show up at my office several years later addicted to a different substance. For this reason, RMT believes that biological containment should never be a substitute for comprehensive treatment nor should biological treatment be the only method of interrupting substance use in Domain A.

Patient Dynamics and Containment Types

When a treatment provider begins applying containment to a patient's addiction, deeper issues of control and past struggles with authority emerge. This dynamic is illustrated in the following example.

John is a bright, thirty-four-year-old male who consumes 144 ounces of beer on average per day. He has done so for the past twelve years with increasing regularity. His alcohol dependence has resulted in several job failures, a crumbling marriage, and deteriorating self-esteem. When seen by his addiction physician, he was in significant alcohol withdrawal. John was adamant about stopping cold turkey. His physician expressed concerns about the dangers of quitting abruptly and told John that he would like him to enter a detoxification center. John became agitated at the thought, stating, "I cannot stand being locked up. No one tells me what to do."

Although it might not have seemed to be the right time to explore psychodynamic issues, John's physician inquired briefly about his vehemence. John reported a childhood where his parents, notably his father, were repressive and controlling. As a boy, John was traumatized by being locked in his room for prolonged periods. He felt trapped and lonely. Using RecoveryMind Training, his physician pointed out that despite his credo against being told what to do, John had let his alcoholism waltz in and take complete control of his life. His physician responded by saying, "Well, at this point in time, your alcohol problem has locked you up in a different way." He then gently added, "Perhaps if you see this as your decision to protect yourself from a menace that has become as cruel as your father, detoxification may feel more like setting yourself free than being locked up." He encouraged John to go to the detoxification center and ask questions that will help address his fears or even tour the facility so that he might get the help he needs and feel safe in doing so.

This example illustrates the importance of understanding a patient's psychological makeup when considering containment. The concepts of RMT help differentiate the control of AddictBrain from the external control of containment. It also underscores the importance of engaging the patient and discussions regarding the intensity and type of containment. Some individuals respond to physical containment with a sense of relief early on in their recovery, uttering, "I felt like I could finally get off the merry-go-round, but I had to be locked up at first to do it." On the other hand, patients with a surfeit of shame might unwittingly construct a self-punishing containment system that has an unconscious purpose of continuing self-flagellation.

Programs that use RMT always explain why containment is necessary. They encourage patients to verbalize difficulties with particular elements of containment in order to assist patients with a wide variety of personality types. The goal for many individuals with alcohol and drug use disorders is to shift from acting out to direct expression of discomfort or defiance. Regardless of personality, AddictBrain will always fight against constraint. In all cases, a therapist's job is to help his or her patient recognize the safety and health produced by carefully balancing addiction containment. The framework provided by containment becomes a blackboard; each patient writes his or her own intrapsychic conflicts upon that board. Containment provides structure for the patient while simultaneously exploring certain aspects of his or her personality structure. The astute therapist learns addiction containment exercises to glean insight into that patient's personality and life issues.

Putting It All Together

Addiction containment varies dramatically depending on the setting, but the four components of containment remain the same. In an outpatient setting, the therapist has more variability but little, if any, social or physical containment. A residential program has limited variability but more physical and social containment. In both cases, the treatment goal in Domain A is temporarily halting substance use so the patient or client can begin to experience medical, physical, and emotional stability; decrease drug cravings; and create a treatment plan for Domains B through F. These differences are highlighted in Table 9.1.

Patients who bond well with others respond handily to social containment. Patients who have difficulties with healthy attachment may need more biological and contractual containment. Such patients might also need intensive and more long-lasting group therapy to increase healthy interdependence with peers and family.

When a patient is in organized treatment less intense than ASAM Level 3, physical containment is not feasible. A physician or therapist relies on biological containment if it is available for a patient's substance(s) of choice. Contractual containment (showing up at therapy sessions, complying with urine drug screens, and attending support group meetings) supplies the bulk of needed addiction

Table 9.1 - Containment at Different Levels of Care

ASAM Level of Care	Containment Type			
	Physical	Social	Contractual	Biological
Level 1 Outpatient Practice	None	Use support groups	Individualized	Independent of level and type of other care
Level 2.1 Intensive Outpatient Program	Low intensity and intermittent	Light	Program driven, light intensity, and intermittent	
Level 2.5 Partial Hospitalization Program	Low intensity and intermittent	Moderate	Program driven, moderate intensity, and intermittent	
Level 3.1 Low Intensity Residential	Moderate intensity and intermittent	Light to moderate	Program driven, moderate, and intermittent	
Level 3.3 & 3.5 Medium and High Intensity Residential	Moderate to high intensity and continuous	High	Program driven, high intensity, and continuous	
Level 3.7 & 4 Medically Monitored or Managed Inpatient Treatment	High and continuous	Low (limited by short stay and acuity)	Program driven, varies but continuous	

containment while building Recovery Skills in an outpatient setting. More recently, several software applications are under development to help with contractual containment and provide contingency management.[52]

Biological containment can be effectively implemented at any time in the treatment or recovery process. For example, a treatment setting may institute biological containment when the elements of social and contractual containment are slipping away. One example of this is the patient who is ready for discharge from a residential, partial hospitalization, or intensive outpatient treatment setting. I strongly suggest such biological containment should not be implemented as an afterthought. Starting a patient on disulfiram or opioid treatment services (naltrexone or buprenorphine) should begin at a point in time where questions can be addressed, the patient can be acclimated to the medication, and any unwanted side effects are managed.

Walk through the list of potential containment types, noting the patient's response to each. Follow the patient's attitude and demeanor closely. Carefully match the patient's needs with the acceptability and intrusiveness of each containment method. Try to focus on containment techniques that are simultaneously acceptable and protective. Avoid implementing insufficient levels of containment because a patient or client resists them. Instead use such maneuvers as an opportunity to explore ambivalence about abstinence.

Containment in Organized Treatment

Containment in an organized treatment setting is determined by program guidelines, at least during initial care. The more organized a treatment system is, the less variability in the types and intensities of containment. If an individual is placed in a residential treatment program, for example, he or she has to abide by the rules of that program. Such rules create a cohesive community where needs and benefits override nuanced differences regarding an individual's needs.

However, even in large communities, some variability is useful. RMT suggests some type of "level system" that tapers physical containment and modifies contractual containment as the patient accomplishes the skills needed to maintain abstinence in the treatment setting. The level system then becomes part or even the centerpiece of contractual containment within the facility. Level systems are especially helpful for adolescents and young adults who need to internalize healthy living skills.

Containment in the Outpatient Practice

Patients who have milder forms of addiction can, and do, recover in an outpatient setting (ASAM Level 1). However, psychotherapy—including the systematic therapies such as cognitive behavioral therapy—should be supplemented with skill building, addiction specific group therapy, or support group attendance. In the outpatient office of a physician, psychologist, or therapist, contingency contracting is a vital element that helps such patients or clients transition from substance use to remission. The caregiver begins work in Domain A by discussing the types of containment available and guiding the patient to containment modes that will prove most effective while simultaneously allowing individual preference. If she opts for the least effective method, the therapist can choose to adopt a "try and see" approach, modifying containment until remission is achieved. The largest drawback to this approach—basing containment upon attempts at successive approximation—is that patients often drop out of care before abstinence is achieved.

Some patients will continue to attend office sessions without any meaningful interruption in their substance use. In my experience, caring for an actively using patient in an outpatient practice and expecting him or her to improve without some type of containment is a pipe dream. At a minimum, the outpatient therapist should establish an initial treatment plan that the patient is expected to work toward and eventually acquire periods of sustained abstinence. If the patient is unable to put together brief periods of abstinence during this level of care, the therapy contract or agreement should state that the patient will, with the help of his therapist, seek out higher levels of care. If a therapist continues to see a patient who is actively drinking and constantly hoping he will eventually stop, the net effect is to reinforce the patient's helplessness and hopelessness.

In over thirty years of work with addiction, I can count on one hand the number of times a patient has arrived in my office out of completely self-driven motives, internally capable of containing his or her addictive behaviors and ready to begin the recovery journey. I often see patients who begin their first encounter with a thinly veiled assertion that they seek care of their own accord. Over time, this declaration becomes hollow; the real drivers are a pending divorce, legal charges, or the possibility of impending medical doom.[53]

It is not helpful to waste precious time searching for recovery motivation in a patient who is actively detoxifying or brought in by loved ones or the law. Once medically stable, I use the Transtheoretical Stages of Change Model[54] to assess his change status. I look for what the patient *is* motivated to accomplish (e.g., a divorced father who wants visitation time with his children or an adolescent who would like to be able to drive the family car). I emphasize that proper addiction containment reassures the ex-spouse or parents that the disease is temporarily at bay. In doing so, it becomes palatable to the ambivalent patient as well. In session, we work through the Recovery Skills in Domain A, selecting containment types that are acceptable to the patient while simultaneously resolving natural resistance. Containment is not, however, acceptable to all patients; it should be considered in the context of the following four-quadrant table.

**Table 9.2 - Relationship between Stage of Change,
Disease Severity, and Containment**

		Stage of Change	
		Precontemplation or Contemplation	**Preparation, Action, or Later**
Disease Severity	**Low**	Addiction containment is difficult, and the patient will react against it or abort treatment.	Contractual or social containment may be sufficient to initiate the recovery process.
	High	Physical containment may induce hostility but may prove necessary. Repeated failures with lesser levels of containment may help move the patient toward the action stage.	Start with physical containment. Patient may express relief. Consider using biological containment.

Frequently, outpatient therapy can be bolstered with biological containment and additional contractual elements. Drug screening is important and most often essential. Family involvement that confirms abstinence should also be used, if available. If the therapist implements a containment contract that subsequently fails, the therapy shifts from outpatient disease containment to preparing the individual for entry into a treatment program with higher levels of containment.

When treating addiction patients, outpatient therapists often wind up neglecting containment tasks. This is unfortunate as many addiction patients can be managed in such a venue. To ensure containment is addressed in each session, the therapist should set aside the first twenty minutes of an hour session to address Domain A skills. Alternatively, a counselor assistant trained in RMT can see the patient to assess containment procedures before a psychotherapy visit. Once containment is stable and effective, work shifts to Domains B through F.

When Should Containment Be Modified?

Tapering addiction containment requires experience and finesse. If the therapist or institution tapers containment too rapidly, the patient will relapse. On the other hand, if the caregiver moves too slowly, the patient will become oppositional or overly dependent. In either case, the recovering individual will fail to learn how to establish his or her own barriers to relapse. Repeated discussions about containment types and timing should be an integral part of care. Such discussions minimize patient resistance while at the same time reinforce the importance of continued vigilance in recovery.

The overall goal of treatment is to hand the reins of recovery over to the patient a bit at a time and for increasing periods. Therapists or physicians who have little addiction experience often hand the reins of a wildly out of control horse (i.e., early recovery) over to their patient and wonder why a relapse occurs so quickly. Other caregivers, who see their patients as too vulnerable or have their own needs for validation, fail to teach their patients how to manage their own recovery. In either case, if a patient fails to learn how to care for his or her addictive disease, he or she winds up feeling ineffective, impotent, or permanently broken. Both are ultimately more vulnerable to relapse.

The art of good care in Domain A comes from balancing the types and intensity of containment over time. The physician or therapist reviews the goals of containment and repeatedly asks for patient input. The knowledgeable caregiver weighs her appraisal against the patient's self-assessment. Wide gaps between the two indicate difficulties with knowledge or insight. This, in turn, leads to additional education and discussion about containment, focusing on how it benefits the patient over the long haul.

Physical containment should be tapered first. Keeping a patient in a locked-down situation for extended periods, unless clinically indicated, sends a message that he is unfixable. On the other hand, if a patient feels relief when physically protected from his disease, the caregiver is best to reflect this back to the patient as a sign that he understands the power of their common enemy, AddictBrain. Physical containment may also vary in intensity during the day or week. For example, a treatment center may have an open campus where patients drive from a residence to the center during the day, but at night, car keys are returned and perhaps the doors even locked. In this example, social containment during the day replaces physical containment at night. Patients who are further along in their care should be given more access to the outside world (e.g., decreasing physical containment by returning car keys or cell phone) as they internalize and explore other modes of containment.

When needs change, the patient and his or her therapist collaborate in reviewing the various methods of containment, choosing one or two that continue to be acceptable and effective. For example, one patient might choose to continue urine drug screens with the results going to his or her spouse. Another may commit to an intimate and mature twelve-step group that checks up on each other from time to time. A third may choose to remain on biological containment during periods of higher stress, stopping the medication when stressors remit and after discussing this with his or her therapist or physician.

When a brief relapse occurs during containment taper, this information is fed back into the treatment plan. When stumbles occur, the patient learns valuable lessons about the types and qualities of containment she will need moving forward. Such a relapse, when handled rapidly and with equanimity, is often the inflection point in recovery. That is, a patient may begin her treatment in earnest when the therapist or treatment center helps her examine what happened before and after a substance use event. It is counterproductive to discharge a patient who has a limited episode of substance use unless she eschews containment completely; her actions have a strong negative effect on the milieu; or the safety of others is compromised.

When Does Containment End?

As a patient completes her initial treatment, it is helpful to remind her that addiction is a lifelong illness; therefore, some sustained attention to the illness will be needed to ensure lifelong recovery. The intensity, frequency, and persistence of AddictBrain-driven ambivalence and relapse hunger remit over time but never disappear completely. Some level of self-guided or externally structured, but internally endorsed, containment is helpful for decades. This is especially true in patients or clients with more severe addiction disorders.

Some therapists may harbor secret desires for their patients to attain an absolute and continuous commitment to lifelong recovery. In their well-meaning drive to help, they run the risk of unconsciously shaming their clients if they are unable to make such a pledge. Such a therapist unconsciously promotes the opposite response. The patient feels his or her own ambivalence, weighing it against the therapist's unconscious need, and winds up making a false promise that disavows his or her ambivalence. This, in turn, furthers his or her belief that he or she is defective and unfixable.

In fact, AddictBrain thinking never completely disappears; therefore, some form of acceptable containment should remain in place for decades or even throughout a lifetime. In time, most patients acquire a sixth sense that their recovery is in jeopardy. Others never seem to do so. In both, but especially the latter case, continued involvement with twelve-step support, especially a relationship with a sponsor, is important. Sponsors who maintain a close relationship with their sponsees can often tell when a sponsee is in trouble, even after the shortest of conversations. Therapists with decades of experience treating individuals with addiction disorders also acquire this skill.

By living with containment and exploring its effect, patients learn that a supple recovery does not demand their internal pilot is impeccably accurate. Instead, containment establishes a series of safeguards against the inevitable lapses in insight or commitment to abstinence. These safeguards become integral to self-guided relapse prevention.

Recovery Skills for Domain A

In order to quantify addiction treatment, each domain in RecoveryMind Training contains a set of Recovery Skills. These skills establish specific behaviors, attitudes, and knowledge acquisition milestones patients acquire through the course of work in that domain. Treatment is focused on accomplishing the Recovery Skills of that domain. Each milestone represents a step along the path to recovery, and a given patient is assigned a number of skills in each domain, according to need. When a recovery skill has been accomplished, the patient moves onto the next assigned skill in that domain. When all assigned Recovery Skills in a domain are completed, the patient moves on to work in another domain. Occasionally, a patient may be working on skills in more than one domain. However, staff members must be careful about creating confusion; completing work in one domain before moving onto the next is preferable.

In some treatment settings, accomplishing a certain Recovery Skill may trigger a change in the treatment plan or level of care. For example, when a patient understands and is compliant with a center's drug screening protocol for contractual containment, she may be eligible to return to the outside world for a brief time (i.e., go on a leave) where she can evaluate her progress.

Remember that containment is the *sine qua non* of addiction treatment. To progress in addiction treatment, substance use must be under control. Even brief relapses are traumatic to patients and their families. When relapses occur, it is best to discontinue other therapies and refocus on abstinence.

The Recovery Skills for Domain A are accomplished in an approximately sequential order. Patients and staff routinely complete a progress assessment form that tracks progress.[55] The progress assessment form lists a domain's Recovery Skills with a three-point status rating (**B**egun, **I**ntermediate, and **C**ompleted). During assessment, the patient completes the form first. This is followed by staff evaluation of the same form. The patient and staff then meet to reconcile discrepancies between the two evaluations. In this manner, the patient and his or her caregivers have a clear understanding of treatment progress.

The Recovery Skills in Domain A are complete when the following tasks occur:

1. The patient understands the four types of containment and has discussed the containment available to him or her in the current treatment setting.

2. The patient understands, in the abstract, that addiction must be contained before any meaningful improvement occurs whether or not he or she believes it applies in his or her situation.

3. The patient is able to describe why he or she needs containment at present and how it will prove helpful in the future to a varying degree.

4. The patient cooperates in developing a containment plan specific to his or her level of care (if in ASAM Level 1 treatment) or agrees to system-wide containment in his or her current level of care (ASAM Level 2.1, 2.5 or any Level 3 program).

5. The patient executes or cooperates with his or her containment plan. He or she openly expresses discomfort or resistance to said plan rather than acting out. When the patient has difficulty with the agreed upon containment plan, he or she remains open to exploring resistance in order to modify or reassert healthy disease containment.

6. The patient recognizes how past experiences, emotions, and personality issues affect compliance and acceptability of one or many containment methods.

7. The patient recognizes and spontaneously reports the benefits of containment on multiple occasions. He or she internalizes the need for containment and expresses relief from, rather than opposition to, its presence.

8.   The patient predicts the need for an adjustment in containment protocols in future high-risk situations. He or she participates with his or her therapist or treatment team in determining the types and qualities of containment that will prove most effective and acceptable.

9.   The patient helps modify containment as need decreases and openly discusses options to taper during extended care lasting over many months.

Remember, a given patient or client may be assigned a subset of this complete skill list based upon need. The Recovery Skills for each domain may extend over months or years. If an outpatient provider or treatment program only has a limited time with a client or patient, he or she will naturally be unable to complete every competency while under the provider's care. After reviewing the listed Recovery Skills in Domain A, for example, it is reasonable to expect that an uncomplicated substance-addicted patient will complete Domain A Recovery Skills 1–7 while in an evening intensive outpatient program for six weeks. Patients will overlap domain work, addressing two or possibly three domains during the same period.

Chapter Nine Notes

1. J. B. Rotter, "Some problems and misconceptions related to the construct of internal versus external control of reinforcement," *J Consult Clin Psychol* 43, no. 1 (1975): 56–67.

2. "Internal versus external control of reinforcement: A case history of a variable," *American Psychologist* 45, no. 4 (1990): 489–93.

3. H. M. Boudin, "Contingency contracting as a therapeutic tool in the deceleration of amphetamine use," *Behavior Therapy* 3, no. 4 (1972): 604–08.

4. K. Carroll, S. A. Ball, and C. Nich, "Targeting behavioral therapies to enhance naltrexone treatment of opioid dependence: Efficacy of contingency management and significant other involvement," *Arch Gen Psychiatry* 58, no. 8 (2001): 755–61.

5. S. T. Higgins, D. D. Delaney, A. J. Budney, W. K. Bickel, J. R. Hughes, F. Foerg, and J. W. Fenwick, "A behavioral approach to achieving initial cocaine abstinence," *Am J Psychiatry* 148, no. 9 (Sep 1991): 1218–24.

6. S. T. Higgins, "Contingency Management," Chap. 27 in *Textbook of Substance Abuse Treatment*, eds. H. Kleber, M. Galanter (Arlington, VA: American Psychiatric Publishing, 2008).

7. N. M. Petry, B. Martin, J. L. Cooney, and H. R. Kranzler, "Give them prizes and they will come: Contingency management for treatment of alcohol dependence," *J Clin Psych* 68, no. 2 (2000): 250–57.

8. N. M. Petry, J. Tedford, M. Austin, C. Nich, K. M. Carroll, and B. J. Rounsaville, "Prize reinforcement contingency management for treating cocaine users: how low can we go, and with whom?" *Addiction* 99, no. 3 (2004): 349–60.

9. J. M. Roll, G. J. Madden, R. Rawson, and N. M. Petry, "Facilitating the adoption of contingency management for the treatment of substance use disorders," *Behav Anal Pract* 2, no. 1 (Spring 2009): 4–13.

10. K. Silverman, A. DeFulio, and S. O. Sigurdsson, "Maintenance of reinforcement to address the chronic nature of drug addiction," *Prev Med* 55, Supplement (2012): S46–S53.

11. A. T. McLellan, G. E. Skipper, M. Campbell, and D. R. L., "Five year outcomes in a cohort study of physicians treated for substance use disorders in the United States," *BMJ* 337 (2008): 1–6.

12. K. M. Carroll and L. S. Onken, "Behavioral Therapies for Drug Abuse," *American Journal of Psychiatry* 162, no. 8 (2005): 1452–60.

13. R. L. DuPont, and G. E. Skipper, "Six Lessons from State Physician Health Programs to Promote Long-Term Recovery," *J Psychoactive Drugs* 44, no. 1 (2012): 72–78.

14. J. Prochaska, The Transtheoretical Model of Behavior Change, in *The Handbook of Health Behavior Change*, Second ed. (New York: Springer Publishing Co, 1998).

15. W. L. White, *Slaying the Dragon: The History of Addiction Treatment and Recovery in America* (Bloomington, IL: Chestnut Health Systems/Lighthouse Institute, 1998).

16. G. Marlatt, "Surfing the Urge," Inquiring Mind, http://www.inquiringmind.com/Articles/SurfingTheUrge.html.

17. G. DeLeon, *The Therapeutic Community: Theory, Model, and Method* (New York: Springer Publishing Company, 2000).

18. ASAM, *The ASAM Criteria: Treatment Criteria for Addictive, Substance-related and Co-occuring Disorders*, Third ed., ed. David Mee-Lee (Carson City, NV: The Change Companies, 2013).

19. M. Galanter, and D. Brook, "Network Therapy for Addiction: Bringing Family and Peer Support into Office Practice, " *International Journal of Group Psychotherapy* 51, no. 1 (2001): 101–22.

20. Please refer to the discussion of A.A.'s effectiveness in Chapter Ten.

21. P. J. Flores, *Addiction as an Attachment Disorder* (Oxford: Jason Aronson, Inc., 2004).

22. J. Wallace, *John Wallace: Writings - The Alcoholism Papers* (Newport, RI: Edgehill Publications, 1989).

23. R. B. Swotinsky and K. H. Chase, "The Medical Review Officer," *Journal of Occupational and Environmental Medicine* 32, no. 10 (1990): 1003–08.

24. D. E. Smith, W. Glatt, D. E. Tucker, R. Deutsch, and R. B. Seymour, "Drug testing in the workplace: integrating medical review officer duties into occupational medicine," *Occupational Medicine (Philadelphia, Pa.)* 17, no. 1 (2002): 79.

25. American Society of Addiction Medicine, "Drug Testing: A White Paper of the American Society of Addiction Medicine (ASAM)," (Chevy Chase, MD: ASAM, 2013).

26. A. Saitman, H.-D. Park, and R. L. Fitzgerald, "False-Positive Interferences of Common Urine Drug Screen Immunoassays: A Review," *J Anal Toxicol* 38, no. 7 (2014): 387–96.

27. Ibid.

28. C. Yuan, D. Chen, and S. Wang, "Drug confirmation by mass spectrometry: Identification criteria and complicating factors," *Clinica Chimica Acta* 438 (2015): 119–25.

29. S. M. Lampert, A. D. Kaye, R. D. Urman, and L. Manchikanti, "Drug Testing and Adherence Monitoring in Substance Abuse Patients," in *Substance Abuse* (New York: Springer, 2015), 621–31.

30. F. M. Wurst, G. E. Skipper, and W. Weinmann, "Ethyl Glucuronide—the Direct Ethanol Metabolite on the Threshold from Science to Routine Use," *Addiction* 98, no. s2 (2003): 51–61.

31. A. Helander, I. Olsson, and H. Dahl, "Postcollection synthesis of ethyl glucuronide by bacteria in urine may cause false identification of alcohol consumption," *Clin Chem* 53, no. 10 (2007): 1855–57.

32. A. Helander, M. Böttcher, C. Fehr, N. Dahmen, and O. Beck, "Detection times for urinary ethyl glucuronide and ethyl sulfate in heavy drinkers during alcohol detoxification," *Alcohol and Alcoholism* 44, no. 1 (2009): 55–61.

33. G. E. Skipper, N. Thon, R. L. DuPont, L. Baxter, and F. M. Wurst, "Phosphatidylethanol: the potential role in further evaluating low positive urinary ethyl glucuronide and ethyl sulfate results," *Alcoholism: Clinical and Experimental Research* 37, no. 9 (2013): 1582–86.

34. G. A. J. Ayliffe, J. R. Babb, J. G. Davies, and H. A. Lilly, "Hand disinfection: a comparison of various agents in laboratory and ward studies," *Journal of Hospital Infection* 11, no. 3 (Apr. 1988): 226–43.

35. See above, n. 23.

36. See above, n. 25.

37. P. H. Earley and G. Skipper, "Medication Guide for a Safe Recovery," http://paulearley. net/download/medication-guide.

38. S. Aradottir, G. Asanovska, S. Gjerss, P. Hansson, and C. Alling, "Phosphatidylethanol (PEth) concentrations in blood are correlated to reported alcohol intake in alcohol-dependent patients," *Alcohol and Alcoholism* 41, no. 4 (July/August 2006): 431–37.

39. See above, n. 11.

40. J. S. Goldkamp, M. D. White, and J. B. Robinson, "Do Drug Courts Work? Getting inside the Drug Court Black Box," *J Drug Issues* 31, no. 1 (2001): 27–72.

41. R. L. DuPont and G. E. Skipper, "Physician Health Programs - A model of successful treatment of addiction," *Counselor* (Dec 2010): 22–29.

42. R. L. DuPont, A. T. McLellan, G. Carr, M. Gendel, G. E. Skipper, "How are addicted physicians treated? A national survey of Physician Health Programs," *J Subst Abuse Treat* 37, no. 1 (2009): 1–7.

43. B. A. Martell, F. M. Orson, J. Poling, E. Mitchell, R. D. Rossen, T. Gardner, and T. R. Kosten, "Cocaine vaccine for the treatment of cocaine dependence in methadone-maintained patients: a randomized, double-blind, placebo-controlled efficacy trial," *Arch Gen Psychiatry* 66, no. 10 (2009): 1116–23.

44. H. R. Kranzler, J. J. Stephenson, L. Montejano, S. Wang, and D. R. Gastfriend, "Persistence with oral naltrexone for alcohol treatment: implications for health-care utilization," *Addiction* 103, no. 11 (2008): 1801–08.

45. S. I. Sideroff, V. C. Charuvastra, and M. E. Jarvik, "Craving in heroin addicts maintained on the opiate antagonist naltrexone," *Am J Drug Alcohol Abuse* 5, no. 4 (1978): 415–23.

46. S. O'Malley, S. Krishnan-Sarin, C. Farren, R. Sinha, and M. Kreek, "Naltrexone decreases craving and alcohol self-administration in alcohol-dependent subjects and activates the hypothalamo–pituitary–adrenocortical axis," *Psychopharmacology (Berl)* 160, no. 1 (2002): 19–29.

47. J. R. Volpicelli, N. T. Watson, A. C. King, C. E. Sherman, and C. P. O'Brien, "Effect of naltrexone on alcohol "high" in alcoholics," *Am J Psychiatry* 152, no. 4 (Apr 1995): 613–15.

48. Part of craving is "perceived availability," a concept so named by one of the giants in the addiction field, Herbert Kleber, MD.

49. M. Connock, J.-G. A, and S. Jowett, "Methadone and buprenorphine for the management of opioid dependence: a systematic review and economic evaluation," in *NIHR Health Technology Assessment Programme: Executive Summaries* (Southampton (UK): National Institute for Health Research, 2007).

50. J. Liberto, "Handbook of Office-Based Buprenorphine Treatment of Opioid Treatment," *Psychiatric Services* 63, no. 5 (2012): 515.

51. In the ASAM Criteria, naltrexone is also considered to be part of Opioid Treatment Services. Naltrexone is pulled out here to emphasize that naltrexone and buprenorphine do produce a subtle but important difference in the treatment experience.

52. Examples of using information technology to improve containment and implement contingency contracting are DynamiCare Health (http://www.dynamicarehealth.com) and Triggr Health (https://triggrhealth.com).

53. Therapists should not use the patient's crumbling proclamation as an opportunity to take the upper hand. Rather, it is helpful to use the patient's previous confusion as a means of illuminating problems with self-insight.

54. J. P. Carbonari and C. C. DiClemente, "Using transtheoretical model profiles to differentiate levels of alcohol abstinence success," *J Consult Clin Psychol* 68, no. 5 (2000): 810–17.

55. Domain skill training, patient worksheets, and progress assessment forms are available in the companion volume, *RecoveryMind Training: Implementation Workbook*.

CHAPTER TEN

Domain B: Recovery Basics

In the previous chapter, we explored the first task in addiction treatment: containing the illness. Containing the illness is nothing more than putting a rabid dog in a cage. It does not repair the damage caused by addiction or create a sustained change—it is only the first part of a longer journey in recovery. The remainder of this text outlines the skills patients or clients should acquire in order to shift from addiction to recovery.

Domain B is a bit of a hodgepodge, designed that way out of practicality. Domain B contains the essential elements for a basic addiction treatment program. Domain A (Containment) and Domain B (Recovery Basics) comprise essential skills every individual with addiction needs in order to engage with recovery and reestablish equilibrium in his or her life. Some patients have not suffered extensive emotional damage (Domain C), lost a healthy self-concept (Domain D), disconnected from others and their spirituality (Domain E), and/or require fewer relapse prevention (Domain F) skills to sustain recovery. Such individuals find success by working in Domains A and B at a lower level of treatment (ASAM Level 2.1, IOP program or even work with a skilled addiction therapist in ASAM Level 1 treatment) and do quite well. They complete their RMT treatment with work in Domain B.

Another group of patients may not have the luxury of a prolonged treatment course. Their treatment resources are often limited to an evening IOP program where work in Domain B predominates. By focusing their work on Domain B, they leave such a program with core Recovery Skills. Note that Domain B does introduce skills that are covered more extensively in Domains C through F. Work in Domain B will feel like a traditional treatment program, organized and systematized by the learning constructs of RecoveryMind Training. Individuals in this second group should continue RecoveryMind Training exercises in Domains C through F through work with an individual or group therapist trained in RMT.

Other patients have more complex needs that mandate a longer course of treatment and continued psychotherapy as they build Recovery Skills in multiple domains. When patients complete work in multiple domains, they obtain a broader base of skills that decrease the probability of relapse, strengthen their recovery, and improve their quality of life. Patients with co-occurring psychiatric conditions, psychological trauma, victims of neglect or abuse, and those who have failed less intensive treatment fall into this category. They often need to build skills in Domains C though F working in a supportive therapeutic milieu. For best results, such individuals may require a supportive living environment at the same time.

Course of Treatment

So how do you determine the best RMT treatment course? First, the length and intensity should match the patient's condition. I recommend all treatment providers use the ASAM Criteria[1] to judge the initial type and intensity of care. Then, consider a patient's needs specific to the addiction illness itself using the domains of RecoveryMind Training. An individual who has more needs in a specific domain should spend more time attaining Recovery Skills there. The domains are arranged in an order that address addiction's most common care needs first. The ordering is not absolute. For example, Domain F (Relapse Prevention) appears at the end of the domain list because relapse prevention work becomes more meaningful near the end of the initial treatment.

Many individuals with addiction begin their recovery journey after a treatment focused solely in Domains A and B, only to stumble later on. They should return to therapy or treatment, revisit their efforts in Domains A and B briefly, and continue work in Domains C through F. Addiction is a complex tenacious illness; the majority of individuals who contract it will experience the lasting change by building Recovery Skills in all six domains. RecoveryMind Training does not suggest that work in all six domains needs to be in a residential or other structured living arrangement away from families or loved ones. The advantage to residential treatment is that it prioritizes the importance and focuses and sustains attention on recovery in an all-day setting. Daylong treatment also builds healthy attachment skills and connectedness (Domain E). These higher levels of care are only necessary in certain cases. Many individuals, once their illness is sufficiently contained (Domain A) and recovery basics are established (Domain B), can continue their recovery work in a less restrictive setting.

Despite decades of research and clinical experience with thousands of patients, it has proved difficult to determine which person will be successful with less care and who will require more care. The length of time the disease has been active, the types of drugs consumed, the age when the illness began, and the family history of addiction all contribute to disease severity and prognosis. Co-occurring medical, psychological, and psychiatric conditions and family conflict are huge factors that make the road to recovery steeper and more tortuous.

Because the treatment industry cannot reliably predict who will succeed with lesser amounts of treatment and who needs more, third party payers (i.e., managed care companies and HMOs) have adopted a "fail-first" approach to addiction treatment. Using fail-first, a patient is placed in the lowest level of care. If he or she cannot attain recovery at a lower level of care, then, and only then, more treatment is authorized. This approach may seem economically prudent, avoiding the higher costs of more complex care where it is not needed. It does have two important and unfortunate side effects. The first comes from the reinforcing downhill spiral that arises when relapse occurs. When relapse occurs, those with addiction become ensnared in an inexorable cycle of using, craving, and finding ways of obtaining and using more substances. Escape from this cycle can seem impossible at times. The second and more vexing consequence of repeated treatment failures is the damage to an individual's self-efficacy. While medical director of a tertiary care facility for addiction (most of our patients had been through three or more treatments before arriving at our door), I noted that most of these patients felt hopeless at admission. They felt they would never be successful at treatment; they had "heard it all before, and it never worked previously." Even the most authoritative and balanced addiction treatment-matching tool, the ASAM Criteria, has a bias toward placing patients at lower levels of care initially. Treatment/disease matching is only partially effective. Starting treatment at lower levels of care can have unintended negative consequences. Better assessment and triage tools are needed.

Are Twelve-Step Programs Effective?

When I train therapists, nurses, and physicians in RecoveryMind Training, I often hear concerns about the efficacy of twelve-step programs. Lately, I've heard many uninformed professionals declaring that the use of twelve-step programs in treatment is not evidence-based. This is simply not true. In the past, twelve-step programs avoided any involvement with science, mostly due to concerns regarding independence and confidentiality. Researchers, in turn, eschewed research into AA, NA, and other twelve-step support systems, partly due to the spiritual or religious elements of these support groups. An academic-AA standoff occurred. In addition, there is more federal and industry-funded research dollars earmarked to evaluate the efficacy of addiction treatment medications. Therefore, by default, more evidence is available to support the use of medications in the treatment of addiction. At the same time, other treatment methods were evaluated for their efficacy, and when deemed scientifically effective, they were placed in the bucket labeled "evidence-based treatment."

Despite these difficulties, significant research concerning the efficacy of twelve-step programs has occurred. Today it is scientifically incorrect to state there is no evidence that the twelve-step support system has not proven to be effective. Beginning with the seminal work by George Vaillant, MD,[2] the bulk of recent research recognizes the clinical efficacy of twelve-step programs in establishing and maintaining abstinence and recovery.[3] Twelve-step treatment has been shown to be effective in improving and maintaining outcomes.[4] Project MATCH (a large multicenter study focused on comparing multiple therapy approaches and medications) concluded that Twelve-Step Facilitation Therapy (TSF), Motivational Enhancement Therapy (MET), and Cognitive Behavioral Therapy (CBT) were of equal effectiveness, although this study elicited a number of cogent concerns.[5, 6, 7] A second large study reported comparable outcomes between CBT and TSF in greater than 3,000 VA patients.[8] A third concluded that CBT was more effective than TSF.[9]

In some studies, TSF has proven superior at increasing rates of continuous abstinence. Specifically, 24 percent of the outpatients in TSF were continuously abstinent throughout the year after treatment, compared to 15 percent and 14 percent in CBT and MET, respectively. Abstinence rates at three years continued to favor TSF with 36 percent reporting abstinence, compared to 24 percent in CBT and 27 percent in MET.[10]

Critics of twelve-step research suggest that the positive effect of twelve-step affiliation is limited to a small demographic. Research suggests otherwise. Twelve-step affiliation seems to be effective for different age groups and varying cultural and socioeconomic groups.[11, 12] Referral to twelve-step meetings seems to be effective regardless of previous religious affiliation.[13]

Although a meta-analysis conducted by the Cochrane Library concluded that there is no definitive proof of the efficacy of twelve-step programs,[14] this assertion is directly contradicted by Lee Ann Kaskutas, DrPH, director of training at the Alcohol Research Group. She applied the six gold standard criteria of effectiveness in epidemiology[15] to determine if AA is indeed effective and concluded

> . . . the evidence for AA effectiveness is quite strong: Rates of abstinence are about twice as high among those who attend AA (criteria 1, magnitude); higher levels of attendance are related to higher rates of abstinence (criteria 2, dose-response); these relationships are found for different samples and follow-up periods (criteria 3, consistency); prior AA attendance is predictive of subsequent abstinence (criteria 4, temporal); and mechanisms of action predicted by theories of behavior change are evident at AA meetings and through the AA steps and fellowship. (criteria 6, plausibility).[16]

Opponents and those who question AA often point to AA's spirituality as nonscientific, ineffective, and coercive, even in light of the organization's open-mindedness in this area.[17] In a review that asks what elements of AA are most helpful, John Kelly, PhD, et al., conclude that AA promotes recovery though common process mechanisms, including enhancing self-efficacy, coping skills, improving motivation, and facilitating changes that build healthy social networks. Although spiritual mechanisms are often cited as central to recovery, little research supports AA's spiritual mechanisms, which are notoriously difficult to study. They conclude their review by saying that AA's "chief strength may lie in its ability to provide free, long-term, easy access, and exposure to recovery-related common therapeutic elements, the dose of which, can be adaptively self-regulated according to perceived need."[18]

Some of the problems with such studies come from the definition of twelve-step treatment; it is a diffuse concept that is taught with varying emphasis and efficacy across a variety of treatment settings. Sending a large number of patients to AA or NA meetings without information or preparation will produce wildly varying results. In response to this need, several researchers have developed a twelve-step psycho-educational training process; one example is the Making AA Easier (MAAEZ) developed by Kaskutas.[19] A second example is the Project MATCH *Twelve-Step Facilitation Therapy Manual.*[20]

Using the MAAEZ, Kaskutas obtained a substantive and sustained benefit over five or more years. The improvement was positively correlated with a high initial frequency or a sustained meeting attendance.[21, 22] It has been shown to be effective in adolescents,[23] including the outcome measure of reducing medical costs.[24] Twelve-step-based treatment has been shown to be effective with disenfranchised populations and those who suffer from co-occurring psychiatric conditions.[25] An intensive (versus advised) referral process decreases drug use and improves psychiatric outcomes with addiction patients who also carry a psychiatric diagnosis.[26] Interestingly enough, a lack of previous religious experience does not predict negative outcomes,[27] but a positive attitude of the referring therapist resulted in higher rates of referral.[28] Psychologists John Kelly, PhD, and Rudolf Moos, PhD, described predictors of twelve-step drop out and interventions to prevent this from occurring.[29] Results suggest that active work on the Twelve Steps by cocaine-dependent patients is more important than meeting attendance alone and that a combination of individual drug counseling and active twelve-step participation is effective for these patients.[30] All this research is covered in detail along with the history of AA by Marc Galanter, MD.[31] This book is a must-read for anyone who treats addiction.

The number of confounding co-variables increases dramatically when one studies any complex and admittedly amorphous organization such as AA. The difficulty research has in studying a phenomenon, however, does not equate to a lack of efficacy. All soft, multifocal interventions in behavioral medicine are much more difficult to study, as is made plain when studies try to understand older schools of psychotherapy. This makes person-centered psychotherapy appear less effective than cognitive-behavioral therapy, for example. More effective tools, primarily through the science of "big data" will help determine efficacy of AA and other psychological interventions in the future.

How RMT Encourages Twelve-Step Programs

RMT believes the best approach to patients with substance-related disorders is to use all known effective techniques. Good treatment utilizes contingency contracting, behavioral management, cognitive behavioral therapy, mindfulness training, family systems approach, relapse prevention training, and the principles of twelve-step recovery. The strength of RMT lies in how it combines all these techniques into a cohesive whole. I cannot emphasize enough the importance of a clear and coherent addiction model. When a patient and his or her caregivers are not clear on the goals and directions of the treatment process, nothing gets done and little, if any, improvement follows.

RMT hangs its framework on twelve-step recovery. The reason for this is twofold. First, twelve-step programming provides a lifelong support network that helps individuals manage their chronic illness. Second, over my many years of experience, I have seen the most substantive change in the personalities of my patients who align with and attend twelve-step meetings and work on the path described by the Twelve Steps, even if they do not endorse the spirituality that is part of the AA program. Individuals who spend time in Alcoholics Anonymous begin to see the world and their place in it in a different light. They spontaneously experience many important elements of positive psychology (especially transcendence, gratitude, and humor).[32] This is not to say other types of treatment do not create change; however, twelve-step recovery, when properly implemented, provides a lifelong support model that encourages emotional and character growth and continued self-exploration.

RMT describes twelve-step support group meetings as effective medicine with lower potency. That is to say, twelve-step support group meetings help people remain abstinent and change their personalities, but they also require frequent and consistent dosing to be truly effective.[33] This is similar to older antibiotics that had to be consumed four times per day for two weeks in order to be effective. Alcoholics Anonymous meetings are effective but require repeated, frequent, and consistent administration, especially during the first one to two years of recovery.[34]

In this chapter, I will describe the initial tools a patient needs to use twelve-step principles and recovery support effectively. Taken in its entirety, all the RMT domains contain some material taken from twelve-step recovery. Its principles overlap with Domain D (Healthy Internal Narrative), Domain E (Connectedness and Spirituality), and Domain F (Relapse Prevention). The content of Domain B (Recovery Basics) introduces the patient to the pragmatic skills one must exercise daily in order to extricate oneself from the AddictBrain trap. In addition, Domain B defines the parts of twelve-step recovery that should be learned—and preferably memorized—to retrain one's brain.

I would also like to cover some of the patient (and therapist) resistances to twelve-step principles. It is the job of the skilled therapist to help patients get what they can out of these recovery basics even when patients show an initial resistance. How many times have we seen resistance, for example, when a patient initially cannot accept that their childhood was less than perfect? We carefully explore this resistance because we know insight into childhood trauma is an important first step in halting self-defeating or self-harm behaviors as an adult. Such a patient may say, "The past is the past; it is over and done with, and there is nothing I can do about it. My parents are dead; they were not perfect. I loved them and still do! All I want to do is learn what I can to move forward, to make my life better. I do not want to make them the villains in my life."

As therapists, we work with this resistance to seeing the world in a more powerful way, guiding through repressed anger at a parent's inadequacy or cruelty, exploring it in detail, and examining how it forged that patient's self-concept. We help patients accept their past and, in doing so, note the diminution of their self-abuse and self-sabotage. Parenthetically, we note that along this journey, our patients do not lose their love for their parents, imperfect as they might have been.

In a similar manner, addicted patients commonly express resistance to AA and its principles. RMT asserts that we should explore this resistance—most of which is driven by AddictBrain. When psychology or medical students are asked to attend AA as part of a class assignment, we often hear them say, "Wow, it was very interesting. Everyone should have a support network like that!" They find the meetings interesting and the message uplifting. In contrast, the majority of addicted individuals do not like AA at first. This is because AA does not fit their view of themselves and the world around them. It is jarring and threatening to the thoughts and beliefs produced by AddictBrain. It is a solution that feels painfully slow to those suffering with addiction who want to change how they feel *right now*. They find the stories depressing because they are a mirror for their hurt and loss. These are indeed the very problems that require repair. To change, individuals with substance use disorder have to become someone else, someone who sees him- or herself in a different way. In the majority of cases, it turns out the "someone else" enjoys AA or at the very least extracts helpful elements from attending meetings and working the Twelve Steps. They discard the maladaptive view promoted by AddictBrain and, in doing so, decrease the probability of future relapse. They learn to accept that meaningful growth takes time. They are set free from the obsessions of their addiction and see the world through a unique lens formed by twelve-step thinking. They seek camaraderie and kinship. They pursue transcendent life goals rather than the mean, stuck, self-centered existence of their disease.

RMT believes the unique skills gathered from the Twelve Steps transform the personality. The small mindedness of AddictBrain always produces a lonely self-centeredness, a bitter meaningless end. In its principles and practices, AA heals the AddictBrain personality slowly and steadily over many years. It teaches that joy is the byproduct of a well-lived life, happiness comes from serving others, and one becomes grateful by adopting a practiced attitude of gratitude, rather than demanding happiness and contentment like an impetuous child.

When a patient arrives with initial resistance to (or downright rebellion from) attending meetings or other components of twelve-step recovery, the best initial response is mutual discovery. The therapy may begin with an exploration of the patient's beliefs about religion or other spiritual pursuits. If patients become stuck here, it is best to roll with the resistance.[35] RMT stresses the pragmatic value of twelve-step meetings first: "I know you have problems with the God thing, let's not try to solve that now. In the meantime, wouldn't it be helpful to spend time with other individuals who have been in your situation, asking for pointers on how they derived benefit despite being agnostic or atheist?" Some patients wind up attending twelve-step meetings for this singular benefit, which should be considered a success.

Once a patient accepts the small benefits of mutual help meetings, I can then tiptoe into his or her dynamic resistance. I stress that the patient's own coping skills did not prove successful at finding a way out of the addiction maelstrom. I ask, "What elements of twelve-step recovery trouble you and why?" This often results in an exploration of earlier life experiences and conflicts. What appears at first glance to be a problem with religion or spirituality often ends up being something entirely different. The recovering individual splatters his or her own issues across the blank canvas of twelve-step recovery in the same manner a patient develops transference to his or her therapist.

Patients who were mercilessly over-controlled as children feel pushed around by the more zealous members, calling them AA bullies. Protection from such members of AA, even if the pressure springs from good intentions, is warranted. Others who feel constant pressure to become the alpha dog in any group situation will become unnerved by the leaderless quality of meetings and may project their need for power dynamics onto others. Each of these AA-transference experiences is discussed in individual and group therapy while in treatment. The RMT therapist should not respond to resistance with more pressure but rather by encouraging curiosity. For example, if a patient says, "I just don't like those meetings." The RMT therapist asks, "What part was especially difficult?" Asking "Why not?" invites push back. In group therapy, other members may chime in with reassurance, "At first, I did not like meetings either, but you just have to buckle down and go." The therapist gently interjects, "That may be true, but I am still curious where problems lie. Was it listening to others problems, the expectation that you had to talk, the fact that the group had no quick fixes for the craving you have been having, or something else?" Group work in RMT encourages dissent as long as it increases mutual exploration.

Difficulties with meeting attendance, step work, or sponsors become windows into the personality. The patient is encouraged to remain curious. Even if a given patient ultimately decides to never set foot in a twelve-step meeting again, a nonjudgmental exploration of his or her resistance to the principles of AA provides important insights to future sticking points that may arise with other support systems such as SMART Recovery, Secular Organizations for Sobriety, LifeRing Secular Recovery, and Celebrate Recovery. Once provided information about twelve-step meetings and given time to acclimate to them, most patients find them helpful, albeit to varying degrees. Some may embrace the camaraderie of recovery but balk at the religious undertones of some of its members. Others will find the step work liberating but struggle with being close to their fellows. Some will find the frank disclosure of other members liberating and, down the road, become unburdened by sharing their darker secrets. I am always heartened when an agnostic or atheist patient finds joy in any of the available support systems.

In this manner, a carefully crafted treatment process that incorporates twelve-step philosophy and meetings never wastes time, even for those who will never step foot in a twelve-step meeting in the future. RMT explores and prods individuals to use twelve-step philosophy and meetings, not out of a particular spiritual or moral belief system but rather out of a pragmatic truth that daily vigilance of a community of like-minded individuals is the best path to sustained recovery. Patients who have deep-seated difficulties with the religious undertones of some of the participants, or even the universal spiritual teachings of Alcoholics Anonymous, may eventually drift away. At this point, a RMT therapist will silently and subtly change tactics, finding other means to provide the extensive support needed to suppress AddictBrain and sustain a life in recovery.

The Five Segments of Domain B

Domain B is a large domain and binds five disparate segments into a cohesive whole. The Recovery Skills in these segments help patients in the following ways:

1. Develop a corrective narration that describes the course of their illness.
2. Effectively use support groups for continued growth.
3. Learn how to understand and use twelve-step literature.
4. Use mindfulness meditation to calm emotional turmoil and impulsivity.
5. Instill discipline by practicing "Recovery Reflection," a tool that cultivates insight and personal growth.

Each of the segments contains individual Recovery Skills. Specific Recovery Skills in each of these areas are important to quantify progress in Domain B and are reviewed in detail within subsequent sections of this chapter.

Segment 1: Addiction Awareness

Most treatment centers have specific assignments designed to increase addiction self-awareness. Such exercises remove distortions and provide insight into the progressive and self-destructive course of the illness in a given individual. The most common exercise has the patient write a narrative that describes that course; the narrative is commonly presented in group therapy. Many centers use twelve-step terminology to describe these assignments, and such an exercise is often called a "First Step Assignment."

The distortions produced by AddictBrain are deep and complex. Therefore, RMT uses more than one linked assignment to correct the twists and turns of thought that build up over time. A patient completes each of the assignments followed by a presentation and discussion in assignment group. When she has a level of clarity about her illness then, and only then, will she "take the first step." This process differentiates the "work" (completing specific assignments) from the desired but not always obtainable results (accepting the power and depth of her disease).

Self-disclosure is one of the key skills patients need to learn to maintain recovery. AddictBrain loves secrecy and vagueness; RecoveryMind requires sharing and accuracy. Most individuals who have suffered from addiction for an extended period have amassed vast quantities of deceit and self-deception. Such falsehoods maintain the illness. What often starts out as an attempt to hide drug or alcohol use rapidly escalates, in the vast majority of cases, to pervasive deception of self and others. It is rare for someone with a substance use disorder to arrive in a therapy office or treatment center without dissimulation. Whatever its extent, dishonesty and vagueness must be corrected in order to recover.

The primary method for correcting the AddictBrain dissemblance is simple: patients disclose past behaviors regularly with their fellow patients and staff members. Once the initial phase of treatment has been completed, honest self-disclosure should continue in support group meetings, with a sponsor, and eventually between friends and loved ones. When a patient has a memory of a past dishonesty, it should be brought to the surface in all therapy sessions and throughout the day. If the current situation is not appropriate (e.g., the memory occurs in a training exercise where another patient is the focus of work), it should be earmarked for discussion at the first opportunity. RMT describes this process as "telling on your disease."

Occasionally, patients present information in a way that produces retaliatory anger by other members of the group. Staff must intercede during these times, and disclosure will only continue if all react with compassion or, at least, equanimity. Other patients will disclose details in a manner that builds a case for continued substance use; therefore, when a patient requests time to disclose about a past addiction-related event, the therapist listens to the details of the disclosure, searching for any unconscious agenda. Within a group therapy session, the therapist might nudge the group to help the disclosing patient find solace and acceptance and concede to the painful truth about his or her past.

Specific worksheets and assignments slowly move the patient from secrecy and delusion to open disclosure and insight. The basic steps are as follows:

1. The patient completes an assignment where he records and discloses triggers that promote substance use, high-risk situations, and negative consequences of substance use.

2. The patient records and discloses secrecies and self-deception used to hide his substance use. Disclosure then occurs in a structured group. Reinforce continued disclosure.

3. The patient completes an exhaustive inventory of past substance use. This helps him see the important role substance use played in his life. The inventory should also include other addictive disorders and at least touch on past traumata, psychiatric conditions, and major life events. This inventory is read in a structured group.

This sequence of assignments provides a stepwise increase in clarity, gently nudging patients to a broader understanding of the illness. They override AddictBrain's vagueness and obfuscation, erasing the cloak that hides the disease from its victim. Patients are encouraged to continue "telling on your disease"—which really means revealing AddictBrain thoughts.

The process of disclosure—be it in a therapy group or a support group meeting—opens the door to autobiographical reasoning. Autobiographical reasoning occurs when concepts of self are attached to personal experiences in order to improve meaning and a favorable self-concept. William Dunlop, PhD, and Jessica Tracy, PhD, suggest that narrating positive self-change in the wake of substance abuse may underlie positive psychological adjustment, and this may account for some of the positive effects that result when a patient revisits his past and discusses it in a group setting.[36]

Addiction traumatizes every patient. Recounting the events of the past may be quite disturbing to some. As the patient moves through the assignment list outlined previously, staff members must watch for deterioration in mood. Individuals who have suffered childhood trauma prior to the onset of their addiction disorder are especially vulnerable to the retraumatizing effect of self-disclosure. In such cases, assignments are set-aside for a while. At times, the process of corrective autobiographical reasoning triggers individuals who have co-occurring post-traumatic stress disorder (PTSD). However, I cannot understate the importance of corrective self-concept in building a substantive recovery. A careful therapist or treatment team deftly threads this needle, helping the patient understand his or her past while minimizing the damage of memory reenactment. Parts of addiction treatment follow the same path as the treatment of PTSD.[37] The excavation of disease behaviors and emotional states bears a striking resemblance to the progressive narrative exposure technique[38] used in PTSD care.

Segment 2: Using Support Groups

A significant percentage of treatment programs in the United States utilize or refer to twelve-step or other mutual support groups to assist in their treatment efforts. Despite this, very few programs train their patients about what to expect when attending a support group meeting. Nor do they describe potential benefits and pitfalls of their attendance at twelve-step meetings. This is a significant error. Like everything else in RMT, if an intervention is utilized in the treatment of addiction, then the treatment process must explain how it fits into the overall structure of the recovery process. And, patients are taught how to use support groups and practice such skills in group training sessions.

The same can be said for the utilization of support group meetings. I fully recognize that some patients may take to support groups like a duck to water. However, others may find sitting in a support group meeting to be nothing short of torture. RMT provides education to both types of individuals. Some of the information may be covered using a brief lecture or through the use of reading materials, such as a glossary of the types of twelve-step meetings available in the area (AA, NA, CA, CMA, etc.) and meeting structure (speaker meetings, open discussion, close discussion, and meetings aimed at a particular cohort, such as women or men only meetings). Alternatives to AA should also be provided.

Using the RMT style of training, patients are introduced to support group meetings through role-play. Group dynamics are described. Patients who tend to "hide out" are encouraged to move in incremental steps from the back toward the front, increasing their contribution slightly with each step. Patients who always seem to garner the spotlight are encouraged to sit and observe. The use of repetition in the structure of meetings is explained. The importance of limiting crosstalk in support group meetings and examples illuminating the difference between group therapy and support groups are also described. Group etiquette is role-played in a skill building session as well.

Different personality types need to practice different skills. Patients with social phobia should practice navigating the unstructured parts of meetings: walking in the door, finding a seat, and the most difficult of all, open sharing. Other individuals who expect profound insight at every turn will be disappointed in twelve-step meetings without expectation management. Such individuals need to learn how to "meta-listen." This process encourages the individual to hear the message beneath the words that are spoken. Here is an example.

> *Patients and a group leader sit in a circle similar to that of an AA meeting. An appointed staff member or more senior patient is encouraged to describe her day now that she is in recovery. Her description should include a few glimpses of inner peace, something about freedom from having to procure drugs or alcohol, and meeting an old friend to whom she no longer has to lie. After about five minutes of sharing, that process is stopped. The group is then queried for the messages conveyed by sharing. The group leader encourages group members to reflect on how it relates to them in their situation. What was the message underneath the sharing? Are there elements of gratitude? How is this different from or similar to their current situation?*

Some patients—especially patients with attention deficit disorder or other difficulties with focus—may become bored during the readings from the recovery literature. RMT suggests several techniques to encourage continued attention. For example, patients are told to listen to an upcoming passage knowing that their unconscious mind will pick out a word or phrase within that reading that is relevant to them at that very moment. A reading occurs, say the beginning of Chapter Five of *Alcoholics Anonymous*. When sharing at the end of the reading, a patient may report being struck anew by the phrase "thoroughly followed our path." Through active listening, curiosity focuses attention. What about this phrase speaks to his current struggles?

Patients new to treatment should learn the difference between psychotherapy and support groups. Patients who are confused about the purpose of support groups will feel misaligned with their flow and leave feeling empty, conflicted, or unfulfilled. I have even seen patients who have attended meeting for many years return to treatment with a chronic misunderstanding of why, for example, "No one ever seemed to talk back to me. I felt like I was ignored after I spoke up." For these reasons, a significant portion of time in early treatment is focused on how to effectively use support groups. Meetings are described as a tool in the recovery toolbox. Just as a mechanic needs to learn how best to use his tools, patients need to learn how to use the tools of recovery.

Although I often hear complaints about the rhetoric of AA, this is often a smokescreen for other problems, such as social anxiety, difficulties with social intimacy, fear of revealing oneself to others, problems with control or authority, and simple jealousy that others are succeeding while one has failed to remain in recovery and take charge of his or her life. A skilled therapist sees AA meetings as a blank canvas onto which each patient places his or her own psychological conflicts and struggles. Like group therapy, meetings provide a test bed for reorganizing one's life, replacing chemical use with healthy interdependence. Using this model, resistance to meetings is similar to resistance in psychotherapy—just another opportunity to grow. If we can get our patients to be curious about their resistance instead of being reactive, they will learn something about themselves.

Many treatment providers effectively use one or more sayings from the twelve-step community to help with meeting resistance, such as the following:

- "It's not important that you believe in God, but it is important to know you're not him."
- "Find some type of higher power, such as the group, that you can learn to trust."
- "We don't have a pill to fix addiction, so we'd best get busy figuring out how to use the tools we do have. This includes learning how to accept help from each other."

In all cases, it is critical for staff members and fellow patients to address their peers who have problems with spiritual matters as their equals and to avoid judgmentalism and condescension. Special attention should be paid to patients who are agnostic or atheist. In helping patients benefit from meetings despite these concerns, it is best to be pragmatic. Discussion with such patients begins with "Recovery requires constant vigilance and a methodical plan. Twelve-step meetings are readily available and free. There is a lot of talk about spirituality, but AA offers much more. We want you to learn how to use every available tool in this difficult fight for survival. If you have difficulties with references to organized religion, let's do what we can to keep it from getting in your way." In the vast majority of cases, I have found that even the most diehard atheist can learn to look past "the God stuff." In the few instances where a patient is unable to use the recovery support networks, he or she is referred to alternative support groups, such as SMART Recovery, Secular Organizations for Sobriety, LifeRing Secular Recovery, and Rational Recovery for needed ongoing support. Involvement in any of the mutual help groups entrains relapse prevention tools, replaces bitterness with gratitude, and encourages connection with others in supportive fellowship.

Segment 3: Recovery Literature as an Agent of Change

Similar to twelve-step meetings, the recovery literature builds a framework around the recovery experience. In many treatment programs, patients are expected to read various sections of *Alcoholics Anonymous*[39] (the "Big Book" of AA) or *Narcotics Anonymous* [40] (the "Basic Text" of NA). Many use *Twelve Steps and Twelve Traditions*[41] (the "twelve and twelve" of AA) for their introduction to the Twelve Steps. While all these resources prove beneficial, it is important to measure knowledge accumulation in this area. Which part of this literature should patients read? What parts are best to know well? What parts (if any) should be memorized? The typical approach of many treatment programs is to expose patients to various parts of the recovery literature, hoping the passages that are meaningful will stick. This approach is well meaning but inconsistent and ineffective. Rather, each facility should set up their study into three categories:

1. Literature the patient should read.
2. Literature the patient should be familiar with, paraphrasing the meaning contained within those passages.
3. Passages that should be memorized and understood in their entirety. The patient should be able to describe how these memorized passages relate (or do not relate) to him or her.

Every addiction therapist, physician, counselor, or sponsor has their own favorite readings they believe should be placed in each of these three categories. It would be presumptuous for this text to insist on certain readings being placed in one category or another. Therefore, I will suggest areas to be considered based upon the initial dose of treatment available. The proposed list serves as a starting point for the development of your own assigned reading list. The important point here is not which items go into which categories, but that such categories are important for quantifiable progress. In RMT, patients are given a clear and concise path.

The learning grid in Table 10.1 is suggestive only; please do not take this as gospel for how readings should be structured at all treatment centers. In addition, please note this grid does not include readings from a "daily meditation" text. This type of reading is part of the Recovery Reflection described later in this chapter. Some centers that specialize in the treatment of cocaine, methamphetamine, or other types of drug dependence might use literature from their respective twelve-step fellowships.

Table 10.1 - Suggested Reading and Memorizing Recovery Literature

	Read	Familiar and Understand	Memorize
Shorter Outpatient	**AA Big Book:** How It Works **AA 12&12:** Steps One through Three **NA Basic Text:** How It Works **NA *It Works: How and Why:*** Steps One through Three	**AA/NA Steps:** One through Three **AA Big Book:** How It Works **AA 12&12:** Step One **NA *It Works: How and Why:*** Step One	**AA/NA Steps:** One **Serenity Prayer**
Longer Outpatient or Intermediate Day Hospital	All the above plus: **AA Big Book:** The Doctor's Opinion, Bill's Story, or **NA Basic Text:** We Do Recovery (Jimmy K's story) **AA 12&12:** Steps One through Five **NA *It Works: How and Why:*** Steps One through Five	**AA/NA Steps:** One through Five **AA Big Book:** How It Works and the Promises (Chapter Six) **NA Basic Text:** Chapter Ten (More Will Be Revealed)	**AA/NA Steps:** One through Three **Serenity Prayer**
Extended Residential	All the above plus: **AA 12&12:** Entire text **NA *It Works: How and Why:*** Entire text	**AA/NA Steps:** All the steps **AA Big Book:** How It Works and the Promises **NA Basic Text:** Chapter Ten (More Will Be Revealed)	**AA/NA Steps:** One through Five **Serenity Prayer**

	Read	Familiar and Understand	Memorize
Long-term Residential	All the above	**AA/NA Steps:** All the steps **AA Big Book:** How it Works **AA 12&12:** Entire text **NA *It Works: How and Why*:** Entire text	**AA/NA Steps**: All the steps **Serenity Prayer** **AA Promises**

Table Legend: AA/NA Steps: The wording of the Twelve Steps in *Alcoholics Anonymous, Third* or *Fourth Edition*, or *Narcotics Anonymous, Sixth Edition*; **AA Big Book**: Chapters in *Alcoholics Anonymous*; **AA 12&12**: Chapters in *Twelve Steps and Twelve Traditions*; **NA Basic Text**: Chapters in *Narcotics Anonymous, Sixth Edition*; **NA** *It Works: How and Why*; **AA Promises**: Passage from Chapter Six of *Alcoholics Anonymous, Third* or *Fourth Edition*; **Serenity Prayer**: The Serenity Prayer, as used in most twelve-step fellowships and modified from the original by Reinhold Niebuhr.[42]

Working the Steps

The most confusing phrase in all of addiction care is the term "working the steps." This phrase is commonly used in the recovery community, and its meaning varies from individual to individual. If a patient states, "I'm working the steps," the receiver has little to no information about what is actually going on. In some cases, this may mean an individual is reading a chapter in AA literature related to a particular step. In others, it may mean an individual is completing a worksheet provided by his sponsor regarding his personal understanding and feelings about a certain step. This phrase is also uttered by individuals in recovery when they are involved in a difficult situation and do not know how to proceed. In this situation, they may use the wisdom contained in one or more steps to guide their actions.

In RMT, the phrase "working the steps" is clearly delimited and defined. A patient is said to be working the steps when he is completing specific paperwork regarding one or more of the Twelve Steps, or he is discussing a particular step with a sponsor or counselor. I believe this eliminates some of the confusion regarding this phrase. More importantly, it prevents patients from sidestepping important internal struggles that everyone must go through to integrate twelve-step recovery into their beliefs and worldview.

Several other terms may be important in this regard. When a recovering individual is caught in a bind and uses the wisdom of one or more steps to guide her actions, this is called "using a step." This may seem self-explanatory, but when an individual is mulling over a certain step (e.g., trying to understand how the word "unmanageable" from the first step applies to him), the phrase "considering" or "thinking about" a particular step is used. As a therapeutic note, if a patient arrives at a therapy session railing against the contents of the first step—"I am not powerless over anything"—I think of this as "considering" or "struggling with" that step. It is important to approach the intense reaction with curiosity, not a hammer.

In summary, I use the phrase "working a step" when someone is discussing or writing about a specific step on the way to integrating that step into his recovery plan. Actions that occur prior to accepting the concept of a step into his life or occur internally or when an individual utilizes the content within a step to solve an external situation are not, in RMT language, working the steps.

Why is this language so important? The most cogent answer is that using concise language produces clarity of thought, which in turn produces clarity of action. I do not expect my patients to understand the subtle differences at first. Rather, by offering clarity we focus action and create measurable responses.

Work in this segment is straightforward. The patient reads assigned pages in the recovery literature and then completes worksheets that explore his or her reaction to the reading. The worksheets are reviewed by staff members and discussed in specific assignment groups. In an outpatient practice, the worksheets are discussed in session. In both cases, a patient's response to readings in a worksheet is reviewed openly without judgment as to correct or incorrect. An air of collaborative exploration helps a patient remain open to the benefits inherent in twelve-step literature.

Segment 4: Mindfulness Meditation

The fourth segment of Domain B is mindfulness meditation. A bit of background may prove helpful in exploring this important skill. During the course of our day, the mind moves among several distinct "brain states." Some of these brain states are obvious to the casual observer, for example, being awake and asleep. Actually, what appear to be two distinct brain states is actually three. They are:

1. Wakefulness
2. Non-REM sleep
3. REM sleep

Sleep research has shown that REM sleep is a distinctly different brain state from simple sleep; wakefulness is different from the other two. Based upon electroencephalographic (brainwave) research, many scientists view meditation as a fourth distinct brain state, different from the other states noted previously. During meditation, practitioners experience a calming of thoughts, but, surprisingly, electrical activity in the frontal lobes of the brain actually increases. When an individual practices meditation for a period of months, the electrical power in the α (alpha) frequency range becomes asymmetric (even when not meditating), increasing in the left brain and decreasing in the right. The brain's gray matter increases in size and density[43] in the executive and memory areas of the brain,[44, 45] helping the mind control emotional dissonance.[46, 47]

Recent research differentiates the three major forms of meditation as practiced in the Buddhist tradition: focused attention, mindfulness, and the meditation of compassion and loving-kindness. Research into one of these meditation types, focused attention, follows the electrical response of the brain as meditation begins.[48, 49] Before meditation, the default mode network (discussed in Chapter Five) is active. The first change in meditation is mindfulness, where the individual notices sensations and thoughts without being carried away by them. This quiets the amygdala and insula (centers activated during high emotional states). This is followed by distraction awareness, where the individual notes the brain following a thought or feeling (the start of DMN activity). When the DMN is thwarted, the dorsolateral prefrontal cortex and the inferior parietal lobe return to the rhythmic electrical oscillation of meditation. Sustained focus leads to stronger activity in the dorsolateral prefrontal cortex, deepening the meditative state. For more information, refer to an excellent review of the neurobiology of meditation by Yi-Yaun Tang, PhD, et al.[50]

Meditation has other effects on the mind and body, including a decrease in baseline anxiety and improvement in immune function.[51] All these effects help the recovering individual maintain an abstinent state. Just as important, mindfulness meditation increases joy and the appreciation of "what is." Preliminary research into the effectiveness of mindfulness meditation specific to the treatment of addiction disorders[52] and addiction relapse[53] is very promising.

There are many different forms of mindfulness meditation. Despite differences in technique, research suggests that all the major schools of meditation seem to produce the same desired effect.[54] However, this does not suggest that we can make up any simple procedure and call it meditation. RecoveryMind Training relies on evidence-based techniques whenever available. Regarding meditation and mindfulness, the best-studied technique is traditional Buddhist meditation, modified for distractible western minds. I recommend the teachings of Thich Nhat Hanh for its simplicity and directness.[55] I strongly recommend therapists and trainers obtain formal training in meditation practices before implementing the practice with their patients.

The meditation trainer should point out that meditation must be practiced for some time to be effective; the benefits are cumulative and realized slowly. Individuals with an addiction disorder may expect an instantaneous "bang" of insight, expressing frustration at the slow measured benefits that accrue from a daily meditation practice. Meditation should occur in a room shielded from extraneous noise. When initially learning meditation, most patients feel the most comfortable sitting upright in a chair. As the practitioner gains experience, he or she may consider other modifications, such as sitting on the floor on a mat or meditating outside. Different meditation schools train in different ways; however, the basic components for the beginner are similar:

1. Remove extraneous objects from your lap.
2. Sit upright in a chair with your feet planted lightly on the floor.
3. Adjust the body to an upright but relaxed posture.
4. Allow the face muscles to relax into the hint of a smile.
5. Let the eyes close and slowly move the mind inward.
6. Begin focusing on the breath as it moves gently in and out.
7. When a thought distracts focus, either acknowledge it by pointing to it in within the mind or labeling it with the word "thinking." Alternatively, one can place each thought on a leaf in a stream and watch it drift away.
8. If distracted for several seconds, gently return to focusing on the breath.
9. Avoid abrupt movements. If possible, avoid any movement with the exception of movements created by the breath.
10. When it is time to stop, keep the eyes closed for a moment while thoughts return to the room.
11. Slowly open the eyes and look at a neutral object. Return to the presence of others in the room and avoid any rapid change of posture, conversation, or other purposeful activity for one minute or more.

During the course of treatment, all patients and staff should set aside a common time within the treatment day to meditate. Meditation can be practiced singly or in groups. Some patients find it distracting to meditate in groups; others find it deepens their meditation almost as if the energy of communal meditation intensifies the experience. Patients who have just completed detoxification may not be able to tolerate sitting still for meditation. The best approach in such cases is to keep the dose of meditation very brief (less than one minute at first). Using the timer and gradually increasing meditation period decreases frustration. Many excellent references are available for mindfulness training. A brief list appears in the Chapter Notes at the end of this chapter.[56, 57, 58–62]

Despite repeated efforts, some patients may be unable to meditate. One effective alternative is sound-based brainwave entrainment. The best studied of these is binaural brainwave entrainment. This procedure applies sounds of slightly different frequencies to each ear. Headphones must be used because the harmonics produced by the interference between the different frequencies in each ear modulates the brain's natural frequencies,[63] inducing a state similar to meditation. Several commercial products produce brainwave entrainments[64] and prove quite useful for those who cannot enter a meditative state.

Once detoxification is complete and the patient is oriented to treatment, RecoveryMind Training recommends starting a daily meditation practice. The recovering individual should set aside a specific time during each day to practice meditation. Nearly any time of day will work; however, it is best not to meditate too close to bedtime.

Addiction destroys one's capacity for self-reflection and restraint; meditation restores both. Early on in the course of RMT treatment, patients are taught simple mindfulness skills to be used throughout each treatment day. In RecoveryMind Training, once a patient has learned to meditate, it becomes part of his or her Recovery Reflection. Meditation prepares the patient for an honest, calm self-assessment that is important for the other parts of Recovery Reflection.

Meditation is taught using concrete, step-by-step instructions. I have found that many clients profess proficiency at mindfulness meditation based upon reading a book or article on the subject. In RMT, diligent and persistent instruction as well as observation and gentle correction of the practice hone the skill.

Training can occur in a group setting. The group leader begins with a brief explanation of the benefits of meditation. A set of simple steps is reviewed, followed by a brief meditation practice. The group concludes with feedback and discussion about the participants' experience. Chemically dependent individuals often expect dramatic changes or cosmic bliss after a few sessions of meditation and become discouraged when it does not occur. It is best to dissuade them of this classically addictive thought: "I want to feel better right now."

Some patients who are healing from the toxic effects of sustained drug use get little out of meditation at first. They are encouraged to go through the motions of meditation even if they perceive no immediate rewards from the experience. Even if no positive effects occur for some time, a patient who goes through the motions of this simple practice will learn an important lesson: one should not discard a healthy pursuit because it lacks immediate rewards. Instead, I suggest staff members limit meditation in such an individual to three to five minutes, or even less, at first. Over time, the length of a patient's meditation can be slowly increased.

Segment 5: Recovery Reflection

RMT is based upon the concept that once addiction has been established in the brain, AddictBrain will continue its self-destructive path unless systematic and methodical steps are taken to thwart its effect. AddictBrain entrains using habits. This is more than the simple habit of using alcohol or other drugs. AddictBrain is a series of habitual thoughts, beliefs, and behaviors that lead the afflicted individual down the primrose path toward eventual substance use. The victim of AddictBrain cannot undo its effects by simply thinking about it. Instead, RMT lays down a second set of thoughts, beliefs, and behaviors that, once properly entrained, disempower self-destructive AddictBrain thinking. One simple tool designed to thwart AddictBrain is a diligent daily inventory and planning process called Recovery Reflection.

Recovery Reflection is taught early on in the treatment process. Recovery Reflection builds a pattern to the day's activities, undoing addiction chaos. Treatment establishes a healthy rhythm to the day and trains the patient how to use Recovery Reflection for continued self-examination. Patients are encouraged to use a daily (or more frequent) Recovery Reflection for the first several years of recovery.

How should treatment programs implement Recovery Reflection? Like everything else in RMT, the Recovery Reflection training is taught using role-play. During the training, staff provides each participant a copy of the Recovery Reflection forms (see the Appendix for an example of this form). The leader provides a brief explanation of its purpose. A patient volunteer might review one example of a completed form with the group. She answers questions and ponders her responses aloud. Other members discuss their answers, searching for depth and meaning. The leader steers the discussion, maximizing understanding of the purpose of the exercise. Then, all members of the group complete the form, asking questions of the entire group along the way—patients learn from each other. The responses to Recovery Reflection questions are reviewed as a group; this too promotes group learning and peer-based self-examination.

In individual therapy setting, the therapist walks the patient through completion of the form, answering questions along the way. The patient is sent home with a supply of reflection forms and asked to bring several completed forms to the next session. The therapist reviews the forms, honing goal setting skills, promoting self-insight, meditation skills, and step work. Recovery Reflection trains RecoveryMind with a defined set of important skills that should be practiced each day on the road to recovery.

Recovery Reflection introduces patients to elements of Domains C through F, providing initial attention to issues addressed in these domains. Each element of the Recovery Reflection relates back to a specific domain, preparing patients for subsequent focused attention in needed areas. When a staff member reviews a Recovery Reflection worksheet, it may reveal areas that need additional work. For example, the Recovery Reflection may reveal that a patient has difficulties recognizing and labeling feelings. Discovering this, the patient's counselor or therapist recognizes that work in Domain C (Emotional Recognition and Resilience) should be added to the treatment plan.

This process also helps delineate a patient's needs in continuing care. For example, if a patient is in an evening intensive outpatient program that meets for three hours, three times per week for four weeks (ASAM Level 2.1), he will not have the time to learn about, catalog, and train in relapse prevention skills. At best, he may only have a brief introduction to relapse prevention training. Through Recovery Reflection, the patient and his treatment team recognize that important work in Domain F (Relapse Prevention) needs attention. Depending on the depth of the need, care may need to shift to Domain F immediately despite his limited time in ASAM Level 2.1 treatment. Or, the patient may be referred to a relapse prevention specialist who uses RecoveryMind Training once his current level of care is complete. In this way, RMT capitalizes on the treatment that is available to each individual, be it three months of residential care or sixteen sessions of an evening intensive outpatient program.

Using the Recovery Reflection

Once or twice each day, the recovering individual is asked to reflect on his or her recovery. The number of reflections per day depends on the type and intensity of treatment. In organized treatment, time for the Recovery Reflection should be hardwired into the treatment schedule. If, however, the patient is attending an evening treatment or a treatment process with even less structure, Recovery Reflection becomes that much more critical. Recovery Reflection uses two different forms because each time of day has different reflection items.

Patients turn in completed Recovery Reflection forms for staff review. The staff culls through the worksheets to guide and focus treatment going forward. It is best for staff members to return these sheets to patients so they may be placed in a treatment logbook that patients use to chart improvements throughout the course of their care.

An overview of the elements of Recovery Reflection appears in Table 10.2. Each element should be completed in the order shown in that table. Note the table uses symbols to delineate the two types of reflection— morning and night. The morning Recovery Reflection is completed at the start of each day, and the evening review occurs at the end of each day. The middle five elements of the reflection are repeated twice per day, upon arising in the morning, during the optional midday break, and some time in the evening. The time to complete a Recovery Reflection is set-aside in the program schedule if a patient is in daylong treatment. If a patient is in intensive outpatient day or evening treatment, the program instructs patients to complete a Recovery Reflection at designated times throughout their day.

Table 10.2 - The Recovery Reflection

Element	Time of Day	Purpose	Domain
Recovery Schedule	☀	Important recovery activities must be scheduled each day to prevent daily activities from being hijacked by AddictBrain.	A
Mindfulness Meditation	☀ ☾	Mindfulness training increases frontal lobe control of strong emotions and drug craving. It quiets and prepares the mind for the other elements of the Recovery Reflection.	C

Element	Time of Day	Purpose	Domain
Emotional Awareness	☀ ☾	Naming and noticing feeling states prevents those with addiction from acting them out unconsciously. Difficult feeling states should be processed in group therapy sessions.	C
Deception Detection	☀ ☾	Recovery requires accurate self-examination. Here the patient catalogs dishonesty with self and others. This breaks the internal and external lies that AddictBrain uses to hide.	D
Healthy Attachment	☀ ☾	Learning healthy attachment to others breaks the self-focused nature of addiction and teaches patients how to use external support.	E
Craving Recognition	☀ ☾	By noting the relationship between events, thoughts, feelings, and the resultant craving, the patient begins building a relapse prevention plan.	F
Step Review	☾	In this element, the patient records which of the Twelve Steps was considered or studied that day and any change in understanding or attitude that occurred.	B
Issue Identification	☾	The patient builds a list of emotional and interpersonal issues that need attention over the next several days.	All

Recovery Schedule

Each morning, the patient plans his daily activities. For highly structured treatment settings, the actual planning of the day's activities might be minimal. If there are specific written assignments or therapy work to be accomplished that day, they are recorded in the patient's schedule. Writing down a task on a schedule crystalizes commitment, which is more powerful than simply thinking about or even verbalizing a goal. Early in treatment, patients are encouraged to keep goals simple, such as "Remain sober and in treatment for today." This in itself can seem like a tall task during those bleak first days. As treatment progresses, the schedule will become more complex; however, addiction recovery must be the first priority during the first year.

Patients are encouraged to place logistical goals (e.g., "Call my wife to ask her to come to the family group."), learning goals (e.g., "Learn the difference between a using thought and a high risk situation."), and therapeutic goals on their schedule (e.g., "Talk in group about how my father's drinking affected me."). Some patients will write little, and others will produce volumes. RMT likes to keep this list to short realizable tasks that can be confirmed at the end of the day. It is best to avoid creating an all-inclusive list (e.g., "eat lunch"). When this information is reviewed, the staff gets a clear idea about the patient's focus and direction. Spending a few minutes each day to realign a patient's list to realistic, obtainable, recovery-based goals goes a long way when teaching a patient how to set the larger goals required for the life-long journey of recovery.

Mindfulness

Mindfulness meditation is part of Recovery Reflection. Once a patient learns the basics of meditation, he or she can now practice it during this time. Refer to the previously discussed mindfulness meditation section for more information.

Emotional Awareness

The next element of Recovery Reflection addresses emotional awareness. Patients who develop addiction disorders have a wide range of understanding and comfort with their feelings. At one end of the spectrum, some patients are unable to recognize feeling states or name them when they emerge. When an emotion occurs, they use a general term such as "upset" or "uneasy." At the other end of the spectrum, there are patients who constantly describe their emotional states in a voluble and erratic fashion, unable to self-regulate but willing and able to describe their moment-to-moment emotional responses with piercing accuracy. In general, the first group needs to recognize feeling states, and the second group needs to be more emotionally resilient when feelings occur. The therapist responds with distinctly different approaches based upon a given patient's emotional style. I will cover emotional regulation and stability in more detail in Chapter Eleven.

Addiction recovery obligates those afflicted to becoming better friends with their feelings. Patients need to manage their feeling states in the same manner they handle meaningful friendships. With our friends, we are careful and respectful because we value what they bring to our life. We need to get to know them better and do what we can to help them live full lives. Sometimes we need to set limits and boundaries with them or tell them they are being too intrusive or hurtful. At times, we instruct them on how to best be with us in our world and respect that we have our own needs, too. Importantly, we look to our friends to provide advice and counsel to help us navigate through life, as well as our feelings. We give proper respect and care, knowing our feelings bring meaning to our world. At times we have to set limits on feeling states, not letting them run rip shod through our life. We look to our feelings to provide advice and counsel in life, to set our priorities, and to give our life meaning. All of this requires a consistent attitude of exploration and openness regarding emotions.

During Recovery Reflection, patients note their current feelings, searching for more subtle feelings at the end of mindfulness meditation. These are recorded with single feeling words or a brief phrase. Patients are encouraged to note they may have multiple feelings simultaneously. They then list one or more feelings that are most troublesome at the current moment. The Recovery Reflection worksheet queries the patient as to why this particular feeling is most uncomfortable, setting up further exploration.

From time to time, patients are encouraged to go back to previous Recovery Reflections, reviewing how they felt during the previous session. They record which feelings have remained consistent over multiple reflections and which feelings come and go. The more persistent feeling states are noted for subsequent exploration during group and individual therapy sessions. The more ephemeral feeling states are also noted. Many patients are shocked to learn a feeling that was so important to them yesterday or earlier in the day is all but gone by the next reflection period. This exercise teaches patients to walk through life, allowing feelings to come and go. They should not have to take action when an intense feeling erupts—sometimes simply watching the feeling as it washes over them is sufficient.

Deception Detection

One of the most maladaptive—and arguably the most maddening— addiction behavior is deception of self and others. Using the understanding of RMT, I describe deception as a tool AddictBrain uses to hide its goals and objectives. AddictBrain must hide its behaviors lest the addicted person emerge from the cloak of its deception only to discover that it is slowly murdering its victim. If a patient deeply understands this truth, he or she would reject AddictBrain immediately. When addiction reaches a full-blown state, it is kill or be killed. AddictBrain, by necessity, hides inside under a cloak of deception. AddictBrain ensures it is not discovered by friends, family, and coworkers, as it uses deception with them as well. Therefore, a critical skill for recovery is deconstructing the deception of self and others.

During each Recovery Reflection, the patient is asked to catalog mendacities he has told himself or others since the last reflection. In the reflection worksheet, the patient writes down factual lies, such as "I told everyone in group today that I have only abused painkillers for the past year. I really have been abusing them for five years." After each deception, the patient writes down a corrective action, such as "Tomorrow in group I will tell them how long I have been using narcotic painkillers." During each Recovery Reflection, the patient is also asked to consider the self-deceptions he has lived with through the years. He may write, "I always told myself I drank because I like the taste of alcohol, but what was more important to me was the alcohol-induced oblivion."

Addicted individuals develop a complex web of deception of self and others. They lose track of prevarications they have told themselves, which makes them befuddled and confused internally. In contrast, others may see them as crafty and manipulative. Whatever the changes, the recovering individual needs to learn a central skill, "telling on AddictBrain." The period of Recovery Reflection establishes a daily inquiry into deception and directs a patient to undo this deception through self-disclosure. Disclosure is best performed in groups but may also be carried out with a therapist or twelve-step sponsor. Disclosure to others is the first step toward rigorous honesty, a prerequisite for a substantive recovery.

Craving Recognition

Craving is a universal experience for patients who develop chemical dependency. At one end of the spectrum, some patients are acutely aware of their craving experiences, and others seem to act out their cravings but have little conscious awareness of them. They may see themselves as plagued by unremitting craving and, through the process of cataloging them, come to realize they are transient events rather than a continuous call to action.

At the other end of the spectrum, some patients sit through treatment without recognizing a single episode of craving. Most of these individuals will begin to recognize cravings when they learn a framework that categorizes cravings, followed by sitting quietly in Recovery Reflection. RecoveryMind Training uses a defined craving scale that improves craving recognition. In this element of Recovery Reflection, patients sit for a time and review the recent past, searching for and grading past craving events. Noticing and validating cravings is the first step in a comprehensive relapse prevention plan.

As preparation for work in Domain F, Recovery Reflection uncovers cravings and validates their presence when they are written down.

Simply writing down a craving often decreases its power. At the very least, writing down cravings will start work for relapse prevention. Specific exercises regarding cravings management and other relapse prevention skills will be covered in Chapter Fourteen.

Healthy Attachment

During Recovery Reflection, the patient takes a brief moment to notice the connectedness between him and others. Events from the past several days are considered: Was everyone healthy, enmeshed, or conflicted? The Recovery Reflection worksheet asks, "Who did you feel connected to today?" and "What caused this to transpire?" The worksheet then asks for a simple analysis of the healthy and unhealthy elements (if any) of this episode of connectedness. Philip J. Flores, PhD, has written extensively on the importance of healthy attachment styles for patients in recovery.[65] In his theory, difficulties with interpersonal attachment make one susceptible to the disease of addiction, and in contradistinction, healthy relationships are a central component of a robust recovery.

Similar to all other elements of Recovery Reflection, recording connectedness to others increases awareness, prioritizes the importance of healthy attachments, and sets a patient on the path of repairing connections with friends and family. Individuals who have addiction disorders need the counsel and support of others to help them see and defeat AddictBrain. Connectedness with others also improves one's self-concept.[66]

Addicted individuals tend to fall into sexualized attachments once the drugs and alcohol have left their system. One simple way of differentiating an inappropriate sexualized relationship from a healthy attachment is to ask the question, "Are you willing to tell others about what you are experiencing and feeling in this new relationship and how it has helped you?" Healthy attachment styles and their importance in recovery will be discussed in Chapter Twelve.

Step Review

During each Recovery Reflection, patients are asked to review their work and thoughts about one or more of the Twelve Steps. This review is not a time where specific reading or written step assignments are completed. Rather, the patient is asked to consider changes in his attitude or understanding of one or more steps. During the early stages of an episode of treatment, a patient is commonly focused on Step One.

When asked about recent insights regarding the steps during the step review section of Recovery Reflection, the patient may write, "In the past when I thought about the word unmanageable, I thought about how my drinking had gotten out of control. Now I see the word "unmanageable" refers to how my illness wreaked havoc in almost every part of my life."

Even when working with areas of resistance, step review is helpful. Patients are instructed to write what they do not like about the Twelve Steps as well. During step review, such a patient may write, "I don't like the word "powerless"; I don't like to think that I'm powerless over anything in my life!" When staff members study the step review, this patient who has valid concerns about the word "powerless" may benefit from additional education about AddictBrain or may need to explore previous wounding promulgated by past authority figures.

Staff members may instruct a patient to focus her review on a particular step as she moves through treatment; however, they should also encourage patients to write extemporaneously about their issues with step work. I often find a patient musing on a previous (or future) step in her Recovery Reflection, which then triggers a review of past step work using her reflection writings as a guide.

Issue Identification

The last item in Recovery Reflection is Issue Identification. As patients go through the each of the previous items, they are bound to discover issues that need additional attention in treatment. When reviewing the day's emotions, a patient might think, "When I heard Carol talk about the grief she felt after her mother died, I was overwhelmed with sadness. Perhaps I need to talk about my brother's death that occurred when I was ten years old. I have not thought about this in years, but now it seems so fresh in my mind!" A forthright patient will supply his or her therapist with many important therapy issues from this last category.

When staff members review the Issue Identification section, they should carefully inquire what the patient would like to do with issues identified here. This is especially true for the first significant issue a patient discloses during Recovery Reflection. When the therapist notices nascent concerns, they are best discussed briefly in an individual session. The therapist might begin by stating, "I see you wrote about your brother's death. What would you like to do with this while you are with us?" By beginning with a nondirective approach, the therapist fosters trust, which in turn encourages further disclosures in Recovery Reflection and treatment in general.

Techniques to Ensure Patient Endorsement

How do we best ensure Recovery Reflection becomes a part of daily life? The answer is surprisingly simple. RMT asserts that setting up and executing Recovery Skills in a rhythm of recovery through each day entrains the mind to an alternate path from the patterns established by AddictBrain. This decreases the probability of relapse. In traditional treatment, each treatment day has a specified schedule. However, as treatment professionals, we often fail to describe why things are set up this way and how they are best incorporated into patients' lives once they have completed their initial course of treatment. Patients wind up walking through treatment accepting the schedule almost like a series of classes they attend at school. Once the "semester" is complete, they return to old habits. When working with RMT, it is critical to explain the purpose of each element of care, including Recovery Reflection. Daily self-reflection should become a habit that is practiced with specific worksheets until self-reflection is internalized.

Finally, I encourage curiosity. Which elements of Recovery Reflection seem the most helpful? Which of these are difficult to do? Which of these does a particular patient seem to repeatedly forget to complete or always remember? What clues does this provide a patient about him- or herself?

The logistics of managing these forms are simple but important. The staff requests and receives the previous day's form and thanks the patient for taking the time to complete it. They should never be thrown into an in-box. These worksheets contain valuable and personal information. If the staff does not treat them in this manner, the patients will not place value on the process either.

Recovery Skills for Domain B

The Recovery Skills for Domain B cover each of the five segments in the domain. Work in Domain B is extensive; therefore, it has the largest number of Recovery Skills. These skills establish specific behaviors, attitudes, and knowledge acquisition milestones that a patient develops through the course of his or her work in this domain. Each milestone represents a step along the path to recovery.

The Recovery Skills within each of the segments are most often accomplished in the order shown in the following sections. However, each of the segments need not be accomplished in any particular order. For example, if a patient feels uncomfortable with meditation, it can be addressed later in Domain B or even later in the treatment process. In Domain B, the patient should accomplish a majority of skills in the following five segments, but certain segments may prove unnecessary for patients with knowledge and demonstrated skill in a given area.

As in Domain A, patients and staff routinely complete an assessment form that tracks progress. The progress assessment form lists a domain's Recovery Skills with a three-point status rating (**B**egun, **I**ntermediate, and **C**ompleted). The patient completes the form first. This is followed by staff evaluation of the same form. Once complete, the patient and staff meet to reconcile discrepancies between the two evaluations. In this manner, the patient and his or her caregivers have a clear understanding the goals of and progress through treatment.

Segment 1: Addiction Awareness

In this segment, the patient explores the depth and breadth of her illness in a stepwise fashion with each competency deepening her awareness of the illness. A recovery skill in this segment is complete when the following tasks occur:

1. The patient develops a list of five triggers that produced substance use, five high-risk situations in which using occurred, and five negative consequences from substance use. This is presented in a group of her peers. Constructive feedback hones the list.

2. The patient constructs a list of falsehoods she told herself, her family, or friends about her substance use or its consequences. This list is presented in group therapy to begin the process of telling on the disease.

3. The patient completes an exhaustive list of the substances used during her life, noting the ages when each substance was used and how that use changed over time. This list is presented in assignment group therapy, building a corrective narration that completely and accurately describes her illness.

4. The patient completes a narrative addiction history using the elements from the above three assignments. This story is presented in assignment group therapy, increasing insight into the depth and breadth of her disorder.

Segment 2: Using Support Groups

In this segment, the patient learns how to use support group meetings to reinforce recovery. As always, patients who have effectively used support groups in the past may skip some or all skills in this segment. A recovery skill in this segment is complete when the following tasks occur:

1. The patient has participated in a role-play of a support group meeting and has identified personal barriers that prevent its effectiveness.

2. The patient has discussed barriers to support group in group therapy and has a plan to overcome the most difficult of them.

3. The patient reports and discusses the benefits of support group attendance (e.g., decrease shame, correct feelings of being uniquely defective, learn drug or alcohol refusal skills) and applies them to her own particular challenges.

Segment 3: Learning from Recovery Literature

The singular recovery skill in this segment is closest to a school assignment. The patient reads assigned material in twelve-step literature and completes forms that test a patient's understanding and challenge its integration into her recovery.

The recovery skill in this segment is complete when the patient has read the assigned reading, completed a worksheet designed to explore her comprehension, and exhibits self-reflection about the reading. In many centers, staff members or group therapy may discuss the worksheet for this segment to promote patient-to-patient learning.

Segment 4: Meditation

The Recovery Skills in this segment are specific to the practice of meditation. A recovery skill in this segment is complete when the following tasks occur:

1. The patient has participated actively in meditation training. She has determined if she is able to practice brief meditation. If unable, she has explored sound-based brainwave entrainment as an alternative.

2. The patient has successfully practiced meditation daily for two weeks and is able to evaluate whether or not it has proved helpful.

Segment 5: Recovery Reflection

The Recovery Skills in this segment relate to the effective use of Recovery Reflection. A recovery skill in this segment is complete when the following tasks occur:

1. The patient has participated in one training group on how to use Recovery Reflection as a self-exploration tool in recovery.

2. The patient has used the tool for two weeks and has responded to staff suggestions for its best use in recovery.

3. The patient has used Recovery Reflection to increase her commitment to self-care, hold herself accountable to discuss an issue in group therapy, note new or different emotions, and disclose self-deception.

Chapter Ten Notes

1.   ASAM, *The ASAM Criteria: Treatment Criteria for Addictive, Substance-related and Co-occuring Disorders*, Third ed., ed. David Mee-Lee (Carson City, NV: The Change Companies, 2013).

2.   G. E. Vaillant, "Alcoholics Anonymous: cult or cure?" *Australian and New Zealand Journal of Psychiatry* 39, no. 6 (2005): 431–36.

3.   R. Fiorentine, "After Drug Treatment: Are 12-Step Programs Effective in Maintaining Abstinence?" *Am J Drug Alcohol Abuse* 25, no. 1 (1999): 93–116.

4.   F. W. Chi, L. A. Kaskutas, S. Sterling, C. I. Campbell, and C. Weisner, "Twelve-Step affiliation and three-year substance use outcomes among adolescents: social support and religious service attendance as potential mediators," *Addiction* 104, no. 6 (2009): 927–39.

5.   R. B. Cutler and D. A. Fishbain, "Are alcoholism treatments effective? The Project MATCH data," *BMC Public Health* 5 (2005): 75.

6.   J. Allen, M. Mattson, W. Miller, J. Tonigan, G. Connors, R. Rychtarik, C. Randall, *et al.*, "Matching alcoholism treatments to client heterogeneity: Project MATCH posttreatment drinking outcomes," *J Stud Alcohol* 58, no. 1 (1997): 7–29.

7.   R. Kadden, J. Carbonari, M. Litt, S. Tonigan, and A. Zweben, "Matching alcoholism treatments to client heterogeneity: Project MATCH three-year drinking outcomes," *Alcohol Clin Exp Res* 22 (1998): 1300–11.

8.   P. C. Ouimette, J. W. Finney, and R. H. Moos, "Twelve-step and cognitive-behavioral treatment for substance abuse: a comparison of treatment effectiveness," *J Consult Clin Psychol* 65, no. 2 (Apr 1997): 230–40.

9.   S. A. Brown, S. V. Glasner-Edwards, S. R. Tate, J. R. McQuaid, J. Chalekian, and E. Granholm, "Integrated Cognitive Behavioral Therapy Versus Twelve-Step Facilitation Therapy for Substance-Dependent Adults with Depressive Disorders," *J Psychoactive Drugs* 38, no. 4 (2006): 449–60.

10. N. L. Cooney, T. F. Babor, C. C. DiClemente, and F. K. Del Boca, "Clinical and scientific implications of Project MATCH," *Treatment matching in alcoholism* (2003): 222–37.

11. See above, n. 4.

12. K. Humphreys, B. Mavisb, and B. Stöffelmayr, "Are twelve step programs appropriate for disenfranchised groups? Evidence from a study of posttreatment mutual help involvement," in *Prevention in Human Services*, 165–79, 1994.

13. A. Winzelberg and K. Humphreys, "Should patients' religiosity influence clinicians' referral to 12-step self-help groups? Evidence from a study of 3,018 male substance abuse patients," *J Consult Clin Psychol* 67, no. 5 (1999): 790–94.

14. M. Ferri, L. Amato, and M. Davoli, "Alcoholics Anonymous and other 12-step programmes for alcohol dependence," *Cochrane Database Syst Rev*, no. 3 (2006): CD005032.

15. J. S. Mausner, S. Kramer, and A. K. Bahn, *Epidemiology: An Introductory Text*, Second ed. (Philadelphia, PA: Saunders, 1985).

16. L. A. Kaskutas, "Alcoholics Anonymous Effectiveness: Faith Meets Science," *J Addict Dis* 28, no. 2 (2009): 145–57.

17. G. Glaser, "The irrationality of alcoholics anonymous," *The Atlantic* 2015, no. 4 (2015).

18.   J. F. Kelly, M. Magill, and R. L. Stout, "How do people recover from alcohol dependence? A systematic review of the research on mechanisms of behavior change in Alcoholics Anonymous," *Addiction Research & Theory* 17, no. 3 (2009): 236–59.

19.   L. A. Kaskutas, M. S. Subbaraman, J. Witbrodt, and S. E. Zemore, "Effectiveness of Making Alcoholics Anonymous Easier: a group format 12-step facilitation approach," *J Subst Abuse Treat* 37, no. 3 (2009): 228–39.

20.   J. Nowinski, S. Baker, and K. Carroll, *Twelve-Step Facilitation Therapy Manual* (Rockville, MD: U.S. Department of Health and Human Services, 1995).

21.   J. Witbrodt, J. Mertens, L. A. Kaskutas, J. Bond, F. Chi, and C. Weisner, "Do 12-step meeting attendance trajectories over 9 years predict abstinence?" *J Subst Abuse Treat* 43, no. 1 (2012): 30–43.

22.   L. A. Kaskutas, J. Bond, and L. A. Avalos, "7-year trajectories of Alcoholics Anonymous attendance and associations with treatment," *Addict Behav* 34, no. 12 (2009): 1029–35.

23.   J. F. Kelly, M. G. Myers, and S. A. Brown, "Do adolescents affiliate with 12-step groups? A multivariate process model of effects," *J Stud Alcohol* 63, no. 3 (2002): 293–304.

24.   M. P. Mundt, S. Parthasarathy, F. W. Chi, S. Sterling, and C. I. Campbell, "12-Step participation reduces medical use costs among adolescents with a history of alcohol and other drug treatment," *Drug Alcohol Depend* 126, no. 1–2 (2012): 124–30.

25.   See above, n. 12.

26.   C. Timko, A. Sutkowi, R. C. Cronkite, K. Makin-Byrd, and R. H. Moos, "Intensive referral to 12-step dual-focused mutual-help groups," *Drug Alcohol Depend* 118, no. 2–3 (2011): 194–201.

27.   See above, n. 13.

28.   A. B. Laudet and W. L. White, "An Exploratory Investigation of the Association between Clinicians' Attitudes toward Twelve-step Groups and Referral Rates," *Alcoholism Treatment Quarterly* 23, no. 1 (2005): 31–45.

29.   J. F. Kelly and R. Moos, "Dropout from 12-step self-help groups: Prevalence, predictors, and counteracting treatment influences," *J Subst Abuse Treat* 24, no. 3 (2003): 241–50.

30.   R. D. Weiss, M. L. Griffin, R. J. Gallop, L. M. Najavits, A. Frank, P. Crits-Christoph, M. E. Thase, *et al.*, "The effect of 12-step self-help group attendance and participation on drug use outcomes among cocaine-dependent patients," *Drug Alcohol Depend* 77, no. 2 (2005): 177–84.

31.   M. Galanter, *What is Alcoholics Anonymous?: A Path from Addiction to Recovery* (Oxford: Oxford University Press, 2016).

32.   C. Peterson and M. E. P. Seligman, *Character Strengths and Virtues: A Handbook and Classification* (Oxford: Oxford University Press, 2004).

33.   L. A. Kaskutas, L. Ammon, K. Delucchi, R. Room, J. Bond, and C. Weisner, "Alcoholics anonymous careers: patterns of AA involvement five years after treatment entry," *Alcohol Clin Exp Res* 29, no. 11 (2005): 1983–90.

34.   Ibid.

35.   The phrase "roll with the resistance" is borrowed from Motivational Interviewing. All addiction therapists should learn MI; its principles prove invaluable when working with addicted patients.

36.   W. L. Dunlop and J. L. Tracy, "The autobiography of addiction: autobiographical reasoning and psychological adjustment in abstinent alcoholics," *Memory* 21, no. 1 (2013): 64–78.

37.   M. Bean-Bayog, "Psychopathology Produced by Alcoholism," in *Psychopathology and Addictive Disorders*, ed.. R Meyer (New York: Guilford Press, 1986), 334–45.

38.   H. Adenauer, C. Catani, H. Gola, J. Keil, M. Ruf, M. Schauer, and F. Neuner, "Narrative exposure therapy for PTSD increases top-down processing of aversive stimuli - evidence from a randomized controlled treatment trial," *BMC Neurosci* 12 (2011): 127–27.

39.   Alcoholics Anonymous, *Alcoholics Anonymous*, Fourth Ed. (New York: A.A. World Services, 1976).

40.   Narcotics Anonymous, *Narcotics Anonymous*, Sixth Ed. (Van Nuys, CA: Narcotics Anonymous World Services, Inc., 2008).

41.   AA World Services, *Twelve Steps and Twelve Traditions* (New York: AA World Services, Inc., 2002).

42.   General Service Office of Alcoholics Anonymous, "The Elusive Origins of the Serenity Prayer," *Box 459* 38 (1992): 1–2.

43.   The increase in size and sensitivity of the gray matter indicates increased interconnection between nerve cells through dendritic growth (dendritic branching). The increased amount of gray matter may indicate an increase in the number of neurons as well.

44.   E. Luders, A. W. Toga, N. Lepore, and C. Gaser, "The underlying anatomical correlates of long-term meditation: Larger hippocampal and frontal volumes of gray matter," *Neuroimage* 45, no. 3 (2009): 672–78.

45.   V. L. Ives-Deliperi, M. Solms, and E. M. Meintjes, "The neural substrates of mindfulness: an fMRI investigation," *Soc Neurosci* 6, no. 3 (2011): 231–42.

46   A. Lutz, J. Brefczynski-Lewis, T. Johnstone, and R. J. Davidson, "Regulation of the neural circuitry of emotion by compassion meditation: effects of meditative expertise," *PLoS One* 3, no. 3 (2008): e1897.

47.   V. A. Taylor, J. Grant, V. Daneault, G. Scavone, E. Breton, S. Roffe-Vidal, J. Courtemanche, A. S. Lavarenne, and M. Beauregard, "Impact of mindfulness on the neural responses to emotional pictures in experienced and beginner meditators." *Neuroimage* 57, no. 4 (2011): 1524–33.

48.   See above, n. 46.

49.   M. Ricard, A. Lutz, and R. J. Davidson, "Mind of the meditator," *Sci Am* 311, no. 5 (2014): 38–45.

50.   Y. Y. Tang, B. K. Holzel, and M. I. Posner, "The neuroscience of mindfulness meditation," *Nat Rev Neurosci* 16, no. 4 (Apr 2015): 213–25.

51.   R. J. Davidson, J. Kabat-Zinn, J. Schumacher, M. Rosenkranz, D. Muller, S. F. Santorelli, F. Urbanowski, *et al.*, "Alterations in brain and immune function produced by mindfulness meditation," *Psychosom Med* 65, no. 4 (2003): 564–70.

52.   B. E. Carlson and H. Larkin, "Meditation as a Coping Intervention for Treatment of Addiction," *Journal of Religion & Spirituality in Social Work: Social Thought* 28, no. 4 (2009): 379–92.

53.   A. Zgierska, D. Rabago, M. Zuelsdorff, C. Coe, M. Miller, and M. Fleming, "Mindfulness Meditation for Alcohol Relapse Prevention: A Feasibility Pilot Study," *J Addict Med* 2, no. 3 (2008): 165–73.

54.   P. Milz, A. Theodoropoulou, S. Tei, P. L. Faber, K. Kochi, and D. Lehmann, "P02-347- Common EEG spectral power characteristics during meditation in five meditation traditions," *European Psychiatry* 26, Supplement 1 (2011): 943.

55. T. N. Hanh, *The Miracle of Mindfulness: An Introduction to the Practice of Meditation* (Boston, MA: Beacon Press, 1976).

56. See above, n. 52.

57. See above, n. 53.

58. See above, n. 55.

59. G. A. Marlatt and N. Chawla, "Meditation and Alcohol Use," *South Med J* 100, no. 4 (2007): 451–53.

60. D. H. Angres, *Positive Sobriety* (CreateSpace Independent Publishing Platform, 2012).

61. D. Lama, *Stages of Meditation* (Boulder, CO: Snow Lion Publications, 2001).

62. J. Kornfield, *Meditation for Beginners* (New York: Bantam Books, 2005).

63. G. Oster, "Auditory Beats in the Brain," *Sci Am* 229, no. 4 (1973): 94–102.

64. BrainSync (http://www.brainsync.com/) and the Monroe Institute's HemiSync (http://www.hemi-sync.com/) are but a few of the available options.

65. P. J. Flores, *Addiction as an Attachment Disorder* (Oxford: Jason Aronson, Inc., 2004).

66. Psychotherapist and founder of psychomotor psychotherapy Albert Pesso would go even further. His theory of ego formation states that the formation of personality occurs at the interface of connectedness between a child and his or her parents and caregivers. Touching, holding, hugging, and nurturing literally create the ego, the self-reflective, and self-understanding parts of our evolving brain.

CHAPTER ELEVEN

Domain C: Emotional Awareness and Resilience

The sense of unhappiness is so much easier to
convey than that of happiness. In misery, we seem
aware of our own existence ... But happiness
annihilates us: we lose our identity.

GRAHAM GREENE

In this chapter, I will describe the steps to emotional awareness and resilience. In many ways, this is a lifelong quest, and one that is never perfected. For many, entering recovery is the start of that quest. Each individual has his or her own particular emotional blocks and difficulties and unique path to healing. The richest and most meaningful life results from an ability to recognize and live in the presence of every deep emotional experience. Sharing together in compassionate connection ensures that one's life is worth living. Addiction robs those afflicted of this experience and leaves the addicted individual hollow, searching, and unsatisfied and with snippets of chemically induced emotions. Abstinence and subsequent recovery are often painful. Teaching patients to sit with uncomfortable emotions is crucial to a robust recovery. When those with addiction describe their turmoil in rich detail, bemoaning the emotional agony, the therapist best responds by congratulating them for all the "heavy lifting" that is a part of the recovery journey.

Emotions are central to what it means to be a human being. Our feelings color and flavor our daily lives, providing meaning and value to our existence. As much as emotions are a part of our joy, they are also at the core of our suffering. Few claim to be at peace with their feelings. Most people spend a considerable portion of their waking life fighting battles with their internal emotional world. Others have learned, unconsciously or consciously, to constrict their emotional response in an effort to avoid painful feelings. Some displace or act out their emotions to avoid having to sit in their presence. Indeed, it is the rare individual who can live his or her emotional life to the fullest in a world rich with emotion—complex and subtle yet peaceful and centered at the same time.

AddictBrain and Emotions

RecoveryMind Training asserts that AddictBrain has two separate agendas regarding emotions. The first agenda is capturing all emotional experience inside of the chemical use and addiction-related behaviors. Emotions produce value in our life; they validate what is important and push aside what is not. As addiction develops, AddictBrain reroutes emotional experience. Drug hunger, drug seeking, the ritual of alcohol and other drug consumption, and the consequences of that use rewire the brain, developing deep emotional connections with the planning, procurement, and use of addicting substances.

Many individuals with alcohol use disorder say, "I knew after my first drink that I was in love." Even when addiction reaches its wretched dead end, such emotions sustain the individual's deep attachment. As one patient put it, "I had a bad marriage to lady cocaine; she would brutalize me every time I was with her but drew me back by promising she would love me the next time. Foolish me, I kept believing it."

AddictBrain can hold emotions unto itself to ensure its survival. It matters not as to whether the feelings are pleasant or unpleasant.

Emotions produce meaning, and AddictBrain is constantly reinforcing the importance of the addiction and profundity of the addiction experience by culling emotions unto itself. The outside world becomes flat and gray. The internal cacophony of addiction seems vital and rich with meaning.

The second AddictBrain agenda regarding feelings is shifting them away from the outside world. The victim's emotional connection to family and life goals fades away, and they become pale and distant in comparison to the addiction experience. As this shift occurs, the interior world created by addiction expands in importance. As one individual explained, "I always knew on some level I was excluding my husband and children. After a time, however, it seemed as if they were calling to me from the other side of a leaded glass door. I could see them waving their hands frantically at me, hoping to reach me, but I could not hear what they were saying or feel their anguish."

Addicted or not, everyone is at odds with their emotions from time to time. Addicted people do not corner the market on emotional suffering. Dependent individuals do have one critical difference from non-addicted individuals regarding their emotions. Those not addicted do not relapse into a maelstrom on self-destructive chemical use when they suffer at the hand of disturbing emotions. On the other hand, individuals with substance use disorders fall back into this maelstrom when they are unable to tolerate disquieting emotion. For this reason alone, such individuals must learn to experience, accept, and prevent maladaptive responses to their emotions. To prevent relapse, the addicted individual must be *more* emotionally resilient than their non-addicted friends and relatives.

Commonly, the qualities of an individual's maladaptive emotional responses predate the onset of his or her addiction disorder. In the early stages of the illness, addiction takes hold of these responses; it uses preexisting emotional discord for its own ends. AddictBrain triggers and exaggerates maladaptive emotional patterns, twisting them in a manner that ensures its own survival. Once addiction is full-blown, minor difficulties create an emotional frenzy. The patient acts like an adolescent, prepubescent, or child. He is unable to sit with a minor emotional discomfort, acting out emotions, projecting them on others, or constantly steaming like an emotional pressure cooker.

One common cultural myth, promoted by modern Western cultures, is that *feeling* better, even for a moment, means we are *doing* better. Our cultural ethos is aimed at pleasure; if we are having fun right now, it means we are succeeding. We live in a culture of the instant fix. Happiness in the moment is success; unhappiness or emotional strife is failure. AddictBrain loves this concept. It promises pleasure and chides the person with drug use disorder for putting off the pleasure of ingesting drugs or alcohol. By the time patients arrive in treatment, they desperately want to feel better. Haven't they suffered enough at the hands of their disease? When treatment providers ask such patients to dig down deep into their past, unearth years of emotional pain, and wallow in it until their recovery becomes meaningful, patients rebel. "Wait a minute, I came here because I wanted to feel better!" they shout.

After years of trying to perfect the instant fix—the feel good in a bottle—the emotional work of recovery is a hard sell to most people with substance use disorders. It is our job as addiction treatment professionals to help patients accept the hard truth that the road to recovery is long and painful at times. There are no quick fixes. Deeper joy will come from the pursuit of self-reconciliation. And, most importantly, AddictBrain's siren song of chemical pleasure is subterfuge and must be ignored.

Addiction and Other Mental Health Problems

Emotional resilience proves especially difficult for those who suffer from psychiatric disorders or mental health problems in addition to their addiction. The most common psychiatric conditions that co-occur with addiction are mood disorders—unipolar and bipolar—and anxiety disorders. I briefly discussed the interplay between mood disorders and addiction in Chapter Two; however, its importance demands additional discussion here.

The mind of *Homo sapiens* constantly searches for the cause of any effect. If two things occur at the same time, the discriminating engine inside our brain automatically labels one as the "cause" and the other as the "effect." This tendency is strengthened even when two events have the weakest relationship.[1] Such is the case with addiction and other psychiatric disorders. When a new client, who has depression and addiction, comes under your care, it is a natural tendency to try to discern which disorder is the "cause" and which is the "effect." A mental health professional who specializes in depression would tend to see addiction as being "caused" by depression. A professional who specializes in addiction tends to see depression as being "caused" by the patient's addiction disorder. This raging battle of ideology is at best irrelevant and at worst detrimental to the health of our clients.

RecoveryMind Training takes the stand that addiction, including all its manifestations, and other mental health problems are not related by cause and effect. This is not to say there is no relationship between them. Both conditions color and contribute to the other. Depression or anxiety exacerbates addiction and vice versa. RMT believes both conditions need to be aggressively treated—preferably simultaneously—for the best overall prognosis. At the same time, it is dangerous and counterproductive to tell an addicted patient that his addiction was caused by his depressive disorder or his depressive disorder was caused by addiction. Such a proclamation immediately drives a patient to dangerous conclusions in either instance. For example, a patient could conclude, "Because my depression caused my addiction, I should be able to drink alcohol once my depression improves." Or if a therapist implies that the patient's substance use caused depression, the patient could conversely conclude, "If my addiction made me depressed, once I have a few weeks of abstinence, I can stop taking my antidepressant medications."

RecoveryMind Training agrees that psychiatric conditions and addiction illnesses are deeply intertwined; both color and intensify the other. If a patient has a significant addiction disorder and a co-occurring mood (or anxiety) disorder, providers must assiduously avoid discussions that attempt to ascertain which disease is *primary*. Once a provider defines one illness as primary and causative of the other, he unintentionally gives short shrift to the other. It is best to see *neither* condition as causative of the other.

Some professionals rely on the presence of depression symptoms that existed prior to substance use (so-called premorbid symptoms) to differentiate a primary mood disorder from a substance-induced mood disorder. I have found this distinction to be sophomoric and distorted by an all too common human trait called "revisionist history." Revisionist history is the peculiar refactoring of our past that occurs every time we reconsider our present situation. Even at our best, our autobiographical memory is deeply flawed. Following addicted patients for years has taught me that I cannot predict which patients who arrive in treatment with symptoms of depression or anxiety require long-term treatment for these conditions and which I will later discover never had the diagnosis in the first place.

Most modern medications used to treat mood or anxiety disorders today have little to no addiction liability; therefore, the default approach is to treat the patient who presents with significant mood or anxiety symptoms as if he or she has the full disorder—to assume it is not a byproduct of addiction. At the same time, the physician should clearly state that the jury is still out on a final diagnosis; time will tell. This may result in overtreating depression and anxiety disorders, but it prevents the more dangerous situation: missing subtle comorbid conditions that disrupt early recovery.

A patient with alcohol use disorder may enter treatment complaining that her anxiety caused her to drink prior to social functions. Some staff members think she has an anxiety disorder; others think her addiction is at the root of the anxiety complaints. In either case, she is best treated with a selective serotonin reuptake inhibitor (SSRI) or other safe medication during treatment. Her social anxiety improves. After her initial treatment dose, she returns home and notes her anxiety is almost non-existent. Over time, her physician tapers and discontinues the SSRI, and she reports she has only occasional mild symptoms of social anxiety. Was this improvement because she has completed detoxification and post-acute withdrawal? Is it because of the medication? Is it because she addressed dishonesties in her marriage? Is it because she learned how to speak in group therapy and support group meetings? The diagnosis, when all is said and done, frequently remains unclear. Over time, it often becomes irrelevant.

A second co-occurring problem in addicted patients is wounding caused by past emotional, physical, sexual, or spiritual trauma. In the first stages of addiction treatment, patients and therapists need to proceed slowly and cautiously when unearthing past trauma. Looking over the long haul, past traumas should be addressed to ensure the most robust and joyful recovery. The pacing of this work depends on many factors, including the level of physical protection from relapse, the emotional safety in the treatment environment, and the patient's emotional stability. A deft hand is important here. The skilled therapist must learn when it is best to delay trauma exploration and when it is best to proceed. If trauma psychotherapy occurs too soon, the therapist runs the risk of triggering addiction relapse. In certain cases, however, a patient may arrive in a safe treatment setting with an intransigent need to explore a long suppressed hurt. In such cases, staff members and the patient should work together to construct therapeutic safety and protection from relapse. Trauma therapy should proceed as soon as both are in place. Although the subtleties and details of this process are beyond the scope of this text, all therapists should validate the patient's emotional unrest and recognize the power of trauma-induced relapse triggers.

Many other psychiatric problems are associated with addiction. Attention deficit disorder, anorexia and bulimia nervosa, binge eating disorders, sexual compulsivity, and a host of other conditions are associated with addictive disease. A large proportion of the chronically mentally ill also suffer from substance abuse disorders. Patients with schizophrenia and certain personality disorders are at risk for substance dependence. Each of these illnesses needs to be aggressively treated simultaneously if one hopes to attain recovery. All addiction programs should have a close relationship with an addiction psychiatrist and psychologists who specialize in such psychiatric disorders. In the best addiction programs, psychiatric care is seamlessly integrated into day-to-day care.

The Science of Emotion

The scientific study of emotions and their relation to facial expression has its roots in Charles Darwin's treatise *The Expression of Emotions in Man and Animals*.[2] Darwin postulated that emotions are universal to primates and man and are expressed through physical movement. When people have an experience they later describe as "emotional," muscle movement occurs. Most of this movement is localized to the face. The facial movements associated with specific emotions is highly cross-cultural.[3] Small, subtle, and often short-lived facial movements communicate our emotions to those around us. This basic communication is aimed outward. Strangely enough, as our sensory system picks up these muscle changes they also provide sensory feedback that helps us recognize our own feelings.[4, 5] Emotions also change vocal tonality. The lack of facial and vocal input explains why we often misinterpret brief written correspondence and the need for emoticons in text messages and email. As therapists, one of our primary jobs is reading nascent feelings in our patients, often before they recognize those emotions for themselves.

Limbic thought (emotion) has several characteristics that differentiate it from cortical thought.[6] When we experience a strong emotion, it seems timeless ("I have felt this way forever and I will go on feeling this way for eternity.") Limbic activity is disconnected with the clocks naturally attached to semantic memory. This sense of timelessness is especially disturbing when emotions are difficult. When overcome by sorrow, it seems as if we have always felt its torment. When in the middle of the rising tide of grief, it seems to stretch forward to the end of time. When our emotions are acknowledged as feelings—become part of our conscious experience—[7,8] the illusion of timelessness is invariably attached to them. Once the most intense parts of the experience subside, we look back on our tears of grief and note that they lasted for minutes, not hours or days. Such episodes of grief recur and in the midst of each new episode, they too seem to last forever—the illusion is impossible to shake. Emotions are also part of cravings, thus the sense of timelessness traps the addicted individual when cravings occur. A craving seems like it will continue forever, and the only way out is to use more chemicals. Just as the phrase "this too shall pass" helps with the anguish of grief, acknowledging this illusion helps one ride through a craving episode.

A second characteristic of emotional experience is urgency. Emotions produced by the limbic brain are hardwired to produce action. When we experience an emotion, it is accompanied by an urge or impulse to move or react. When overcome by anger or loss, we feel compelled to *do* something about it. We experience an urgency to act or change how we feel, which is the perfect formula for relapse or continued use.

There are many ways of categorizing emotions. Some cognitive neuroscientists[9] suggest that we have seven fundamental emotions, expressed on the face in characteristic ways. This theory has its critics,[10] but proves helpful clinically. The following is one such list of discrete emotions:

1. **Happiness/Joy:** A natural smile produces wrinkles around the eyes, whereas the social smile only engages the mouth. In a genuine smile, the area between the eyebrow and the eye decreases, and the cheeks rise, producing crow's feet.

2. **Surprise:** Involves the raising of the eyebrows and eyelids and sometimes a dropping of the jaw.

3. **Contempt:** This is identified by a half-smile, a half-dimple, and/ or a one-sided rise in the lip.

4. **Sadness:** The most reliable indicator of sadness is the raising of the inner corners of the eyebrows.
5. **Fear:** Fear is similar to surprise; however, the brow lowers in fear.
6. **Disgust:** Recognized most by the wrinkling of the nose or the raising of the upper lip.
7. **Anger:** The main ingredients of anger include the lowering of the eyebrows and raising and tightening of the eyelids. This can also include any number of other factors such as clenching the jaw, gritting teeth, or tightening the lips.

Beyond these basic emotions, there are many schemes for outlining and relating emotional states. One system, developed by psychologist Robert Plutchik, PhD,[11] is shown diagrammatically in Figure 11.1. When teaching patients emotional awareness and accuracy, I like to use a long list of feeling words, such as the Feelings Inventory provided by the Center for Nonviolent Communication.[12]

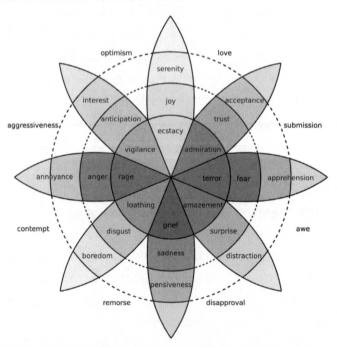

Figure 11.1 - The Emotion Categories of Plutchik

Western society tends to equate rationality and wisdom with the dispassionate intellect. When we say, "I know how it feels, but you really should make the best choice anyway," we place our emotions in a subservient role. We can trace this bias back to the Greek Stoics who placed reason above emotion.[13] In the latter part of the twentieth century, the concept that intelligence is limited to cognition was called into question.[14]

RecoveryMind Training incorporates newer models of intelligence that combine the rational intellect with the wisdom from intuitive and emotional thought. Antonio Damasio, MD, PhD, provided a profound and science-based deconstruction of the false reason/emotion dichotomy in his 1994 book, *Descartes' Error: Emotion, Reason, and the Human Brain.*[15] His treatise, backed by neuroscience, suggests the brain uses a vast collection of emotional and somatic representations when making the best life decisions. His work is consistent with more recent developments in psychology that champion the belief that a combination of emotional intelligence and cognitive skills create the healthiest long-term decisions.

In contrast, those with substance use disorders wind up acting out upon the whim of false and distorted emotional states. AddictBrain manufactures a whole host of emotional responses that ensure its survival—to the detriment of the addicted individual. Every one of us working in the addiction field has had patients who swear, "My husband drives me to drink." Once sober that same individual may discover her husband, although flawed, is committed to strengthen their bond and support her recovery.

Many of the techniques used in Domain C are based upon the work of John D. Mayer, PhD, Peter Salovey, PhD, and David R. Caruso, PhD. These psychologists proposed the concept of "Emotional Intelligence" (EI) in the 1990s.[16, 17] They proposed that emotional intelligence is a standard type of intelligence.[18] The concept was popularized by a best-selling book by Daniel Goleman in 2006.[19] Subsequent public interest in this concept overgeneralized its impact and importance, and emotional intelligence became a passing fad.[20] Nonetheless, central concepts in EI prove helpful in addiction treatment.[21] RecoveryMind Training implements the central components of the original EI model, which states emotional intelligence is a skill that everyone can learn to varying degrees of proficiency. This model states that emotional intelligence helps us

- Accurately perceive emotions in oneself and others;
- Regulate emotional states effectively;[22]
- Use emotions to facilitate thinking and maximize properly prioritized and well-rounded solutions to life's problems. This includes flexible planning, creative thinking, redirecting attention when needed, and motivating toward important goals;[23]
- Understand emotional meanings, connecting them to interpersonal connection and awareness of attitudes and perceptions of others. This skill is important for empathy.

Inherent in EI is the notion that the emotional content of our memory and current emotional state are vital to a healthy, meaningful life. RMT adds to this, stating that a successful recovery is maximized when we accurately perceive and regulate our emotions and combine emotional content with rational thought when making decisions about recovery. Work in Domain C is aimed at helping those with substance use disorders acquire emotional intelligence, improving chances of a solid recovery and a rich, fulfilling life.

Finally, part of Domain C could be conceptualized as a simplified version of several components of Dialectical Behavioral Therapy (DBT).[24, 25] This is not a coincidence. Much of the fine-tuning of RMT occurred in a center that housed a robust DBT program, which heavily influenced the concepts contained in Domain C. I think of Domain C as an abbreviated version of DBT, dissimilar in that it is applicable to all addiction patients. In addition, work in Domain C leads to a critical appreciation of how AddictBrain alters emotional states and feelings, creating distorted and false emotions that the addiction's hapless victim misinterprets as real and significant.

The Four Segments of Domain C

I have divided Domain C into four segments, knowing that with each client the work will not be linear or predictable. Any given patient may be assigned work in one or more of these segments, based on need. The goal of Segment 1 is the correct identification of one's own emotions. Segment 2 focuses on identifying emotions in others. In Segment 3, a patient works to strengthen his emotional resilience; that is, learning how to sit with, accept, and lean into emotions as they occur throughout daily life. In Segment 4, a patient works on identifying how AddictBrain produces and alters certain emotional states for its own benefit. As with everything that has to do with feelings, your client's progress will occur in fits and starts; slow improvement will be peppered by periods of regression.

A hackneyed and stereotypical statement is "Men have problems identifying emotions, and women have problems with emotional resiliency." In reality, each patient or client is different. Men often have problems with emotional resilience once they discover they have emotions. Individuals with substance use disorders of both sexes often repress, act out, or project emotions onto others. In the area of emotional health, every human being has at least some difficulty.

When beginning work in Domain C, I commonly hear, "Why do I need to know more about my feelings? I know a lot of people who would not know a feeling if it hit them in the face. They don't have problems with addiction." To this I respond, "That is true, many people lead successful lives without ever developing emotional familiarity and agility, but *they* are not addicted. A friendly relationship with your feelings strengthens recovery and helps prevent relapse. People with addiction disorders do not have the luxury of emotional ignorance."

Segment 1: Emotional Self-Awareness

Before you go further here, you may want to refer to the section about the triune brain in Chapter Five and refresh your memory about the limbic area. Although emotions are created by interactions between many parts of the brain,[26] the limbic area stands at the center of our emotional life. Feelings are simply the thinking that occurs in our limbic brain. Remember, the limbic area of the brain operates in a parallel process with limited control from our conscious cortex. Feeling states come and go, often without regard to the active thought that commands our attention. It is all too human to register an overheard, fleeting spiteful comment on a subliminal level. It slips past our notice, and we return to our previous ongoing activity. Later, we feel sad or angry but remain at a loss as to why. The insensitive comment, barely acknowledged by our conscious brain, churns about in our limbic area only to surface minutes or even hours later, perhaps coloring an unrelated event. The parallel and loosely connected processes in the limbic and cortical brain create a cacophony of thoughts, memories, and emotions that characterize human existence.

Most people, those with addiction included, are thrashed to and fro by their emotional brain. Individuals with alcohol use disorder try in vain to control their emotions, ignore them, or drink them away. Many have said, "I don't have a problem with my feelings; I simply want to manage which ones come at what time. Oh, and make them go away sometimes as well." This is hopeless folly. Human beings have only a few stereotypical ways of managing their emotions. Each particular patient will have his or her preferred mechanisms of defense. Our job as therapists is to help our patients recognize, relinquish control, sit in the presence of, and experience their emotions for what they are. We should discover each patient's mode of feelings management, dismantle his maladaptive responses, and teach him to live with his limbic brain. When a powerful sorrow appears, it is best to lean into the experience rather than running away.

Over the years, I have noted that patients who develop addiction disorders have a wide variety of self-knowledge regarding their emotional states. At one end of the spectrum, some patients are unable to recognize feeling states or name them when they emerge. When an emotion occurs in such a person, she can only summon a vague descriptor such as "upset" or "uneasy." The technical term for this inability to know or name feeling states—borrowed from the analytic literature—is **alexithymia**.[27] Such individuals should spend as much time as needed to develop the first recovery skill in Domain C to the best of their ability.

At the other end of the spectrum, you may have patients who constantly describe their emotional states—voluble and hectic—and are unable to self-regulate, but they are always willing and able to describe their experiences with piercing accuracy. Such individuals can bypass work in Segment 1. Another subset of patients is able to identify their own feelings, but they constantly misread what others are experiencing. These individuals do not need work in Segment 1 but do need to learn how to identify emotions correctly in others.

For those who suffer from varying degrees of alexithymia, Segment 1 begins by learning one's own feeling states as they occur. During a therapeutic encounter, when the therapist senses emotions in such a patient, the therapist gently interrupts the therapeutic process, asking, "What are you feeling right now?" Each time a therapist inquires about or makes note of feeling states, they become more real as the individual searches to name and know them. Individuals who are unable to put one or more feeling words to their situation should be given a "feelings chart" or similar aid that helps them assign words to their internal experience. Not surprisingly, these aids always show cartoonlike faces depicting emotions. Caricatures exaggerate subtle facial movements that signal emerging emotions, dragging them into conscious awareness.

Therapy with patients who suffer from larger degrees of emotional disconnect may proceed slowly. They often misconstrue or appear completely unaware of others emotions. Patients who suffer from a deep disconnect from their emotional states (and are not too far along the autism spectrum disorder) may benefit from more specific training in recognizing affect.[28] Here is a brief example:

> *In group therapy, Judy describes the terror she experienced during her preteen years when her father would come home intoxicated. Although she was rarely the object of her father's rage, she knew her mother frequently ran the risk of physical injury. In her childhood, she delayed going to bed so she could be at her mother's side should her father return home in a violent state. During the group session, she enumerates the delay tactics and excuses she would push upon her mother so that she could be readily at hand. As she moves into describing one particularly disturbing event, the group falls into silence but remains sharply attentive. The group leader pauses at the end of her story, allowing all to experience deep compassion for Judy. After a long pause, the therapist, carefully studying each face within the room, asks, "How does Judy's story touch each of you?" Members reflect upon times in their life when they experienced fear or worried about the safety of loved ones. Several patients share their feelings, relating them to Judy's past. Out of the corner of her eye, the therapist notes intense, almost violent ticks rolling across the face of Randall, another group member. Randall is tight lipped and silent. The leader gently prods Randall, "Something important is happening to you right now, Randall. Are you willing to talk about it?"*

In this instance, the group leader is reading strong emotions moving across Randall's face. The therapist may not know exactly what Randall is feeling or experiencing, but she does recognize something important. Responding to these subtle movements, the group leader urges Randall's disclosure. In doing so, the leader is reconnecting Randall to his emotional world. The therapist draws Randall's attention to his feelings, using subtle clues that appear on his face. These movements can be quick, subtle, and indistinct. A talented therapist, having observed patients over many years, can often read such signals and create a hypothesis about his internal emotional world. The therapist interrupts the ongoing group process, encouraging Randall to sit quietly and pay attention to his body. Is there tightness across the chest? Is there a sense of hollowness in the belly? Are the muscles in his legs twitching as if to jump and run from the room? Are his eyes becoming moist? Is there fullness in his head or are his thoughts spinning wildly out of control? Each of these questions are looking for the correlates of emotions, reconnecting the noticing cortical brain to the emotional brain.

AddictBrain reaps the benefits of patients who are deeply disconnected from their emotions. Such individuals report the only time they feel alive is when they are using alcohol or other drugs. In such cases, using these substances fabricates chemically induced emotions; in moments of intoxication, they feel alive. The emptiness produced by alexithymia pressures such individuals to relapse "in order to feel anything." Relapse can also occur when such individuals misread others, producing unintended conflicts. Many such patients feel alone and misunderstood simply because they cannot connect with others through interlacing feeling states. Because of this disconnect, they fall back on the only friend they know: the substances they use. AddictBrain uses the low emotional intelligence and blunted emotional experience to ensure its own survival.

RecoveryMind Training has specific Recovery Skills for patients who have difficulty recognizing and correctly naming their own emotions. This begins with Recovery Reflection (see Chapter Ten), where patients record emotions experienced throughout the day. Within their journal, they comment on feeling states that were surprising, distressing, or difficult. Patients are also encouraged to notice and name pleasure and joy when it occurs. RMT encourages patients to compare the feelings they catalog on a given day with those they have experienced in previous days. Such a comparison underscores how feelings are slapdash and ephemeral. Recurrent emotional themes are identified for additional exploration in individual or group therapy.

Patients who have assignments in Segment 1 complete an emotional recognition worksheet and describe their past emotions in group therapy. Such a worksheet is designed to delineate feelings that are common and uncommon, comfortable and not. The process of reviewing emotions increases awareness. This is followed by repeated attempts to identify emotions in ongoing therapy sessions.

Segment 2: Identifying Emotions Correctly in Others

Once patients have learned to recognize their own emotions as they occur, they should turn their gaze outward, learning to identify feelings in others. Knowing what others feel is the first step in building empathic connection. AddictBrain is well served by an inability to read the emotions of others. If the addicted individual has lost the ability to experience empathy with friends and family, he or she can walk all over them without concern or regret. This sustains the addiction illness. In a given individual, it is unclear if AddictBrain disconnects existing empathy when constructing an addiction disorder or if this defect proceeds the onset of the disease. Whatever the mechanism, addicts seem to walk all over friends and family. This aspect is so striking that it led early theorists to diagnose all addicted individuals as sociopaths. In reality, the vast majority of addiction patients, once they relearn empathy skills, shift rapidly into a meaningful connection with friends and family; the previously misdiagnosed "sociopathy" disappears.

Note there are three subtypes of individuals who have difficulty reading the emotions of others. The first is the individual with varying levels of alexithymia. We have discussed them previously. A second type of patient recognizes his or her own feelings but misread others. Many in this second group are "strong feelers." If their emotional experience is strong, they may be unable to see past their own affect turmoil. They rarely require training in identifying internal emotional states. Therefore, this second group need not complete tasks in Segment 1; they already have such skills. Instead, individuals in this group should concentrate their Domain C efforts in Segments 2 and 3 (emotional resilience). The third group, like the second, also includes strong feelers; however, individuals in this group project their feelings onto others. Although the origins of their difficulties differ, all three groups need work in Segment 2, identifying emotions correctly in others.

A smaller subset of the "strong feelers" suffers from a more extreme malady. This group sits in a tiny rowboat riding out violent storms created by a roiling emotional discharge—rising, falling, and always on the verge of capsizing. Individuals in this group are often diagnosed as having borderline personality disorder. AddictBrain relishes such chaos and uses the emotional upheaval as a reason to continue substance use. Unlike alexithymic patients who need to expand their emotional bandwidth, these individuals must temper and regulate feeling states. Recovery requires them to re-catalog negative feeling as noncatastrophic. Their goal is to ride the wave of their emotions without using their drug of choice. Such individuals benefit greatly from Dialectical Behavioral Therapy (DBT)[29] or should at least complete Recovery Skills in Segment 3. All components of DBT, including mindfulness meditation and distress tolerance, help such individuals learn to regulate their emotions without resorting to drugs and alcohol.

Of course, not every addicted individual lies on either of these two extremes of the bell curve of emotions management. All patients should be studied as to their particular relationship with their emotional world, and, once this is known, the proper RecoveryMind skills should be acquired. For decades, group therapy has been seen as the singular best modality for the treatment of addiction. Group therapy is effective for many reasons, but among the most important is to correct emotional problems with identification of emotions and the interpersonal attachment that comes from this knowledge.

Let's continue the session described previously, looking for empathetic connection in the group process.

> *As Randall describes his own childhood with an alcoholic*
> *father, his head drops forward, he looks to the floor, and a*
> *few tears squeak out of the edges of his eyes. He continues*
> *to look down, ashamed of his weakness and tears. The*
> *therapist encourages others to remain quiet, increasing the*
> *sweet tension that emerges out of shared sorrow. Sensing*
> *Randall has gone as far as he is able to go in that session,*
> *she turns to the group quietly and ask, "What do others see*
> *in Randall at this moment and how does that affect you?"*
> *Several patients describe sadness and loss. One patient*
> *quietly sighs and responds, "When Judy talked about her*
> *childhood, I thought of the times I needed protection as*
> *a girl. Then when Randall described his own problems, I*
> *remembered many more things that I had pushed aside*
> *for most of my adult life. If Randall is like me, maybe he is*
> *longing for the things he needed but never received."*

When another group member describes Judy and Randall's feelings, they reactivate lost brain circuits responsible for empathy. Empathic connection overthrows AddictBrain's selfish agenda. If another member, David, misconstrues shared group emotions, the therapist gently takes a poll of group consensus correcting and reconnecting his emotional sensitivity. When David is off track, the therapist can pursue his difficulty in knowing shared feelings or continue to amplify and resonate the sorrow brought forth by Judy's story and Randall's inchoate emotional response. In a group session focused on increasing interpersonal emotional awareness, the therapist often chooses to interrupt group process by asking patients to interpret emotions in others. In more advanced groups, a therapist may choose to amplify and deepen the sorrow, expanding each patient's ability to sit with painful emotions without resorting to chemical use.

Patients share their feeling journals within the group, exploring whether or not their perceived emotions are congruent with emotions expressed to their peers. It is not uncommon for an addicted patient to repeatedly report one emotion (e.g., sadness) only to have his peers report that he exudes another (e.g., anger).

Segment 3: Development of Emotional Resilience

The third segment in Domain C deals with emotional resilience. The components of emotional resilience for those addicted are the same as for every other member of the human race. Emotional resilience allows one to

- Experience a full range of emotions without having to suppress, repress, act them out, or use chemicals in reaction to them;
- Permit feelings to color his or her life experiences and, at the same time, prevent those feelings from producing knee-jerk reactions that disrupt personal goals or life direction;
- Set aside judgments about emotions. Anger, disgust, compassion, love, and anguish are neither good nor bad;
- Accept that he or she cannot preferentially eliminate uncomfortable emotions without destroying the more pleasant ones;
- Connect with others through all emotional states, including the so-called "negative" emotions;
- Experience pleasure without the use of chemicals or addictive behaviors;
- Accept that he or she will always fail at achieving happiness if he or she deliberately seeks it (as in substance use).[30] Happiness is a byproduct of a well-lived life.[31]

This list is certainly a best-case scenario. We might set more humble goals at first, such as "be able to experience emotional states without self-harm or addiction relapse." For those readers who teach or incorporate DBT into their work with clients, you may consider Segment 3 of Domain C to be "DBT-lite." I have incorporated some of the skills from Dr. Linehan's powerful set of skills into this section. If you are already familiar with DBT, you have more than enough training to teach the Recovery Skills in this segment. The DBT concept of Wise Mind is somewhat analogous to RecoveryMind. However, in the case of RecoveryMind, we have the added burden of fighting brain circuits that are distorted and redirected by substance use. Please refer to training in DBT for more information.

The first skill in Segment 3 is mindfulness meditation. In patients with an identified need to bolster emotional resilience, staff members should spend extra effort maximizing the meditation practice that was introduced in Domain B. Meditation provides a respite from the emotional roil that accompanies the activation of the default mode network (see Chapter Five). Mindfulness helps patients notice emotions without reacting to them and deepens contemplation so that if action is called for, it is appropriate and measured.

The second Recovery Skill is self-soothing. Self-soothing, without using substances, evolves out of mindfulness. Patients are taught to be mindful of this exact moment. Then careful attention to each of the five senses induces a serene pleasure that soothes disquieting emotions. With time spent in contemplation of one or more senses, emotional discord takes its place as one of many experiences to observe, and the patient is no longer lost in a storm at sea.

A third and more advanced Recovery Skill is emotion surfing. This skill originated with G. Alan Marlatt, PhD, who developed it to temper drug craving ("surfing the urge"). While working with an addicted patient who was also a surfer, Dr. Marlatt asked his patient to describe his passion for the sport. He applied his patient's in-the-moment joy of surfing to his client's drug cravings.[32] Marsha Linehan, PhD—primary author of DBT—and colleagues adapted Dr. Marlatt's work to surfing emotional states. RecoveryMind Training uses this technique for both purposes, in this instance to learn tolerance of difficult emotions. The skill is best learned using less powerful emotions. With practice, it can be used to manage all levels and types of emotional discord. Once the patient uses this skill with emotions management, it can easily be applied to alcohol and other drug cravings. I will review it in more detail in Domain F (Relapse Prevention) for that purpose.

RMT's surfing technique has been collated from several sources; variations on this technique are part of validated treatment protocols.[33–36] As with all skills, they are best introduced in skills groups. Here are the steps to learn emotion surfing:

1. Begin the session with the patients sitting in a quiet room without distractions. Describe the process to the participants. Reassure them by reiterating, "Although our reactions to emotions may be harmful, emotions by themselves carry no harm. They can only cause harm by driving us to act."

2. Have participants scan recent emotions to find one that is difficult but manageable. If a participant has worked on less intense emotions, encourage him or her to consider a feeling that is slightly more intense than his or her last session. If a participant is new, have him or her select a mildly irritating emotion, avoiding any feeling that could prove immediately overwhelming.

3. Quiet and center the participants. You may choose to use breath work for a few minutes for centering.

4. Have participants say the word of the feeling they selected for this exercise. Tell them, "Name the feeling. Be as precise as possible." There may be a tendency to build a story, such as "I feel hurt because my husband rejected me with that curt, cruel tone of his." Encourage them to avoid replaying the incident by stating, "Avoid thinking through possible scenarios, retributions, or corrective measures. Stay focused on the feeling. Notice its qualities. Do not push it away."

5. Instruct participants to "Take several slow deep breaths; have each breath-in and breath-out phase last for a count of four. Scan your body. Where does the feeling live? What muscles hold its

tension? Does it cause any other sensations? Are they constant or varying? Does it move in your body or stay in one place?"

6. Next, tell your participants, "For a moment, pay attention to how the feeling pushes you to act. Note what happens when you do not react to the feeling; its intensity will crest and fall down the other side like a wave. Then watch it rise again, note its intensity and urgency. Remain still. Pay close attention to how it crests and falls down the other side."

7. If you note a patient struggling with especially troubling and intense feelings, try a new approach by saying, "Inhale the feeling slowly, pulling it into your lungs with your breath. Expand your chest to take in every little bit of this difficult emotion. When your chest is full, slowly and smoothly exhale over a period of ten or more seconds. As you do so, imagine yourself pushing the emotion out with the exhaled air. Breathe in the feeling again with your next breath. Repeat this procedure until the feeling loses its power. If you would like, imagine your breath is a surfboard riding on the crest of the emotion to see if this helps you experience the emotional wave more clearly."

8. Watch your participants. When most have felt the feeling subside, tell them, "If the feeling subsides, try pulling it back. Watch it rise in intensity and crest and fall naturally on its own. Let it be. Notice that it no longer controls you; it just is."

9. After some time, have participants slowly return to the room. Instruct them to note the sounds within the room, the air on their face, sounds off in the distance, or other soothing sensory experiences.

If these three Recovery Skills are insufficient in helping a patient become more emotionally resilient, I recommend the individual participate in a more comprehensive course of dialectical behavioral therapy.

Segment 4: Understands How AddictBrain Uses Emotions

Addiction twists, substitutes, distorts, manufactures, and short circuits emotions. In an effort to catalog these perturbations, I use the AddictBrain concept to create clarity in an otherwise indecipherable mess. Massive disruptions in emotional circuits occur during the course of the illness and in the first several years of recovery. How can we help patients find a way out?

The best singular method to help is to note the many ways AddictBrain disrupts the emotions of addicted individuals. What happens may seem confusing, but AddictBrain's agenda is not. Consider how a particular emotional perturbation helps AddictBrain survive. I will start with a non-exhaustive list of the ways addiction distorts and manipulates emotions, which, in turn, helps AddictBrain survive. The antidote of each dilemma then becomes clear. To complete the Recovery Skills in Segment 4 of Domain C, patients review these emotional contortions, noting the tricks that apply to those emotions. They then write down a solution that is specific to their situation and practice that solution during treatment to gain competency.

Using a prepared worksheet, the patient writes down one or two times when the specific trick occurred. He or she then writes out a specific plan to thwart AddictBrain's skullduggery. This is reviewed with staff members, and the antidote is best practiced in a group session.

AddictBrain Emotional Trick 1

If a patient has an existing mood disorder or other psychiatric condition, AddictBrain uses that illness to promote continued use.

Discussion: I have discussed this problem previously, but it bears mentioning again. For example, if a patient suffers from a unipolar depression, AddictBrain suggests using substances will help relieve depression.

AddictBrain Agenda: Substance use makes every other psychiatric condition worse. If the condition deteriorates, AddictBrain chimes in, suggesting additional substance use.

Patient Recovery Skill: Recognize how continued substance use worsens the mood disorder. This realization tends to come after a period of addiction remission. As this insight seems to be easily lost, a patient might ask family and friends to remind him or her of this simple but elusive truth from time to time.

AddictBrain Emotional Trick 2

AddictBrain learns which emotions trigger substance use and pokes and prods at them to induce relapse.

AddictBrain Agenda: The more a patient suffers with an emotion, the more substance use will seem like a solution rather than a problem.

Patient Recovery Skill: Most patients come into treatment thinking they use substances in response to certain emotional states. The patient should start by cataloging emotions that trigger strong cravings. Then, when such feelings come up, patients are taught to question whether AddictBrain is promoting the feelings rather than the other way around. Open-mindedness is important here. With repeated inquiry, a perceptive patient will start to notice times when AddictBrain is heartlessly instigating the emotion for its own benefit.

AddictBrain Emotional Trick 3

When substances are used to ameliorate difficult emotions, it cripples the individual's emotion management skills. Other emotions management skills soon atrophy. Substance use becomes "the only thing that works."

Discussion: Very few of us learn how to effectively manage difficult emotions in our youth; most acquire the skill through trial and error. We talk things out with our parents and other family members; that is, until adolescence, when our parents are often deemed irrelevant, and friends become the source of all wisdom. We naturally explore techniques, such as exercise, putting our mind on something else, or rationalization.

When a person with substance use disorder begins using chemicals to manage disquieting affect, it appears so effective that his or her other skills atrophy from disuse. If a person begins using as a teenager or earlier, he or she may have never developed any meaningful tools for emotions management. Substance use is all such individuals have.

AddictBrain Agenda: Makes substance use indispensable.

Patient Recovery Skill: Each patient should discover the emotions that are most difficult to feel. With the help of peers, he can walk through these emotions and learn to manage them through emotional resilience skills. Over time, he will realize that he can experience emotions without using.

AddictBrain Emotional Trick 4

With continued use, substances become intensely associated with positive emotional states. Once addiction is full-blown, positive feelings do not occur without drug or alcohol use.

AddictBrain Agenda: "The only way to feel good is to use alcohol or other drugs."

Patient Recovery Skill: The patient should pay careful attention to brief moments of mirth, pleasure, and joy. He can reinforce them by taking note of them when they occur and by thanking others for non-chemical fun.

AddictBrain Emotional Trick 5

The signal salience (reward response) that occurs during substance use overpowers the subtle positive emotions making natural rewards seem flat or second rate.

Discussion: This process was reviewed in Chapters Three and Five. Remember substance use produces a signal of false importance that swamps the reward center and artificially activates reward. True pleasure quickly abates once an addiction disorder has taken hold. However, the promise of pleasure remains, luring those with addiction disorder into trying it "one more time."

AddictBrain Agenda: "Substance use always seems like the best possible thing to do. Why would you want to do anything else?"

Patient Recovery Skill: The reward system takes time to return to normal. Two things will help nudge it along: a commitment to doing things that produce healthy rewards (e.g., helping out others or being open to fun and laughter) and reflecting back on any pleasurable event when it occurs (e.g., "I haven't laughed like that in a long time"). I tell my patients it may take months or even years for the flatness to go away and real pleasure and joy to return.

AddictBrain Emotional Trick 6

The addicted person becomes tolerant to how drugs assuage negative emotions, requiring increased doses. Unfortunately, substance use paradoxically induces the opposite of the desired effect. A viscous cycle ensues.

Discussion: One of the most interesting paradoxes of addiction is that those with substance use disorders wind up with the exact opposite of what they sought during their first use. The person with alcohol use disorder who is anxious and wants to relax arrives in the therapist's office filled with anxiety and restlessness. The individual with a cocaine use disorder, seeking excitement and euphoria, arrives depressed, complaining how her life is uninteresting. The person addicted to opioids who seeks the warm blanket of peace and serenity shows up in treatment agitated by the constant strife from fighting incessant drug withdrawal. Addiction promises one thing and delivers its opposite. Blinded by AddictBrain's mental contortions, she cannot appreciate that see she is the recipient of a cruel trick that has made difficult emotions much worse.

Nowhere is this as clear as in how AddictBrain uses emotional issues to justify continued use. Worried about appearances, the person with alcohol use disorder is socially anxious so he has a few too many drinks before an important work-related social event. He acts inappropriately and realizes his worst fear; his work peers are talking about his drunken display. His embarrassment serves only to promote continued drinking.

AddictBrain Agenda: "I know you feel bad, but you *know* what will make you feel better."

Patient Recovery Skill: Staff members and other patients, if available, need to repeatedly and methodically reinforce this paradox whenever the moment arises. Unwinding the maladaptive response to protracted drug withdrawal and triggering emotions takes time. Once a patient comprehends this paradox and has it pointed out to him on multiple occasions, he will catch himself sooner and eventually be able to prevent entry into the viscous cycle.

AddictBrain Emotional Trick 7

Substance use generates artificial feelings that seem qualitatively distinct. If these feelings are sufficiently rarefied and exalted, the addicted individual spends the rest of his using career chasing them to no avail.

Discussion: In my experience, drug use creates certain emotional experiences that cannot be replicated without substances. Some people who use alcohol and other drugs seem particularly attached to these emotional events. In listening to my patients, they seem to be divided into two groups: substance euphoria and substance meaning.

Substance euphoria occurs with many drugs but is most closely associated with the stimulants (e.g., amphetamines, cocaine, and stimulant analogues, 3,4-Methylenedioxyamphetamine (MDA), 3,4-Methylenedioxymethamphetamine (MDMA), and with intravenous opioids, such as heroin and fentanyl). Users of these drugs report intense and sustained somatic and emotional memories that persist for years after last use. Many experience grief at the loss of this potential experience. The deeply euphoric event occurs early in their usage timeline and becomes increasingly elusive as drug consumption continues. The promise of recapturing several past euphoric events promotes continued use during a binge, especially with drugs like cocaine. The drug promises euphoria but fails to deliver. In frustration, the individual with addiction uses more and more, "chasing the elusive high."

Substance meaning is associated with a wider class of addictive drugs. Alcohol, marijuana, hallucinogens, opioid drugs, and nitrous oxide are commonly mentioned in this regard. A patient addicted to opioids summed it up like this: "I would take a handful of hydrocodone and sit in my chair listening to the quiet hum of the house. A few of those times, I felt as if I was the holder of exclusive knowledge as to the meaning of life, what mattered and what did not." Another description of this type of event appears in Chapter Three. The "deep meaning" that occurs turns out to be hollow. When asked to share the truth that occurs in such revelations, the addicted individual is at a loss for words. Whatever the revelation was, it is ineffable and detached from useful import.

One illuminating example of this comes from the work of a brilliant scientist and chemist Sir Humphry Davy whose research occurred in the late 1700s and the early 1800s. After synthesizing a more pure form of nitrous oxide, he experimented on inhaling the drug himself. Soon, his laboratory became a meeting place for friends who would partake in gas inhalation experiments.[37] Many men of note used the gas. William James, in an 1874 essay that appeared in the *Atlantic Monthly*, proclaimed that when coming out from under the gas "The genius of being is revealed."[38] James was, arguably, the founder of psychology in the United States. His words written while coming out from under the gas were as follows:

What's mistake but a kind of take?

What's nausea but a kind of -ausea?

Sober, drunk, -unk, astonishment ...

Agreement—disagreement!!

Emotion—motion!!! ...

Reconciliation of opposites; sober, drunk, all the same!

Good and evil reconciled in a laugh!
It escapes, it escapes!
But—
What escapes, WHAT escapes?[39]

I am at a loss at determining the revelation in these writings, but he himself seemed to think nitrous oxide inhalation induced important insights.

AddictBrain Agenda: "If only I (AddictBrain) can create this experience, you cannot give me up!"

Patient Recovery Skill: In a controlled environment, the patient should recall these moments and see them for what they really were—intense, yes; truly meaningful, no. More importantly, these events of euphoria and meaning have long since passed and will probably never recur with continued substance use.

The Recovery Skills in Domain C

The following Recovery Skills cover each of the four segments of Domain C. It is best to have each patient consider his or her competence at each of the skills defined in this domain. For example, a patient who has always understood his emotions and is able to correctly label them will consider the first competency complete (understanding one's own emotions) and mark them as such. If the patient has "tested out" of this Recovery Skill, the staff and patient should agree and move on. In this manner, patients differentiate their strengths and weakness in this all-important domain. If more than one segment is to be addressed, they normally do so in the order shown in the last sections of this chapter.

As in all domains, patients and staff routinely complete a progress assessment form that tracks progress.[40] The progress assessment form lists a domain's Recovery Skills with a three-point status rating (**B**egun, **I**ntermediate, and **C**ompleted). The patient completes the form first. This is followed by staff evaluation of the same form. Once complete, the patient and staff meet to reconcile discrepancies between the two evaluations. In this manner, the patient and his or her caregivers have a clear understanding of his or her progress in treatment.

Segment 1: Emotional Self-Awareness

A Recovery Skill in this segment is complete when the following tasks occur:

1. The patient has completed a feelings list and marks emotions that are commonly experienced, difficult to experience, ones that he or she would use substances in order to experience, and emotions that he or she would use substances to decrease or quash.

2. The patient correctly identifies his or her personal feelings in group therapy and individual sessions when they first emerge.

Segment 2: Identifying Emotions Correctly in Others

The Recovery Skill in this segment has been accomplished when the patient can accurately report feelings that others are experiencing in group therapy or other group activities.

Segment 3: Development of Emotional Resilience

A Recovery Skill in this segment is complete when the following tasks occur:

1. The patient has experienced and shared a difficult emotion with others without repressing it, acting out, or projecting it onto others.

2. The patient uses mindfulness or meditation to sit through one or more periods of strong emotion.

3. The patient has learned and implemented self-soothing to tolerate difficult feelings.

4. The patient has learned how to surf a feeling that is problematic and has implemented this technique one or more times.

Segment 4: Understands How AddictBrain Uses Emotions

A Recovery Skill in this segment is complete when the following tasks occur:

1. The patient is able to describe how AddictBrain uses his mood disorder or other psychiatric condition, if applicable, to promote continued alcohol or other drug use.

2. The patient has listed and discussed how AddictBrain has used strong emotions, both positive and negative, to keep him sick.

3. The patient recognizes several key emotions that triggered past use and how AddictBrain promoted this emotion to ensure continued use. The patient has developed a specific plan to recognize and not relapse when such feelings recur.

4. The patient reviews the list of AddictBrain's emotional tricks to see if any apply to him. He then describes specific instances where this occurred and a sequence of thoughts and behaviors that will prevent the trick from promoting use.

Chapter Eleven Notes

1. This is sometimes referred to as a "false cause fallacy," first discussed by David Hume in *A Treatise of Human Nature, Part III*, §6.

2. C. Darwin, *The Expression of the Emotions in Man and Animals* (Minneapolis, MN: Filiquarian, 2007), 370.

3. J. A. Russell, "Is there universal recognition of emotion from facial expression? A review of the cross-cultural studies," *Psychol Bull* 115, no. 1 (1994): 102–41.

4. J. I. Davis, A. Senghas, F. Brandt, and K. N. Ochsner, "The effects of BOTOX injections on emotional experience," *Emotion* 10, no. 3 (2010): 433–40.

5. D. A. Havas, A. M. Glenberg, K. A. Gutowski, M. J. Lucarelli, and R. J. Davidson. "Cosmetic use of botulinum toxin-a affects processing of emotional language," *Psychol Sci* 21, no. 7 (Jul 2010): 895–900.

6. M. R. Roxo, P. R. Franceschini, C. Zubaran, F. Kleber, and J. W. Sander, "The Limbic System Conception and Its Historical Evolution," *Scientific World Journal* 11 (2011): 14.

7. Antonio Damasio in his latest book, *Self Comes to Mind*, creates clarity of language by differentiating "emotions" from "feelings," stating, "Emotions are the complex reactions the body has to certain stimuli. When we are afraid of something, our hearts begin to race, our mouths become dry, our skin turns pale, and our muscles contract. This emotional reaction occurs automatically and unconsciously. Feelings occur after we become aware in our brain of such physical changes; only then do we experience the feeling of fear."

8. A. R. Damasio, *Self Comes to Mind: Constructing the Conscious Brain* (New York: Vintage Books, 2012).

9. S. S. Tomkins, *Affect Imagery Consciousness: The Complete Edition*, 2 vols. (New York: Springer Pub., 2008).

10. L. F. Barrett, M. Gendron, and Y.-M. Huang, "Do discrete emotions exist?" *Philosophical Psychology* 22, no. 4 (2009): 427–37.

11. R. Plutchik, "The nature of emotions," *American Scientist* 89, no. 4 (2001): 344–50.

12. Center for Non-violent Communication, "Feelings Inventory," CNVC, http://www.cnvc. org/sites/default/files/feelings_inventory_0.pdf.

13. R. C. Soloman, "The philosophy of emotions," in *Handbook of Emotions*, eds. M. Lewis, J. M. Haviland-Jones (New York: Guilford Press, 2000), 3–15.

14. H. Gardner, *Frames of Mind: The Theory of Multiple Intelligences*, 10th anniversary ed. (New York: Basic Books, 1993).

15. A. R. Damasio, *Descartes' Error: Emotion, Reason, and the Human Brain* (New York: Penguin Books, 2005).

16. P. Salovey and J. D. Mayer, "Emotional intelligence," *Imagination, Cognition and Personality* 9, no. 3 (1990): 185–211.

17. Ibid.

18. J. D. Mayer, P. Salovey, D. R. Caruso, and G. Sitarenios, "Emotional intelligence as a standard intelligence," *Emotion* 1, no. 3 (2001): 232–42.

19. D. Goleman, *Emotional Intelligence*, 10th Anniversary ed. (New York: Bantam Books, 2006).

20.　N. Gibbs, "Emotional Intelligence: The EQ Factor: New brain research suggests that emotions, not IQ, may be the true measure of human intelligence," *Time Magazine* 146 (Oct. 2, 1995): 44.

21.　J. D. Mayer, P. Salovey, and D. R. Caruso, "Emotional intelligence: Theory, findings, and implications," *Psychological Inquiry* (2004): 197–215.

22.　J. D. Mayer and P. Salovey, "Emotional intelligence and the construction and regulation of feelings," *Applied and Preventive Psychology* 4, no. 3 (1995): 197–208.

23.　See above, n. 16.

24.　M. Linehan, *Cognitive-Behavioral Treatment of Borderline Personality Disorder*, Diagnosis and Treatment of Mental Disorders (New York: Guilford Press, 1993).

25.　M. M. Linehan, *Skills Training Manual for Treating Borderline Personality Disorder*, First ed. (New York: The Guilford Press, 1993).

26.　See above, n. 8.

27.　I. M. Lesser, "A review of the alexithymia concept," *Psychosom Med* 43, no. 6 (1981): 531–43.

28.　P. Elman, *Emotions Revealed: Recognizing Faces and Feelings to Improve Communication and Emotional Life*, First ed. (New York: Holt Paperbacks, 2004).

29.　See above, n. 25.

30.　This is referred to as the "paradox of hedonism," which states that constant pleasure-seeking may not produce the most actual happiness. The act of consciously pursuing pleasure interferes with one's ability to experience it. We often gain more pleasure by pursuing other meaningful life goals. Henry Sidgwick first described this phenomenon in *The Methods of Ethics*, Book II, Chapter 3.

31.　This is a variation on the original words of Viktor Frankl in *Man's Search for Meaning*: "For success, like happiness, cannot be pursued; it must ensue, and it only does so as the unintended side-effect of one's personal dedication to a cause greater than oneself or as the by-product of one's surrender to a person other than oneself." V. E. Frankl, *Man's Search for Meaning* (Boston: Beacon Press, 2006), 16–17.

32.　G. Marlatt, "Surfing the Urge," Inquiring Mind, http://www.inquiringmind.com/Articles/SurfingTheUrge.html.

33.　A. B. R. Center, "Mindfulness Based Relapse Prevention," University of Washington Department of Psychology, http://www.mindfulrp.com/default.html.

34.　S. Bowen, N. Chawla, S. E. Collins, K. Witkiewitz, S. Hsu, J. Grow, S. Clifasefi, *et al.*, "Mindfulness-Based Relapse Prevention for Substance Use Disorders: A Pilot Efficacy Trial," *Substance Abuse* 30, no. 4 (2009): 295–305.

35.　S. Bowen, N. Chawla, and G. Marlatt, *Mindfulness-Based Relapse Prevention for Addictive Behaviors: A Clinician's Guide* (New York: Guilford Press, 2010).

36.　A. B. R. Center, "Urge Surfing," University of Washington Department of Psychology, http://depts.washington.edu/abrc/mbrp/recordings/Urge%20Surfing.mp3.

37.　M. Jay, *Emperors of Dreams: Drugs in the Nineteenth Century* (Gardena, CA: Dedalus, 2000).

38.　W. James, "Review of 'The Anaesthetic Revelation and the Gist of Philosophy'." *The Atlantic Monthly* 33, no. 205 (1874): 627–28.

39.　D. Tymoczko, "The Nitrous Oxide Philosopher," *The Atlantic Monthly* 277, no. 5 (1996): 93–101.

40.　Domain skill training, patient worksheets and progress assessment forms are available in the companion volume: *RecoveryMind Training: An Implementation Guide*.

CHAPTER TWELVE

Domain D: Internal Narrative and Self-Concept

"I've been beating up on myself so much
I feel like hurting myself."
ANONYMOUS

In Domain D, the modes of thinking that reinforce addiction will be examined. The primary tools in this domain are Cognitive Behavioral Therapy (CBT),[1] psychodynamic constructs,[2] and narrative therapy.[3] When combined together, work in this domain repairs language and cognitive distortions; examines how addiction uses innate defense mechanisms; and provides a clear life story for recovery. Goals are divided into three segments that

1. remove language and modes of thought created by AddictBrain;
2. deepen appreciation of the defenses that keep a patient from accepting and addressing his or her illness; and
3. examine and rewrite one's life story, replacing a story of self-sabotage with a narrative that promotes health.

While in treatment, clinicians help patients focus on areas where the most help is needed. For example, a patient who has a deep appreciation of her disease may have very few defenses that prevent her from acknowledging her illness, making work on the second segment is unnecessary. However, that same person may be plagued by a conviction that no matter how hard she tries she will ultimately relapse. She should, therefore, focus on the third segment in this domain.

Language and Addiction

Throughout this text, I have emphasized the importance of exact terms and clear language in addiction treatment. Patients should learn the meaning of terms related to their treatment and staff members should strive for their exacting use. Over the course of the past thirty years, the addiction treatment industry has witnessed the labeling change from "drug misuse" (1960s) to the "disease concept" (1970s and 1980s) and a clarification of addiction as a "brain disease" by Alan Leshner, PhD, in the late 1990s.[4] Today, most therapists and clinicians hold that truth, albeit with varying levels of conviction. I believe it is important to be more accurate—if a bit more long-winded—describing the illness as the "chronic disease of addiction,"[5] although some naysayers continue to balk at that term.[6, 7]

When treatment centers assert that their patients have an illness, it does not provide an excuse for the patients' actions; instead, it defines their current condition—they are ill—and clarifies the path of change they have to work in order to become well. Many of those who oppose the science that validates addiction as a brain disease react with moral outrage: "It gives these people an excuse for their behaviors!" This is an absurd notion; the public holds diabetic and hypertensive individuals responsible for managing their illness from the moment they fully comprehend their situation and have the skills to manage their illness: "It's a shame Rafael had a stroke, but you know he never took his blood pressure medicine." The same should be true for those who suffer from the illness of addiction.

RecoveryMind Training adds the yin and yang of AddictBrain/ RecoveryMind to the daily language of treatment (see Chapter Two).

Language shapes reality. Even the simplest word choices work to prevent or encourage insight. Insight is a rare and precious commodity early in recovery. How we direct our thoughts and actions—and how we chose our words—can move the addicted person toward relapse or recovery. My mentor, Dr. Butcher, used to ask clients who were considering their next life choice, "Is this decision in the service of your addiction (AddictBrain) or your recovery (RecoveryMind)?"

Once a patient has moved into the action stage of change (see Chapter Two), I begin using the term "addiction" when referring to the illness, even though addiction has the potential to carry a pejorative connotation. When a significant substance use disorder is present (*DSM-5* diagnosis moderate or greater), I believe using lesser terms (e.g., substance problem, alcohol abuse, chemical use, and drug habit) trivializes this deadly disease and subtly colludes with our patients' tendencies to hide their illness from themselves. As with all communication, the word "addiction" can be interpreted as supportive or derisive, depending on the speaker's tone and level of compassion. It is best to explain to every new patient why we use this term; it gives serious weight to a serious disease and is but one of the many ways we give respect to this life-threatening illness. However, the search for clarity does not stop there. In Domain D, I ask patients to search out euphemisms and minimizations that protect their illness.

Pathological Euphemisms

Pathological euphemisms are simple phrases used to minimize addiction. Each patient has his or her own set of pet phrases that make light of his or her condition. One might say, "I just took a nip in order to relax at the end of a day." Another patient may say, "I borrowed my mother's hydrocodone." Healthcare professionals will use the phrase "divert medications" rather than "steal drugs." Those addicted to taking pills use euphemistic terms for their drugs, such as "my medication," "my pills," or "my helpers." (Note how the word "my" is spoken with possessiveness and affection). The list of language distortions is voluminous, proportional to the height of a patient's intellect and the depths of his or her defenses. Such subtle contortions of language block insight while discovering and removing them deepens insight and speeds recovery.

Every patient arrives in treatment with a list of wordplays designed to "soften the blow"—cloak the nightmare and prevent close examination. Our job is to help them identify these turns of a phrase that keep them sick. Never pass up a moment to question euphemisms.

When gathering intake information, one of my patients used a euphemism for a life-altering medical event that occurred during a long bout of intoxication. When asked about his medical history, he said, "And there was the time I went to the hospital because I fell." Feigning confusion about this event I asked, "Is this the time you were up on a tall ladder painting your house while intoxicated?" The patient replied, "Yes, that was the time I fell and hurt myself." Gently asking for more clarity, I asked, "If I remember, you fell twenty feet, fractured your leg, and suffered a traumatic brain injury. Do I have the right incident?" The skill here is encouraging curiosity without a trace of hostility. With careful equanimity, I asked, "How did the traumatic brain injury change your life?" Clarification and curiosity opens the door to self-examination.

In this segment, patients compile a list of pathological euphemisms and carefully restate the more accurate truth that lies beneath. The euphemism "Have a little drink to calm my nerves" might mean "Drink three stiff drinks, go to work, and try to function while intoxicated." Once compiled, patients read their list in group therapy. Others may comment, "I have heard you use the phrase 'my medication' for your drugs several times with us here in treatment." The leader should avoid hostile feedback and encourage lighthearted flair during such sessions. Laughing at one's tomfoolery also deepens insight indirectly.

AddictBrain is predictable. If the illness returns, these same twists of language predictably reappear. After reading and discussing her list of pathological euphemisms, the patient should share the list with family members, friends, and members of her recovery support system.

A return of these phrases portends trouble, alerting the individual with an addiction disorder and her support system that her illness is creeping back in.

A Deeper Appreciation of "Denial"

In Domain B, patients explore how they hide their disease from themselves. In Domain D, this obfuscation will be explored more fully. The use of the term **"denial"** has a rich history[8] but unfortunately has devolved into a catchall phrase for all types of distorted thinking. Treatment staff may use it so often and so inaccurately that patients become confused saying, "I know you think I am in denial but I think I am ready to go to that family function." After hearing the term thrown at them haphazardly, patients eventually confuse denial with a questionable decision. Denial has become such an overused cliché that it has been dropped from the American Society of Addiction Medicine's standard definition of addiction;[9, 10] however, there is nothing positive about covert agreement with dangerous modes of thinking and acting. The confusion around the term "denial" and a desire to help patients adopt positive thinking has given the concept of denial an undeserved bad rap. The human mind is by nature a discriminating engine. We have to know where we *are* before we can set a course to where we are *going*. Therefore, RecoveryMind Training retains the term "denial," placing it alongside a longer list of defense mechanisms of the ego that circumvent insight.

More important than the choice of words is compassion. Those suffering with addiction are deeply sensitive to the judgment of others, in large part because they already judge themselves harshly. Nonverbal clues convey intent, attitude, connection, and broad meaning.[11] When a physician or therapist has sufficient experience treating addiction and a complete understanding of addiction as a brain disease, he or she is able to say the hard truth free of negative, nonverbal content. Patients respond to the truth about their condition, appreciating a clear diagnosis that is delivered directly and with kindness.

In its original analytic meaning, denial is literally a "denial of external reality." In denying external reality, the individual has rearranged his or her perception of the external world, which is more exacting than the offhand lingo we see used in addiction treatment. It is more valuable to see denial as one of the many defenses those with addiction exhibit. Also it is important to note that denial is different from repression, where individuals experience a sense of change in their internal world (e.g., "Even after he said all those terrible things to me, I am not angry at all").

In RecoveryMind Training, any maneuver AddictBrain employs to keep its hapless victim sick is a defense mechanism and one part of a larger "defense complex." Defense mechanisms are common contortions humans employ every day in an effort to manage disquieting affect. We employ multiple defense mechanisms to cope with the vicissitudes of life; taken together, they compose a defense complex. When working with addiction patients, these mechanisms are called an Addiction Defense Complex. Remember, these mechanisms are ever present with all of us, varying only in their number and depth of distortion.

To build a more exacting understanding of defense mechanisms, I encourage you to read *Adaptation to Life.*[12] In this groundbreaking work, George E. Vaillant, MD, expanded and categorized existing defense mechanisms from the psychoanalytic literature. I have extracted the most common ones in use by individuals with addiction disorders for use in RecoveryMind Training. In addition, several mechanisms were added to Vaillant's original list.[13] The elements of the Addiction Defense Complex are as follows:

- **Rationalization:** "I deserve a drink after my terrible day at work," or "I know I have many DWI/DUIs but I am a good driver. In fact, I am a better driver drunk than most people are sober!"
- **Minimization:** "I only had three beers before the accident. And the accident was not that bad." In reality, he totaled a car while blindly intoxicated and with two passengers in the car.
- **Blaming:** "My husband is so controlling; he drove me to drink," or "My doctor is at fault because she prescribed the medications."

In reality, the patient went from one doctor to another to obtain needed pills.

- **Going vague:** "I started drinking in college but I didn't drink that much. I only drank at parties." When asked how the drinking progressed, the patient responded, "You know I drank now and then, sometimes more and sometimes less." As the need to obfuscate lessens, use history changes dramatically. AddictBrain loves vagueness; RecoveryMind requires clarity.

- **Intellectualization:** "You say I have a drug problem. Tell me again about which parts of my brain are causing this to happen. I want to understand this better." Intellectualization provides emotional distance from the painful truth.

- **Projection:** "You have the wrong person in treatment. You should see my wife drink. *She's* the real alcoholic," or "I think you are labeling me as an alcoholic because *you* have had alcoholism in *your* family."

- **Hostility as defense:** "Why are you asking all these questions?" or "You are just trying to tell me what is the right and wrong way to live!"

- **Denial:** "I can quit anytime I feel like it," or "The incident my son told you about did not occur. I do not know why he makes up such things about me." People with alcohol use disorder use the unconscious mechanism of denial to prevent themselves from appreciating medical, legal, social, or other complications. Several years ago, I was struck by a statement from a patient who was very unsteady as he shuffled about in a detoxification unit after having many dangerous falls. He said, "I do not have any problems walking and do not need that wheelchair!" The depth of denial may be related to problems with executive functioning caused by neurotoxic substances, such as alcohol.[14]

- **Dishonesty:** Although dishonesty is not commonly labeled a defense mechanism, I include it here. When working in the addiction field, a fine line exists between denial and dishonesty.

Treatment providers are often left wondering, "Does he really believe what he just said, or is he just not telling the truth?" Even when brain functioning is compromised in other areas, people with substance use disorders retain the ability for subterfuge. Dishonesty starts out as a way of covering one's tracks and becomes increasingly automatic, moving from conscious manipulation to automatic reaction. When referring to those who are unable to attain recovery, Chapter Five of *Alcoholics Anonymous* states "They are naturally incapable of grasping and developing a manner of living which demands rigorous honesty."[15] The spectrum of denial and dishonesty is a smooth and seamless product of AddictBrain; however, the ability for honest self-reflection is critical for recovery.

The more patients understand how they use psychological defense mechanisms to fend off the pain of their situation, the sooner they can spot and correct pathological distortions and increase their long-term prognosis. Patients often recognize elements of their own defense complex by observing it in others first. Most treatment centers have traditionally used this technique to move their community into health. Patients who are further along can accelerate their own improvement by recognizing defense mechanisms in others and, in doing so, help their peers and themselves. When a patient becomes agitated after pointing out an element of the Addiction Defense Complex in a fellow patient— who dutifully fails to acknowledge it—it indicates the identifier has residual self-hostile feelings about previous blindness. This irritation is a goldmine and should be explored as the group process evolves. In group therapy, we often hear patients say, "You spot it, you got it."

In RecoveryMind Training, conventional group techniques scrape away pathological AddictBrain defenses. In addition, each patient should complete a worksheet that helps identify specific mechanisms he or she uses most often. Defenses are normalized by staff; they are a normal part of life. However, they are also signposts that direct our attention to needed therapeutic work. Every element of the defense complex is placed on a poster in the group therapy room. The group therapist encourages all the group's participants to gently point out when a member—including the therapist—uses a psychological defense. The therapist ensures that the discovery of defense mechanisms remains lighthearted and mutually exploratory. Accusations and any hint of hostility are dealt with swiftly. When a RMT group is really cooking, you hear deep sharing peppered by other patients' quiet interlocutions: "Minimization!" or "Going vague!"

One's defense style is usually well honed in childhood, long before addiction arrives on the scene. AddictBrain adopts the existing and most effective defenses—ones that most fit an individual's worldview—using them for its own purposes. Once assigned, the defense style worksheet[16] helps a patient identify and compile mechanisms he commonly uses to self-regulate. After completing this worksheet, he may discover the one or two "favorite" defenses that serve as his "go to" reality reorganizers. After reviewing these defenses in group or individual therapy, the patient and staff gently unhinge these maladaptive responses.

The defense style worksheet is best suited for individuals who have the psychological insight needed to parse through their psychological barriers. It is commonly assigned to patients with one or more "sticky" defense mechanisms that AddictBrain is mercilessly exploiting for its own use. Patients with unconscious but recalcitrant blaming defenses, for example, would benefit from completing this assignment and, even more importantly, reviewing it during a group therapy session. They ask their therapist, family, and peers for help in recognizing when they fall back into blaming; work to pull themselves out of this nonproductive pit; and seek a better understanding of their dilemma.

It is important to note that work in this area also helps remove barriers to interpersonal effectiveness, improves mood, and increases insight in general. Even after entering a substantive recovery, patients will continue to use these defense styles when dealing with other life issues. Therefore, a thorough examination of an individual's favored defense mechanisms will help maintain recovery and increase satisfaction in day-to-day interactions with others.

The Denial Rating Scale

RecoveryMind Training uses another tool based upon the work of Jeffrey Goldsmith, MD. Dr. Goldsmith and his colleagues developed and validated the Alcoholism Denial Rating Scale (ADRS) many years ago,[17, 18] which is readily available for download and free to use.[19] Despite its age, the ADRS communicates important aspects of a patient's status quickly and helps staff members quantify the stages of transformation a patient crosses during his or her recovery journey. I have adapted the instrument for patient use in a worksheet form. Patients track their status by sequentially self-administering the ADRS and completing the eight-point scale once or twice a week. This simple self-assessment takes about ten minutes the first time it is used; after several administrations, it can be completed in seconds. The accumulated ADRS scores are periodically brought to therapy for review and discussion.

Many patients view their denial as a binary phenomenon, a light switch that is either off (in denial) or on (completely self-aware). The ADRS helps them realize that their insight is on a dimmer switch; insight waxes and wanes throughout a week or even a day. The ADRS teaches them to recognize when they are sliding into dangerous territory. They begin to understand that recovery is a process of change, not a single location in psychological space. In this manner, the ADRS helps patients develop a nuanced understanding of recovery.

Internal Narrative and Life Story

In the previous section, I discussed how psychological defenses block the development of an accurate self-narrative, which prevents a healthy self-concept. Work in this segment of Domain D corrects the long-term thematic problems created by that narrative.

Internal narrative has two components. The first component is the moment-to-moment internal assertions, or statements we make to ourselves that alter our mood and thought. The second component is the longer-term life stories that refine and harden our self-concept. AddictBrain misdirects both types of narration. In Domain D, the focus is on thematic issues and how negative self-talk keeps the soil fertile for AddictBrain to grow and survive. In contrast, Domain F addresses how short-term thoughts promote or dissuade relapse.

Every one of us has "voices" in our heads; most experience them as thoughts, ideas, or a motivational pressure. Such voices redirect thoughts, nag us to correct our actions, cajole us to improve, and tempt us to eat that dessert. Anthropologist Andrew Irving describes it in this manner:

> The capacity for a multifaceted, imaginative inner life—encompassing internally represented speech, random urges, unfinished thoughts, inchoate imagery, and much else besides—is an essential feature of the human condition and a principal means through which people understand themselves and others. Simply put, without people's inner expressions and imaginative lifeworlds there would be no social existence or understanding, at least not in a form we would recognize.[20]

Internal dialogue is inextricably linked with consciousness. Such dialogue begins in the latency and preadolescent years when parental messages are internalized. During adolescence, we add our own voice to messages from earlier years. As the adolescent narrative emerges, its content stands in direct contradistinction to previously internalized parental voices (e.g., "It feels great to strike out and try new things" countermands preexisting internalized parental phrases, such as "Be careful, you might hurt yourself"). As we mature, we struggle to integrate these polar opposites and, in doing so, strive to form a robust and balanced self-concept.

Our internal narrative is a critical part of the experience of being human. It defines who we are and how we relate to others in a social community.[21] Many schools of psychotherapy posit that parental guidance, abuse, and excessive constraint or control alter the internal narrative.[22, 23] Over many years, this narrative builds an ongoing story that is honed into a coherent self-identity.[24] By the time we reach early adulthood, much repeated phrases and patterns of thought and the resultant self-identity tend to lock us into automatic responses to the outside world.

When developing Cognitive Therapy, Aaron T. Beck, MD, described "automatic thoughts" as spontaneous streams of negative interpretations about self, the world in general, or the future.[25] Many behaviors have preconditioned responses. Cognitive therapy posited that rearranging thoughts and behavior patterns circumvents maladaptive behaviors and eventually reconditions the patient to better self-concept and self-care. RecoveryMind Training borrows from and is very similar to CBT in this manner. RecoveryMind Training notes that AddictBrain produces "automatic thoughts," identical to those first described by Dr. Beck. AddictBrain produces automatic thoughts in all three areas— those about self ("You are weak-willed and will never get sober"), the world ("I am no different; everyone is addicted to something"), and the future ("You may try hard for a while, but something will happen that will eventually cause you to relapse").

The concept of evolving internal narrative is especially important when working with adolescent or young adult addiction patients. Initial alcohol or other drug use in adolescents or young adults is often driven by a reactive or even oppositional, defiant voice in a misguided attempt at self-definition. This voice by necessity defies parental definitions of right and wrong, constraint and control. AddictBrain uses such conflicts to escalate substance use, break away from parental control, and foster attachment to the alcohol or drug use culture. The young adult, in a failed attempt at self-definition, has moved from one constraining force (parents) to a harsher taskmaster (AddictBrain).

This psychodynamic conflict erupts to varying degrees when alcohol or other drug use escalates. At some point, the young adult's illness deteriorates to the point where treatment is necessary. Once in treatment, the treatment center is seen as another voice of senseless authority, and he rebels from it reflexively. If drug use is severe, the only narrative voices in his head are the internalized voice of constraining parental figures and AddictBrain. This, I believe, accounts for a large percentage of the transference/countertransference issues and subsequent difficulty treating this population. A talented therapist watches for this unconscious entrapment and avoids becoming ensnared into either of these polar opposites as much as possible.

Among addicted individuals, internal narrative is deeply interlinked with shame. When embroiled in the battle to control their chemical use, people with substance use disorders "are strongly influenced or controlled by a destructive thought that both seduces the person into the addictive behavior and punishes them for indulging."[26] This invariably leads to self-castigation and shame, which accelerates feelings of helplessness. Critical voices from parental figures and negative self-talk are reinforced by the inevitable maladaptive aspects of living with an addiction disorder, including lying, theft, deceit, and violation of personal values.

Some patients label this critical inner voice as their conscience. The lay public, when opining about addiction, often describes those with addiction as people who "need more will power" and "lack a conscience." Literature and mythology equate our inner voice with our conscience (baby boomers will recall Jiminy Cricket flitting about the ear, singing, "Always let your conscience be your guide"). One important task in Domain D, borrowed from Narrative Therapy and Voice Therapy, is making a distinction between this inner voice and our true moral guide.[27] What most distinguishes the inner voice from a conscience is its degrading, punishing quality. Its demeaning tone tends to increase our feelings of self-hatred instead of motivating us to change undesirable actions in a constructive manner.[28]

This inner voice shows up when the mind is not involved in task-oriented behaviors. When thoughtful action stops, the default mode network activates (see Chapter Five). Thoughts produced by the DMN show up with a critical flair and integrate themselves into one's self-identity over time. We internalize and tacitly accept this harsh internal voice; however, those with addiction are at great danger when they do so—excessive self-hostility promotes reactive relapse or a continuation of current drug use.

Therapists walk a tightrope here, attempting to increase self-insight without exacerbating self-hate. The recovery journey starts by accepting hard truths; such realizations induce shame. Persons with drug use disorders tend to flog themselves with the self-truths gained along the way. Most begin their recovery journey alternating between AddictBrain-driven thoughts and shame-driven internal controls. One example might be alternating thoughts, such as *A drink is the only thing that will make these feelings better,* and *You told yourself you were going to stop. You cannot even make a commitment to do something as simple as not take a drink!* The goal is in finding a different dialogue and discovering an internal voice that promotes self-care without a harsh decree or continual recrimination.

Twelve-step and other similar groups support this process by providing a nonjudgmental mutually supportive network that supports abstinence and personal growth and combining it with unconditional acceptance and love. Using thoughts are accepted as a natural part of the illness. They are normal, one of the long-term sequelae of the disease, and naturally abate over time. Shame is also a normal consequence of addiction-related thoughts and actions. It gradually dissipates thanks to the love received from others, working the Twelve Steps, and, in some cases, a relationship with a self-designated higher power. One's internal dialogue shifts from self-castigation to loving kindness and self-acceptance as a flawed but not defective human being.[29]

Individuals with addiction disorders begin treatment minimizing their illness, even when it is fulminant. As they improve, they begin to say, "I was (or am) sicker than I thought." As insight accelerates, they may even argue with their peers about "who is sicker," asking staff to resolve a friendly argument about which patient wins the grand prize as the sickest person in treatment. Of course, it is best to avoid anything but the most lighthearted of such discussions. However, I have found the transition to accepting the breadth and depth of one's illness to be a good prognostic sign, one that makes its appearance soon after the largest chunk of the defense complex falls away. The astute therapist will notice this as one of the many paradoxes in addiction treatment: as those with addiction move from being sick to acquiring mental and emotional health, they identify themselves as more and more sick, certainly in their past but occasionally in the present as well. Our job as treatment professionals is to prevent this insight from quickly deteriorating into negative automatic thoughts and deprecatory self-appraisal.

Three assignments build Recovery Skills in this segment. In the first assignment, the patient completes a life history that describes her childhood experiences, searching for themes that built her current internal narration. For example, a patient might discover a self-defeating theme; perhaps, her parent unconsciously subverted success by repeatedly telling her as a toddler, "Don't do it that way; you always mess things up!" During the life history, patients are instructed to provide a chronological narrative or timeline, making note of the events that stand out as pivotal or altering their life course. Such events commonly contain thematic material. Staff could ask the question, "Looking back at this event, what did you learn about life?" This clarifies themes in her internal narration.

The patient then tells her story to an individual therapist or in a group therapy. Group members consider possible themes that come from the story. Therapists, group members, and the assigned patient then engage in a collaborative search for life themes. Other members will relate and validate common themes, which simultaneously normalize and increase insight into their negative effect. Caught in their own head, a few group members may project their own themes onto the protagonist, who shrugs off misguided attempts to help. At the conclusion of the session, the protagonist returns to the assignment with a deeper understanding of how thematic internal dialogue continues to wound and block psychological growth.

The second assignment in this segment emerges from the first. Worksheet in hand, the patient reviews her life history, making note of important life themes that were discovered or affirmed by the preceding exercise. Next, she ranks the power and importance of these themes. A brief self-reflection appears at the conclusion of this worksheet, asking, "What did you learn? Did anything surprise you? What new feelings came up as you worked on this assignment?"

The third assignment relates self-concept and internal narrative to AddictBrain. Once addicted, AddictBrain employs themes and stories from the patient's past, using them for its own benefit. If the patient was told she would ultimately fail despite her best efforts to succeed, she should consider whether AddictBrain has coopted this to "You will work at this recovery thing but eventually you will relapse." AddictBrain uses whatever themes are available, manipulating and twisting them in order to thwart recovery.

This exercise may not be fruitful for all patients. An individual who is a concrete thinker may struggle with the metaphoric concepts contained in this assignment. An individual who has not resolved thick defenses prior to this exercise will come up empty-handed. Individuals who are deeply wounded should put off this assignment if self-exploration proves traumatizing. When properly timed and carefully pursued, however, work in this area helps addiction and its co-occurring disorders simultaneously. Depression will lift when hostile interior dialogue recedes; decreasing negative self-talk is one of the central goals of cognitive behavioral therapy. Thus, work in Domain D is especially important for patients with comorbid psychiatric disorders. By design, the therapeutic work in Domain D precedes Domain E, interpersonal connectedness and spirituality.

Recovery Skills for Domain D

As in all domains, a given patient is assigned tasks for a given Domain D Recovery Skill if assessment indicates it will prove useful. Patients and staff routinely complete a progress assessment form that tracks progress in assigned tasks.

The progress assessment form lists a domain's Recovery Skills with a three-point status rating (**B**egun, **I**ntermediate, and **C**ompleted). The patient completes the form first. This is followed by staff evaluation of the same form. Once complete, the patient and staff meet to reconcile discrepancies between the two evaluations. In this manner, the patient and his or her caregivers have a clear understanding of his or her progress in treatment.

Recovery Skills in this domain are complete when the following tasks occur:

1. The patient is able to describe how the AddictBrain concept does and does not apply to him.
2. The patient completes a list of "pathological euphemisms" and catches himself when he uses such words or phrases to minimize his addiction disorder.
3. The patient has successfully identified components of his defense complex.
4. The patient recognizes and gently points out defense mechanisms from the defense complex when others exhibit them.
5. The patient has determined one to three "go to" defenses that he uses most often to avoid painful emotions or insight.
6. The patient has explored how AddictBrain has adopted and twisted his "go to" defenses to sustain addiction.
7. The patient has explored how his favorite defense mechanisms have been used to defend against other emotional issues in his life.

8. The patient has completed a written life story that delineates important life themes and has articulated and examined that story with his therapist and peers (if applicable).

9. Using the life story, the patient has identified one or two important themes that persist in his life journey.

10. The patient has identified how AddictBrain used or modified these themes for its own purposes.

Chapter Twelve Notes

1. A. T. Beck, "Cognitive Therapy. A 30-Year Retrospective," *Am Psychol* 46, no. 4 (1991): 368–75.

2. G. E. Vaillant, *Adaptation to Life*, First ed. (Boston, MA: Brown Little, 1977).

3. M. White and D. Epston, *Narrative Means to Therapeutic Ends*, First ed. (New York: Norton, 1990).

4. A. I. Leshner, "Addiction Is a Brain Disease, and It Matters," *Science* 278, no. 5335 (1997): 45–47.

5. W. L. White, M. Boyle, and D. Loveland, "Alcoholism/Addiction as a Chronic Disease," *Alcoholism Treatment Quarterly* 20, no. 3-4 (2002): 107–29.

6. S. Peele, *Diseasing of America: Addiction Treatment out of Control* (Lexington, MA: Lexington Books, 1989).

7. S. Peele, *Diseasing of America: How We Allowed Recovery Zealots and the Treatment Industry to Convince Us We Are out of Control*, First ed. (New York: Lexington Books, 1995).

8. P. Dare and L. Derigne, "Denial in Alcohol and Other Drug Use Disorders: A Critique of Theory," *Addiction Research & Theory* 18, no. 2 (2010): 181–93.

9. ASAM, "The Definition of Addiction," ASAM, http://www.asam.org/docs/public-policy-statements/1definition_of_addiction_long_4–11.pdf?sfvrsn=2.

10. M. Miller, The Definition of Addiction: Why We Left Out the Word Denial, 2012.

11. J. K. Burgoon, L. K. Guerrero, and V. Manusov, "Nonverbal Signals," in *Handbook of Interpersonal Communication*, eds. M. L. Knapp, J. A. Daly, (Thousand Oaks, CA: Sage, 2011), 239–82 .

12. See above, n. 2.

13. A. Freud, *The Ego and the Mechanisms of Defense*, Revised ed.: 1966 (US) ed. (London: Hogarth Press and Institute of Psycho-Analysis, 1937).

14. W. Rinn, N. Desai, H. Rosenblatt, and D. R. Gastfriend, "Addiction Denial and Cognitive Dysfunction: A Preliminary Investigation," *J Neuropsychiatry Clin Neurosci* 14, no. 1 (2002): 52–57.

15. Alcoholics Anonymous, *Alcoholics Anonymous*, Fourth ed. (New York: A.A. World Services, Inc., 1976).

16. Domain skill training, patient worksheets, and progress assessment forms are available in the companion volume *RecoveryMind Training: An Implementation Guide*.

17. H. H. Breuer and R. J. Goldsmith, "Interrater Reliability of the Alcoholism Denial Rating Scale," *Substance Abuse* 16, no. 3 (1995): 169–76.

18. R. J. Goldsmith and B. L. Green, "A Rating Scale for Alcoholic Denial," *J Nerv Ment Dis* 176, no. 10 (1988): 614–20.

19. J. Goldsmith, "Denial Rating Scale Descision Tree," University of Washington, http://adai.washington.edu/instruments/PDF/Denial_Rating_Scale_94.pdf.

20. A. Irving, "Strange Distance: Towards an Anthropology of Interior Dialogue," *Med Anthropol Quarterly* 25, no. 1 (2011): 22–44.

21. A. Irving, "Dangerous Substances and Visible Evidence: Tears, Blood, Alcohol, Pills," *Visual Studies* 25, no. 1 (2010): 24–35.

22. L. L. Firestone, "Breaking Free from Addiction," Glendon Association, http://www.psychalive.org/breaking-free-from-addiction/.

23. R. W. Firestone, *Voice Therapy: A Psychotherapeutic Approach to Self-Destructive Behavior* (Santa Barbara, CA: Glendon Association, 1988).

24. D. P. McAdams and K. C. McLean, "Narrative Identity," *Current Directions in Psychological Science* 22, no. 3 (2013): 233–38.

25. See above, n. 1.

26. See above, n. 22.

27. See above, n. 23.

28. See above, n. 22.

29. E. Kurtz and K. Ketcham, *The Spirituality of Imperfection: Modern Wisdom from Classic Stories* (New York: Bantam Books, 1992).

CHAPTER THIRTEEN

Domain E: Connectedness and Spirituality

If you go off into a far, far forest and get very quiet, you'll come to understand that you're connected with everything."
ALAN WATTS

We are not human beings having a spiritual experience.
We are spiritual beings having a human experience.
PIERRE TEILHARD DE CHARDIN

Connectedness

Homo sapiens is a social and spiritual creature. Research suggests that social interconnections are deeply wired in our brain and have been critical for the survival of our species.[1] Addiction erodes one's ability to maintain healthy connections with others. Relationships are destroyed by dishonesty, deception, and the self-serving characteristics of the illness. Because addiction destroys healthy social connections and we need interconnection to heal, it makes sense that the road to recovery includes a recalibration of human connectedness.

Coaches in team sports have intuitively recognized when a team works together with mutually reinforcing members, they have a higher probability of success. Research verifies that collective efficiency and team performance have mutually reinforcing effects; that is, teams with high cohesion and collective efficiency increase the probability of success, which further promotes cohesion.[2] This, in turn, increases the psychological health of all teammates.[3] In contrast, the bulk of our educational system is based upon individual achievement and grade performance and social Darwinism.[4] Our job is to help every patient attain recovery; therefore, we must act more like coaches than examiners handing out grades. We focus on the collective milieu and not individual patients. This is especially true in Domain E. The current batch of patients under our care should be viewed as a team not a collection of individuals.[5] The team is a single, live organism focused on collective health of its constituents.

Many addiction treatment models focus on healing within a community. Twelve-step groups are highly structured communities that nurture change in younger members and sustain the recovery of its older members through service to the newcomer. Once a member gains a modicum of stability in his or her recovery, he or she is asked to help others. Ernest Kurtz, PhD, describes this well when delineating one of the four core ideas of AA as "a conversion from destructively total self-centeredness to constructive, creative, and fully human interaction with others."[6]

Healing within a community is the central focus of the Therapeutic Community (TC) treatment model, best described by one of its founders George De Leon, PhD.[7, 8] In the TC model, all patients and staff are seen as a collective, dedicated to interpersonal growth and recovery. Most organized treatment systems use elements of the therapeutic community to foster healthy interdependence, provide mutual insight, and normalize the horrific personal and interpersonal consequences of addiction. Every therapist who works in organized treatment should be familiar with Dr. De Leon's writings on the therapeutic community.

In RecoveryMind Training, patients learn and adopt skills that improve the quality of their interpersonal connection. Similar to the previous team sports example, a team of individuals learns how to develop high cohesion and collective efficiency, which increases the probability of abstinence and recovery for all its members. Continued recovery further promotes cohesion within that group. The first half of Domain E focuses on skills that improve interpersonal connection. This starts with training on how to connect and contribute to a healthy group. Once these individual skills are accomplished, each member examines the qualities of different types of group health, be it a marriage, family, twelve-step group, church congregation, or bowling league. Multiple communities of support help the recovering individual repair and rebuild his or her sense of belonging and purpose.

Clinical experience has shown that addiction recovery is best accomplished by linking individual skills with a healthy interdependence on a cohort dedicated to abstinence and personal growth. Because community healing is powerful—and can be continued long after formal treatment is complete—healthy interdependence provides an important foundation for lifelong health. In Domain E, patients build the skills that engender this interdependence. Unfortunately, quite a few addicted individuals have difficulties connecting, trusting, and learning from others. In such individuals, even a small amount of interconnection can be lifesaving. RecoveryMind Training uses the principles of attachment theory when helping such individuals bond with peers in a manner that supports group-based healing.

Attachment Theory

Attachment theory, as defined by John Bowlby, PhD,[9] and Mary Ainsworth, PhD, provides the most lucid framework for defining this healthy interdependence. Philip J. Flores, PhD, has an excellent book that summarizes how understanding attachment theory is best implemented in addiction treatment.[10] Attachment theory posits that an infant's first connection with a primary caregiver lays a foundation for all future life connections. As animals that are deeply dependent on each other, our interpersonal styles are critical for our well-being. We depend on our relationships for emotional regulation and self-care.[11] Daniel J. Siegel, MD, describes the importance of an infant's first bond: "At the level of the mind, attachment establishes an interpersonal relationship that helps the immature brain use the mature functions of the parent's brain to organize its own processes."[12] He goes on to say, "Repeated experiences become encoded in implicit memory as expectations and then mental models or schemata of attachment, which serve to help a child feel an internal sense of what John Bowlby called a 'secure base' in the world." Using a laboratory setting called the "strange situation," Ainsworth defined three types of childhood attachment: secure (B), avoidant (A), and ambivalent/resistant (C).[13] Later work by Mary Main, PhD, added the disorganized/disoriented classification (D).[14] These patterns are expressed later in all adult relationships, including romantic relationships. Difficulties with healthy attachment in early childhood are associated with later life difficulties.[15] Attachment patterns express themselves in treatment settings and affect a patient's ability to use interpersonal support and guidance both during and after treatment. Maladaptive attachment styles exacerbate many other psychological and psychiatric conditions as well.

If you work in a treatment setting, you may already intuitively recognize adults with healthy attachment. Consider the patient who consistently reports positive feelings toward staff members and peers. She is grateful for new friendships and all she learned from others. She reconnects with her family while under your care. When such a patient comes to the end of her initial treatment (whether it be an ASAM level 2.1, 2.5, 3.1, 3.5, or 3.7 level of care), she may state—to her own surprise—that she is sad to leave, "I have developed meaningful relationships here." She has attached to others and used that connection to guide internal growth. It is natural that she describes reluctance in discontinuing her treatment experience. She has healthy attachment.

In contrast, perturbations in early attachment wreak havoc in later relationships, including those in treatment and recovery. Individuals with avoidant, ambivalent/resistant, or disorganized/disoriented attachment styles may have difficulty connecting and trusting insight that comes from staff members or peers. They may learn the information contained in RMT but have difficulties using human connection to recognize and redirect past addiction behaviors. In treatment, patients mirror one another, and the interconnection between patients provides models for growth and change. When reflected inward, these changes redefine self-concept, creating a new personality: a recovering person. On this deeper level, patients with attachment problems may be unable to empathetically connect at a level that stimulates a piecing together of others' growth experiences, incorporating helpful elements when constructing a new self.

Treatment involves a dismantling of the old self, twisted and crippled by AddictBrain and past neglect. In its place, the individual constructs a new self from the principles of Alcoholics Anonymous (or other support organizations) and RecoveryMind Training. This transition requires a coherence of ego and the clarity that comes from self-discovery. Individuals with all types of attachment problems will have problems with this task; however, those with disorganized or disoriented attachment (D) have "the most seriously impaired capacity to integrate coherence within the mind."[16] Therefore, such individuals may need the slow, persistent repetition of Recovery Skills applied with a compassionate and consistent hand that repairs past ruptures of healthy bonding with others.

The following is a modified list of community-based treatment guidelines for attachment difficulties, based upon the work of Beverly James,[17] who asserts

- Individual therapy has been shown to be inadequate to treat attachment problems;
- The treatment milieu must be rich and supportive;

- Only after a relationship has been developed can treatment be effective;
- Individuals should not be asked to say good-bye to a loss without having something to take its place;
- Treatment must provide support, hope, and guidance;
- Treatment providers must provide a nurturing environment where a relationship of safety, consistency, and emotional closeness is encouraged.

Surprisingly, James has defined the elements of the best residential addiction treatment. Lesser degrees of attachment difficulties may be treated in a lower intensity milieu such as an ASAM level 2.1 or 2.5 program. Individuals who have more severe problems—especially those with a history of early trauma that prevented or ruptured healthy attachment—may need a more knowledgeable and structured setting provided in a residential (ASAM Level 3.3, 3.5, and 3.7) program with substantive psychological sophistication. Unfortunately, inexperienced clinicians and third party payers often neglect this need.

During the initial assessment phase, staff members should consider a patient's attachment style, assisting him or her in beginning the journey from maladaptive attachment (anxious-resistant, anxious-avoidant, and disorganized) to secure attachment to others and a peer group. Many patients who are challenged as to their attachment will do better in connecting to a group rather than individuals within that group. Orderly, structured groups bound by psychological rules of interaction are safest. Twelve-step support groups with their defined meeting times, a predictable sequence of events, and structured interaction are remarkably effective at repairing past, fractured attachment styles with slow, steady progress. Consider studying Dr. Flores's book *Addiction as an Attachment Disorder*[18] for an in-depth examination of this topic.

One underappreciated aspect of a sustained involvement with a twelve-step sponsor is the repair of attachment difficulties. After ten or more years of consistent involvement with a twelve-step sponsor, many addicted individuals with maladaptive interpersonal attachment will report, "My sponsor is the first person I truly trusted; he knows when I am heading in the wrong direction long before I have a clue. I know my sponsor is always there, looking out for my best interest, but he also recognizes when to give me room to grow." Such a relationship repairs damaged attachment and helps the sponsee experience healthy interdependence. Such individuals eventually build an internal model of self, connecting this new self to others.

Recovery Skills in Domain E related to connectedness are divided into two subsets: those related to interpersonal connection and those related to connecting with support groups.

Recovery Skills Related to Interpersonal Connection

In Domain E, RecoveryMind Training Recovery Skills engender healthy interpersonal connection. They help a patient
- Focus on commonality rather than retreating into uniqueness;
- Stay emotionally present during constructive criticism;
- Learn to self-disclose and ask for help;
- Recognize and validate when others provide help;
- Discover meaning that comes from compassion and selfless giving to others;
- Trust external advice, especially when it contradicts faulty internal guidance (i.e., AddictBrain thinking);
- Decrease shame by sharing moral and ethical violations and realizing such violations are a central and universal part of addiction.

You will note many of these skills are implicitly integrated to varying degrees into the fabric of addiction care. RMT makes these skills concrete, teaching patients why the skills are important and providing specific training on how to acquire these goals. Like all RMT Recovery Skills, a specific patient will focus on selected goals in the list based upon his or her needs. The needed skills and the steps to implement them comprise the actual patient-specific treatment plan.

Interpersonal Recovery Skill 1 helps a patient focus on commonality rather than retreating to uniqueness. RecoveryMind Training sees a patient's retreat into uniqueness as a defense mechanism. Patients previously wounded by caregivers who ignored or discounted their specialness are particularly adept at this defense. Such patients are taught to use a balancing technique that preserves their individuality while opening the door to shared experience.

When sharing about another patient's history, current story, or feelings, the patient should use the following verbal framework for assigned work in this skill: "I feel different (or I am unlike you) in that _____ but I am similar to you in how I _____." This structured feedback system retains autonomy but requires connection. When so assigned, staff and other patients gently redirect such an individual to use this tool when he or she unconsciously retreats into dissimilarity.

Interpersonal Recovery Skill 2 involves staying present when constructive criticism occurs. Patients who have difficulties in this area are seen as either "touchy" or "dismissive." When a patient is assigned this skill, she is asked to listen quietly when feedback occurs, knowing she will be required to provide a synopsis immediately after. Staff members should monitor feedback, adjusting the directness and emotional content to the receiver's level of tolerance.

After feedback, the receiver is asked to use the following format to paraphrase the concern of another patient: "When listening to your feedback I felt _____ (feeling word(s)) If I heard you correctly, your feedback to me was _____." The group moves on to helping such an individual balance and correct the information and process her emotional response to them.

Interpersonal Recovery Skill 3 helps patients disclose issues from their past, seeking support and learning to be vulnerable around others. Individuals who have problems with this skill are often the victims of trauma (mild or major), have been ridiculed for past weaknesses, have been taught to expect perfectionism, or suffer from varying degrees of shame. Almost every addiction patient falls into one or more of these categories. Thus, nearly every patient should work on this Recovery Skill.

In group therapy, asking for help misfires when other patients or staff members are unaware that a request is in process. To correct this, patients are given the following assignment early in their course of treatment:

> *List five problems with which you need help. These problems should be past events you are ashamed to discuss, emotions you feel are "not right," or things about you that are painful to consider. In this assignment, you should not list pragmatic issues (e.g., "I need help figuring out how to get a better job").*

Patients are taught to open their requests for help with a signaling sentence that places others on notice, such as "I would like to ask for help with an issue that is hard (or painful) for me to discuss, which is _____." When staff and group members hear this phrase, all move into a mode of empathetic listening. Too often, patients who are reluctant to discuss a difficult issue slide a request in sideways and are hurt when proper attention is not paid to their needs.

Interpersonal Recovery Skill 4 encourages recognition and validation of help provided by others. This skill is often paired with Interpersonal Recovery Skill 3. Patients who have a problem being noticed and cared for are especially vulnerable in this regard. After asking and receiving help, the protagonist in the discussion is encouraged to internalize and synthesize the emotional support provided. He singles out one or more peers from whom he experienced recognition and support and says, "Jim, thank you for noticing how painful my father's rejection was for me and how he should have backed me up at a young age."

When spoken aloud, the provided support is reinforced in the protagonist; it becomes substantive and *real*. If a patient suffers from a sufficiently maladaptive interpersonal style, he or she will not be able to attain Recovery Skills in the first months of recovery. Such individuals should remain in group therapy for the first several years of their recovery to deepen healthy interdependency.

In **Interpersonal Recovery Skill 5**, patients discover meaning that comes from compassion and selfless giving to others. Two different types of individuals have difficulties with compassion. The first is an individual who lacks empathy. Extremes cases of this occur in psychopaths. In addiction treatment, therapists and other treatment professionals more often see individuals who are self-absorbed, immersed in their own emotional upheaval, or have a disorder that falls along the Asperger spectrum. However, most patients with prolonged addiction careers have also lost the ability for selfless compassion. RecoveryMind Training asserts that some degree of compassion can be learned in all but the most difficult cases.

Patients working on Interpersonal Recovery Skill 5 are given an assignment to note instances where they feel an empathetic connection with others. They keep track of this experience on a daily basis for an assigned number of weeks. They are instructed to provide small, anonymous, nonmaterial gifts to these individuals as a way of expressing their compassion. The act of empathy, when combined with selfless giving, reactivates dormant compassion. At some point in the later stages of treatment, such an individual should share a list of these moments of empathy and compassion in a group setting. This furthers the reemergence of healthy interconnectedness.

Interpersonal Recovery Skill 6 teaches patients to learn how to trust others, especially when their intuition is patently incorrect and often different from how others see a situation. AddictBrain, for its own survival, induces a false sense of certainty when it detects an opportunity to reinforce addictive thinking or behaviors. Statements, such as "That may be right for you, but I know myself—it will not work for me," lead to a type of rigidity that prevents emotional growth and blocks new ideas that promote change. Such distortion of beliefs is prevalent in every addicted individual and is especially problematic in those with frequent relapses.

When a staff member recognizes an individual with this trait, the patient is informed of potential problems in this area. The therapist should not insist that the patient agrees with him or her at first. It is much more helpful for the patient to discover AddictBrain's subterfuge over time and with the help of others in treatment. Rather, the therapist brings this distortion of thought to the patient using a question, such as "Have you ever thought that some of your best ideas actually kept you sick?" If the patient acknowledges one or more examples of false certainty, he is given the following assignment:

1. Write down several past examples of beliefs you thought were in your best interest and turned out serving AddictBrain rather than RecoveryMind (e.g., "After three months of not drinking anything, I came to the conclusion I could drink one glass of wine with dinner.").

2. Write down several current beliefs about yourself and your addiction, which others have voiced concern (e.g., "I do not think it is necessary to ask my wife to remove alcohol from the house; I would like to serve guests when they come to visit.").

3. The next part of the assignment is to review thoughts or beliefs with other group members and write down their recommendations.

4. The next step of this assignment is the most difficult. The patient agrees to follow the advice provided by the group diligently and methodically, ignoring his own instincts.

5. After an amount of time, he reviews what he experienced going against his intuition or beliefs. He notes what was easy and difficult as well as pleasant and irritating.

Half of this exercise is an experiment; the patient goes against personal intuition and listens to others, even if he does not agree. This exercise prepares the patient for future tasks in treatment in recovery, where doing the right thing is often counterintuitive. The other half of the exercise opens a patient's mind to the possibility that AddictBrain manufactures many false beliefs that subvert the recovery process. Individuals who are frequently at the mercy of a powerful AddictBrain might do best to continue this exercise, cataloging each time they "act as if the group was right" and looking for patterns when seeking insight into AddictBrain's nefarious deception.

Interpersonal Recovery Skill 7 addresses a universal wound created by addiction: shame over past behaviors. AddictBrain undermines an individual's value system, systematically violating his or her ethical and moral values. This is so commonplace in addiction that it is successfully used in the differential diagnosis of addiction disorders from other disease states. Therefore, secrets and shame about past behaviors should be part of every treatment plan.

Once a patient has developed a modicum of alignment with the treatment team and his peers, he is ready to construct a list of past shameful behaviors related to substance dependence or a behavioral addiction. The list should remain private at first. He then prepares for disclosure, building trust and watching other patients disclose their secrets and shame in group therapy sessions. An astute psychotherapist will sense when that patient is ready to confront his own secretive and shameful past. The patient who discloses these hurts provides a good opportunity for others—especially those working on Interpersonal Recovery Skill 5—to express his or her compassion.

Recovery Skills Related to a Healthy Connection to a Group

In many ways, group connection skills are an outgrowth of the interpersonal skills described in the previous section. In most treatment settings, patients learn and practice interpersonal and group skills simultaneously because these two sets of skills are closely interlinked.

The Domain E skills that lead to healthy group connections are acquired when a patient

- Learns how to use twelve-step meetings to sustain recovery and deepen spiritual growth;
- Finds and bonds with a healthy peer group that practices nonchemical fun;
- Uses guidance from sponsor, therapists, and members of a support group;
- Finds meaning in the wisdom of a group and feels part of that group;
- Is able to help others and experience gratitude from his or her volunteerism;.
- Provides hope to others and in doing so rediscovers hope him- or herself.

In **Group Recovery Skill 1**, patients learn how to use twelve-step meetings effectively. When surveying treatment programs that utilize twelve-step groups and philosophy in their treatment, one of the most surprising findings is how few of these programs actually *teach* patients how to use meetings to heal. In RecoveryMind Training, meetings are considered a tool. Similar to any complicated tool, instruction is necessary for correct use. RMT participants learn what happens in a twelve-step meeting, the meaning of working steps, and how to address important concerns, such as determining when a meeting is not fulfilling recovery needs.

The complete details of twelve-step support systems training are beyond this text; however, several systematic twelve-step training manuals are available. One example is the Making Alcoholics Anonymous Easier (MAAEZ) system developed by Lee Ann Kaskutas, DrPH.[19] A second example is the Project MATCH *Twelve-Step Facilitation Therapy Manual*.[20] These manuals teach the philosophy and introduce the basic elements of twelve-step programs. Many of the staff members whose role it is to introduce patients to twelve-step principles have deep and long-lasting connections to twelve-step philosophy. Paradoxically, this can make it difficult for them to provide introductory training. Years of study can distance the teacher from introductory concepts, missing what a new student needs to know. Manualized training ensures that every patient learns the basic principles of twelve-step recovery in a predictable and systematic fashion.

Manuals that teach the foundations of twelve-step philosophy are a great start but should be supplemented with experiential tools that internalize important concepts. Individuals with social anxiety, an excess of shame, concerns about anonymity, and difficulties connecting with support groups benefit most from this type of training. RecoveryMind Training augments this introduction by role-playing the components of a twelve-step meeting.

In this role-play, outside volunteers, staff members, or senior patients form a small circle in the center of the room and are labeled as the actors. Newer patients sit outside the circle to observe and comment. The actors walked through each of the components of a meeting, beginning with entering the room, finding a place to sit, and settling in to the environment. The therapist leader of the group describes a scenario typical for a twelve-step meeting. The actors enact that phase, stopping frequently to describe their internal experience. Patients with social phobias should be encouraged to process their reactions extensively. Patients and the group leader interrupt the flow frequently. At one such interruption, the leader might ask, "What just happened when Ed shared about his alcohol craving?" The actors and patients discuss feeling states, interpersonal connection, and transcendent truths that emerge from this process. The "meeting" is then restarted. Using this stop-discussion-restart process, patients will deepen their understanding of what it means to "go to a meeting." The group leader, knowing the interpersonal dynamics of the individuals involved in this training might ask, "What part of this discussion would be difficult for you, Joan?" In this manner, patients observe and integrate the healing tools present in the unique AA healing process.

Group Recovery Skill 2 encourages patients to consider ways of having fun that protect them from high-risk alcohol and other drug situations. Most individuals early in recovery live with the delusion they cannot have fun without substances. This cognitive distortion is a normal part of recovery. When asked to consider alcohol- and drug-free fun, most patients come up empty-handed. The future looks bleak and disagreeable.

For this Recovery Skill, staff members may provide a list of ways to have fun while remaining abstinent. Mechanisms for nonchemical social fun are divided into two types. The first is events that are naturally alcohol and drug free, such as a church picnic or a hike in the woods with sober friends. The second type is events that are associated with substance use but made safe by adequate planning. An example of this might be attending a music festival with a large group of friends in NA or AA.

Using group discussion and a subsequent worksheet, patients commit to nonchemical fun after treatment. It is important for staff to validate that nonchemical fun will seem awkward at first. Social events, where drinking occurs, will have to be faced without alcohol. This awkwardness is especially difficult in intimate situations, such as dating and physical intimacy. Preparing patients for this future normalizes their anxiety and provides a roadmap for an enjoyable recovery.

In **Group Recovery Skill 3**, patients learn how to listen and experiment with the advice of others. Group Recovery Skill 3 is similar to the aforementioned Interpersonal Recovery Skill 6. Therapists can use either, or both, of these approaches to promote growth. Patients begin to work on this Recovery Skill when observing the previous role-play and attending twelve-step meetings. Using a worksheet, patients who need to deepen Group Recovery Skill 3 record advice they are given throughout their treatment day, including advice provided at outside twelve-step meetings. In this worksheet, they record their natural resistance to following this advice and formulate a plan to implement the external advice, despite their resistances to it. The fourth column on this worksheet is filled out after executing external advice and provides space for reflection on the outcome. Let's consider an example that illustrates this Recovery Skill.

> *Jamie is a thirty-six-year-old man whose drug of choice is alcohol. In his childhood, he was taught to "keep his business to himself." He arrives in treatment very resistant to outside suggestions about how to rebuild a life of recovery. Staff members and his fellow peers ask him to "try on external advice like an experiment." He is given a worksheet on which he records external guidance. While attending an intensive outpatient program (ASAM Level 2.1), Jamie's wife asks him to attend her annual corporate picnic. At last year's picnic, Jamie drank excessively and made a fool of himself in front of his wife's coworkers. He does not want to go to the picnic this year but is ashamed to tell his wife why. When discussing this in group therapy, several of his peers suggest that he talk it over with his wife. Together, they can plan how to manage his embarrassment. Jamie admits he has never "talked things over" with his wife in fourteen years of marriage. His upbringing has trained him to take care of his problems by himself.*
>
> *In group therapy, Jamie's peers suggest alternatives, for example, informing close friends at the picnic that he has entered treatment. This would explain his past behavior and prevent others from offering alcoholic beverages. Jamie balks at every suggestion. The group leader instructs Jamie to record his initial reaction, the reasons for his resistance to implementing external advice, and a plan that includes one or more of the suggestions he received in that group session. He is to report back with which suggestions he will implement "like an experiment." Jamie decides to tell his wife of his anxiety and ask her to team up with him. He implements this plan. Jamie's wife, relieved at his admission, suggests they stay close to one of her best*

> *friends from the company who, interestingly, is in long-term recovery.*

After the picnic, Jamie records the results of his "experiment," noting any new or surprising consequences of handling a high-risk situation using external direction instead of intuition. He brings his worksheet to therapy group. The group processes his "experiment," cataloging its successes and failures. While many treatment centers do this type of processing, what makes RecoveryMind Training different is the structured processing after the event. Staff members deepen the learning by using a worksheet for each new recovery experiment. This encourages contemplation and promotes change.

RMT also focuses on the meta-message. In the worksheet, Jamie is asked to reflect on what this says about him, his inability to take external advice, and how this is counterproductive for a sustained recovery. Such a discussion should then lead to a deeper examination of the maladaptive consequences of his childhood training and how they were nurtured by AddictBrain.

Group Recovery Skill 4 asks patients to derive meaning from group wisdom, and in doing so, patients experience and acknowledge gratitude for the group. Individuals may have difficulty with this skill for many reasons. Some have difficulties with trust and are reluctant to incorporate collective wisdom; they fear it is misguided at best or dangerous at worst. Others may suffer from excessive arrogance, discarding group-based wisdom as beneath them. Whatever the cause, group-based wisdom is essential for correcting distortions of thought and planning created by AddictBrain. Individuals who need to build skills in this area should discuss their resistance, whatever the etiology. They may benefit from recording group advice as described previously in Group Recovery Skill 3. A worksheet may compare and contrast the patient's self-guided decisions from group-based decisions, analyzing the outcome of both. No matter what the cause, an individual forms a psychological bond with that group when he or she recognizes wisdom in "groupthink." This proves to be an essential element when building a healthy attachment to others.

Group Recovery Skill 5 asks patients to help their peers through volunteerism. Individuals who are severely beaten down by their disease often gain the most from this exercise. In RecoveryMind Training, patients and staff develop and post a list of volunteer activities within the center. Patients sign up for tasks anonymously. They track their volunteer activities and, on a regular basis, record their experiences in carrying them out. The general response is an increase in gratitude and interpersonal connections within the center. One of the most unusual aspects of gratitude is that defining and describing it serves to amplify its intensity. When a patient records and verbalizes her gratitude that comes from volunteerism and giving to others, the depth and breadth of her gratitude increases proportionally.

Group Recovery Skill 6 is a derivative of Group Recovery Skill 5. Unlike Skill 5, this exercise cannot be practiced anonymously. Patients who are further along in the course of treatment should be assigned to others who are just arriving. They become a "buddy" to the newcomers, helping them sort through myriad assignments, rules, names of peers and staff, and the treatment schedule. They may also provide hope by sharing their story and relating to newcomers' fears and anxieties. Patients who are working on Group Recovery Skill 6 record their experience in the Recovery Reflection or other worksheet, providing hope to others in one column and searching for ways the experience increases their own sense of hope in a second column. Through providing and receiving hope, they learn an important skill that can be used for years to come. "Providing hope" is often incorporated into a patient's newfound recovery personality. Many recovering individuals find that providing hope is one of the pillars of their newfound self. Service is also a central component of twelve-step recovery.

Spirituality

The term "spirituality" means different things to different people. Various definitions have been proposed, but ultimately the definition of spirituality is as diffuse as the concept itself. Several concepts help define the elusive nature of spirituality. Leland R. Kaiser, PhD, proposed "Spirituality is about the relationship between ourselves and something larger."[21] Spirituality involves "the search for transcendent meaning."[22] One dictionary defines spirituality as "the experience or expression of the sacred." Spirituality often involves a metaphoric journey where the individual searches for meaning.[23] That journey seems to be driven by an innate yearning to connect with a power greater than the self, even the universe itself. Many individuals and groups equate spirituality with their religion and religious practices. The pursuit of one's faith is profoundly helpful for recovery, but experience has shown that religious faith is not a prerequisite for solid sobriety/recovery. However, the pursuit of spiritual growth energizes and adds sublime significance to recovery that cannot be obtained with abstinence and psychological growth alone.

Spirituality and religious experiences have neurophysiological correlates. Mario Beauregard, PhD, demonstrated that during mystical and religious experiences, the brain shows strong activations in the right medial orbitofrontal cortex, right middle temporal cortex, right inferior and superior parietal lobules, right caudate, left medial prefrontal cortex, left anterior cingulate cortex, left inferior parietal lobule, left insula, and left caudate nucleus. The temporal lobe[24] has long been correlated with religious experience as has the insula.[25] We are hardwired for spiritual hunger.[26] Such an assertion does not mean that God, Allah, Yahweh, and Bhagavan—as well as other names religions use for the Supreme Being— are figments of neuronal firing. It does assert that neural circuitry ignites a drive and subsequent quest for spiritual meaning for the vast majority of human beings.[27]

Looking back over more than a century of humankind's battle with addiction, a religious or spiritual quest lies at the center of nearly every early victory over addiction before and after Alcoholics Anonymous arrived on the scene. In fact, a prescient statement about "transforming experience of the spirit"[28] by Carl Jung indirectly shaped the foundation of AA itself.[29] Although an interest in spiritual pursuits is by no means required, every patient should at least explore their thoughts and feelings and question their attitudes about this important constituent of recovery. Therapists in the field have long recognized that a "spiritual awakening" seems to predict a positive long-term outcome.

But where is the scientific proof of the benefit of spiritual or religious experience in recovery? The breadth of research here is limited by medicine's move to empirical data that has reflexively discarded treatment protocols that involve spiritual activities. Despite this move, research indicates that a spiritual pursuit in recovery does improve long-term prognosis.[30-35] AA members who report a spiritual awakening were over three times more likely to be abstinent three years later than those who did not.[36] A more recent study reviewed the NIDA DATOS dataset and found that those with low spirituality have higher relapse rates whereas those with high spirituality have higher remission for most substance use disorders (excluding cocaine use disorder).[37]

The opposition to adopting spiritual growth as a founding principle of addiction recovery comes from several camps. Some pundits balk at the mistaken notion that treatment centers shackle resistant patients with unwanted religious dogma. Others desire addiction care to be based on science; spirituality defies scientific logic by its very nature—and may do so for centuries to come. A third, smaller group is driven by religious antipathy that arises from many quarters. RecoveryMind Training is pragmatic in its position. Because so many have made peace with their past through spiritual questioning and religious pursuit, I encourage all patients to use their current faith, revisit their past faith, or explore nonsectarian spiritual options in their quest for a substantive recovery. The worst outcome from trying on spiritual ideas is that an individual will find no solace there and walk away. Research strongly supports spirituality as a tool for adjusting to the perceived life threat of cancer.[38] I do find it interesting that many who oppose the use of spirituality in addiction are less opposed to its application to other chronic illnesses, such as cancer.

Continued Work on the Steps: Steps Two and Three

RecoveryMind Training also returns to twelve-step work in Domain E. Patients who are open to spirituality can complete Steps Two and Three of the AA program[39] while they are in their initial treatment. However, it is immensely important to ensure a patient is open to spiritual pursuits and is at peace with his or her faith (if present) before embarking on these two steps. Toward these ends, all patients should complete a questionnaire about their spiritual beliefs that examines points of resistance, past spiritual trauma, past practices, and current attitudes. Most programs have the expertise to develop this questionnaire; research-validated instruments are also available.[40] A staff member reviews this questionnaire with the patient, working with her to ascertain whether she is ready to begin Steps Two and Three. Pushing patients who are unwilling or unable to "believe that a Power greater than ourselves could restore us to sanity" results in a backlash that repels patients from AA. If a patient has internalized Step One and gained needed Recovery Skills, she should be able to maintain sobriety while she continues her personal spiritual quest.

Individuals who have completed Step One (Domain B) are ready to focus on Steps Two and Three. By this time, most patients have accepted their problem as real and need help formulating a path out of their illness. Step Two and Step Three begin the journey. The combination of interpersonal connectedness and connection with a Higher Power of their choosing constructs the spiritual component of a solid recovery. I will assume that the reader has experience with the Twelve Steps of Alcoholics Anonymous and will not expound upon them here, but you may wish to refresh your knowledge by reading any number of books on this matter.[41] Many guides to step work are available for consultation as well.[42]

Table 13.1 - Principles behind Step Two and Step Three

Step		Character Defect	Principle	Action
2	"Came to believe that a Power greater than ourselves could restore us to sanity."	Self-will and Disbelief	Hope	Realization
3	"Made a decision to turn our will and our lives over to the care of God as we understood Him."	Self-will and Fear	Faith	Ask for and accept help

Many patients will rediscover or explore the religious or spiritual teachings of their youth during this period of treatment. It is important for staff members to withhold any pressure in this regard because spiritual and religious beliefs are personal and powerful things. Staff members who hold strong beliefs have the potential to nudge their patients subtly into one belief system or another. The patient, in an effort to "do the correct thing" in treatment, may respond with false compliance that hinders a more genuine examination of his or her personal spiritual path.

Additional Spirituality Skills

Although Step Two and Step Three are the central components of spirituality work in Domain E, additional Recovery Skills should be considered. For patients whose spirituality is not based on a Higher Power, these skills are especially relevant and help build spiritual connectedness through secular humanism.[43] RecoveryMind Training sees spiritual exploration as a goal in and of itself rather than a quest that must end in a spiritual or religious conviction. The AA text describes it in the following manner: "We claim spiritual progress, rather than spiritual perfection."[44]

Staff members may ask a patient to complete one or more of the following assignments to improve spiritual health. The additional assignments for Spiritual Recovery Skills include the following:

1. Recognizing Transcendence
2. Noticing Coincidences
3. Building a Gratitude List
4. Sense a Presence during Meditation
5. Distinguishing the Voice of RecoveryMind
6. Using a "God Box" to Manage Worries
7. Writing an Obituary to Clarify Values

There are two important prerequisites for Spiritual Recovery Skills; both are simple in concept but difficult in practice. The first prerequisite is to make sure the client or patient is ready to benefit from the exercise. Individuals who are in the midst of post-acute withdrawal, suffer from neurocognitive problems from their substance use, are in the acute phases of a mood disorder, are deeply conflicted about recovery, or are in other distressed states should focus more on the pragmatic tasks of early recovery. Individuals who have returned after a brief relapse and need to rethink their recovery program, on the other hand, are excellent candidates to work one or more of these Recovery Skills.

The second prerequisite is to make sure staff is not "punishing" a patient with this exercise. This may seem simple but proves difficult in practice. Let's consider an example.

> *Ashley is a twenty-nine-year-old female who returns to the treatment center after a dramatic relapse. She was the model patient in her previous treatment, working hard at Recovery Skills, completing step assignments, actively sharing with her peers, and being rigorously honest about her drug use history. In that treatment episode, she unearthed past sexual trauma, reluctantly at first and*

later in some detail with her individual therapist. Like many trauma victims, her history cast a pall over the future. However, her mood improved substantially during her course of treatment. She developed friends in recovery. The entire team pronounced her treatment a success. After treatment, she attended twelve-step meetings regularly and came back to the center to tell her story to others. During those times, staff developed a fondness for Ashley and her perseverance against adversity.

After about a year, Ashley disappeared. Her husband called three weeks later. Ashley was in the ICU at the local hospital after a near-fatal overdose. The treatment center staff was saddened by her relapse but grateful she was alive. Once stabilized, Ashley returns to the treatment center to process her relapse to reengage in recovery. When she arrives, other patients remember her story and begin expressing hopelessness about their recovery ("If Ashley cannot maintain her recovery with all she has done, what hope do I have?"). Ashley is negative herself, frustrated about her relapse and pushing to go home so she can "work her program."

After a week in treatment, Ashley's case is dissected in a treatment planning conference. The staff has positive memories about Ashley and her recovery but is unconsciously irritated that their star patient has returned a "fallen star." Her attitude of over-familiarity with the staff is irksome. Her effect on other patients is causing trouble. After reviewing her relapse and her work on several basic assignments, one member of the staff says, "Ashley seemed continuously disheartened by her trauma. She worked hard on the damages cause by her hurt but could never seem to find gratitude in her recovery. Maybe we need her to work on the assignment Build a Gratitude List." The rest of the staff agrees. Ashley dutifully works on the assignment.

Surprisingly, her attitude worsens. After several weeks, she demands discharge with only marginal improvement.

In this case, countertransference stimulated an unconscious hostile response by the staff. Ashley would benefit from gratitude, no doubt about it. However, her past trauma, familiarity with the center's therapists, and her current emotional condition ensure that the assignment of this Recovery Skill will fail. Work on other skills will be the best avenue in this case, especially those in Domain F. With this caveat in mind, I will describe additional Spiritual Recovery Skills in Domain E next.

The first supplemental Spiritual Recovery Skill is **Recognizing Transcendence**. A transcendent event extends beyond the limits of ordinary experience. Most spiritual experiences involve transcendence, and each of us experiences this phenomenon from time to time. It may occur when watching a movie or play that affects you in an unusual manner, often in a way you were not expecting. It may come from listening to music or experiencing a work of art. Transcendence connects seemingly unrelated events, thoughts, or memories in unusual ways. It causes us to quiver and may be accompanied by an odd or full sensation in the head.

Transcendent experiences are common in addiction treatment where people share deep moments in their lives. One patient may begin to disclose an event in their past, pause, and then say, "I am sure no one in this room has ever gone through *this!*" They tell a tale of bizarre and systematic childhood abuse, filled with pain and sorrow. The room remains silent for a moment and then a second group member, who has not spoken a single word in treatment, utters in a hoarse monotone, "Now I know why I am here, in this treatment. When I was a boy, my best friend told me exactly the same story. I watched him wither away. He eventually died, and I did nothing to save him. I have blamed myself for his death my entire life." The room returns to a ringing silence punctuated by expectation.

Although other members of the group therapy may have not gone through such horrors, they connect through empathy and compassion. Just behind the empathy, a second wondrous transcendence emerges. The seemingly happenstance connection between these two members of the group creates a transcendent truth. One member, who has to date not spoken a word, discovers deep meaning as to why he is present in that group at that very moment. This truth takes hold of the past hurt sweeping it into a higher purpose.

Transcendent events are random, intermittent, and unexpected. They are touchstones along a spiritual quest. While working on this Recovery Skill, I ask the assigned patient to "be on the lookout" for transcendent experiences. In doing so, I am preparing her for the experience. Small events that might have passed by unnoticed may take on transcendent qualities. The exercise widens her field of view and invites wonder.

The second supplemental Spiritual Recovery Skill is **Noticing Coincidences**. This assignment is similar to the first assignment but may be more palatable to the spiritual skeptic. The patient is given a worksheet where she records events that strike her as coincidences. Coincidences that alter the course of her treatment are especially valuable. An example might be "My husband is furious, at his wits end, because of my alcoholism. Just yesterday, he happened to run into a friend he has not seen in years. This friend talked about his alcoholism and how much better his life is now that he is in recovery. Somehow, he is now more open to the possibility of my recovery and the repair of our relationship." After entering each "coincidence" on her list, she describes (in writing and in group therapy) her reaction to these events and the lessons learned from them.

The third supplemental Spiritual Recovery Skill comes from **Building a Gratitude List**. When given this assignment, the patient is charged with verbalizing and recording gratitude at least twice per day. The goal here is to encourage a patient to find gratitude in the small things that occur every day. Most people believe gratitude spontaneously erupts when good things happen to them. They believe they will feel better when *things* are better. Wise individuals know that finding and expressing gratitude engenders happiness and contentment.[45] Over time, this exercise reorients the patient; he begins to use gratitude as a means of reframing life experience. This shifts gratitude from a reaction to an action and offers a healthier, more positive way of approaching recovery.

The fourth supplemental Spiritual Recovery Skill arrives when a patient is able to **Sense a Presence** during meditation exercises. The presence may be a feeling that others are with them (e.g., deceased or distant loved ones or a benevolent force in the universe). This exercise should only be assigned to a patient who is ready to consider that outside forces may provide healing. Patients who are resistant or ambivalent to this notion should never be given this assignment. At the point in time when this assignment occurs, the patient should also be comfortable with the mechanics of meditation. He should be practicing daily and report that meditation helps him feel centered and present.

The most common technique is to try to experience the presence of a benevolent presence in the pause between the inhale and the exhale of the breath. During meditation, one inhales slowly and evenly. In the brief moment, the quiet second before an exhale, he opens himself to this presence. Some individuals experience this as a quiet spot or a connection with the hum of the universe. A smooth exhale follows. The staff member describes the technique to the patient, asking him to incorporate the sensing function into his meditation slowly and explicitly stating, "Do not try to force it." The patient records his responses and reviews them with the staff member when needed.

The fifth supplemental Spiritual Recovery Skill asks a patient to **Distinguish the Voice of RecoveryMind** differentiating it from AddictBrain thoughts and concepts. Patients who are given this assignment should be reasonably well established in recovery. They should be comfortable with the concepts of AddictBrain and RecoveryMind. The goal of this exercise is to help patients recognize how difficult it is to distinguish thoughts and plans that are in the service of recovery from those that are in the service of their disease. The ability to accurately discern this difference will not be realized for years to come. Rather, the goal is to help the patient recognize that some thoughts are clearly diseased, some are uncertain, and few are emphatically in the camp of RecoveryMind. Therefore, it should never be assigned to a patient who "has it all figured out." It is best reserved for the thoughtful patient or the patient who lacks confidence in his or her recovery despite the staff's evaluation that he or she is doing well.

This assignment may run in the background for several weeks. When evaluating a two-column list (one for AddictBrain and one for RecoveryMind), the staff avoids direct answers. A patient may ask, "Does this sound like a recovery thought?" The staff member replies, "How might you figure this out?" Along the way, a patient who is comfortable with prayer may ask this question during a contemplative moment of prayer.

The fifth supplemental Spiritual Recovery Skill is achieved by **Using a "God Box" to Manage Worries**. This venerable AA technique is quite helpful for patients who are in uncertain times, suffer from excessive worry, or have difficulties managing anxiety. It connects psychological difficulties with spiritual answers. The patient should have a defined and comfortable relationship with a Higher Power for this assignment to work. Staff members should have a supply of small wooden boxes or plush drawstring bags. When assigned, a patient is provided a box or bag. When she feels troubled or overwhelmed with worry or anxiety about a current or future trouble, she writes the concern on a small piece of paper. She then folds the paper tightly while revisiting the worry and places it in the box or bag. She may choose to say, "I am giving this worry over to God." Please note the God Box is not a place to put one's desires, hopes, or wishes about the future.

The sixth supplemental Spiritual Recovery Skill comes from **Writing an Obituary**. This assignment helps realign life goals and clarifies values that create a life that is worth living. The patient writes his obituary as he would like it to read in the local paper after his death. This is a simple but powerful values clarification exercise. Give clear instructions to the patient; the obituary should be how the patient would *like it to read* not what it will contain based upon his current situation. An example might start similar to the following:

> *James T. Smith was born January 4, 1984, to June and Robert Smith in Franklin, Ohio. He departed this life in the early afternoon of November 17, 2016.*
>
> *At his deathbed were his beloved wife Joan and two children, Sara and Joshua. James was a man committed to his family, always supporting them in times of need . . .*

The patient's obituary should emphasize what was important in his life, projecting into the future (e.g., love of family, commitment to community sports, or a job where he worked for the common good). It should not contain small-minded things that occupy his mind so much of the time (being slighted by the boss, wanting a new car, etc.). It should not be based on his current life situation. In writing the obituary, the patient will reset life goals, setting aside the unimportant and focusing on the important. Once the obituary is complete, the patient reads it in group therapy. He then returns to his composition, rewriting it as necessary. Once complete, the patient lists three important life goals gleaned from this exercise. Some patients will find a deeper connection with their Higher Power during this exercise.

Recovery Skills for Domain E

This domain contains more skills than could ever be accomplished in a single course of treatment. The staff picks the areas that need the most work, making the respective assignments for each patient and matching them by acceptability and need.

As in all domains, patients and staff routinely complete a progress assessment form that tracks progress. The progress assessment form lists a domain's Recovery Skills a with three-point status rating (**Begun,**

Intermediate, and Completed). The patient completes the form first. This is followed by staff evaluation of the same form. Once complete, the patient and staff meet to reconcile discrepancies between the two evaluations. In this manner, the patient and his or her caregivers have a clear understanding of his or her progress in treatment.

The Interpersonal Recovery Skills in this segment include the following:

1. The patient seeks commonality rather than retreating to uniqueness.
2. The patient is able to stay emotionally present during constructive criticism.
3. The patient can self-disclose and ask for help.
4. The patient can recognize and validate when others provide help.
5. The patient experiences meaning from compassion and selfless giving to others.
6. The patient trusts external advice, especially when it contradicts faulty internal guidance (i.e., AddictBrain thinking).
7. The patient experiences a decrease in shame after sharing personal, ethical, or moral violations. The patient realizes such violations are a central and universal experience in addiction.

The Group Recovery Skills in Domain E include the following:

1. The patient learns how to use twelve-step meetings to sustain recovery and deepen spiritual growth.
2. The patient is able to bond with a healthy peer group that practices nonchemical fun.
3. The patient uses guidance from sponsor, therapists, and other members of a support group.
4. The patient finds meaning in the wisdom of a group and feels part of that group.
5. The patient helps others and experiences gratitude from volunteerism.

6. The patient provides hope for others and in doing so rediscovers hope for himself.

The Step Work Recovery Skills in Domain E are complete when the following tasks occur:
1. The patient has completed the Step Two worksheet and received feedback in his group therapy.
2. The patient has internalized Step Two.
3. The patient has completed the Step Three worksheet and received feedback in his group therapy.
4. The patient has internalized Step Three.

The additional Spiritual Recovery Skills in Domain E are complete when the following tasks occur:
1. The patient has used the Recognizing Transcendence assignment to increase spiritual awareness.
2. The patient has used the Noticing Coincidences assignment to open up to the possibility of a spiritual life.
3. The patient has used the assignment Building a Gratitude List to foster hope for the future.
4. The patient has added sensing his Higher Power to his meditation practice to improve conscious contact with that Higher Power.
5. The patient has practiced distinguishing the voice of RecoveryMind to deepen self-understanding.
6. The patient has used a "God box" to manage worries about the future and to increase his faith.
7. The patient has written an obituary to help him clarify the values he will strive for in his life of recovery.

Chapter Thirteen Notes

1. R. Adolphs, "The Neurobiology of Social Cognition," *Curr Opin Neurobiol* 11, no. 2 (2001): 231–39.

2. J.P. Heuzé, N. Raimbault, and P. Fontayne, "Relationships between Cohesion, Collective Efficacy and Performance in Professional Basketball Teams: An Examination of Mediating Effects," *J Sports Sci* 24, no. 1 (2006): 59–68.

3. D. W. Johnson, R. T. Johnson, and M. L. Krotee, "The Relation between Social Interdependence and Psychological Health on the 1980 U.S. Olympic Ice Hockey Team," *The Journal of Psychology* 120, no. 3 (1986): 279–91.

4. D. W. Johnson, R. T. Johnson, and E. Holubec, *Cooperation in the Classroom*, Eighth ed. (Edina, MN: Interaction Book Company, 2008).

5. G. D. Leon, "Therapeutic Communities for Addictions: A Theoretical Framework," *Subst Use Misuse* 30, no. 12 (1995): 1603–45.

6. E. Kurtz, *Not-God: A History of Alcoholics Anonymous* (Center City: Hazelden Publishing, 1991).

7. G. DeLeon, F. Tims, and N. Jainchill, "Therapeutic Community: Advances in Research and Application, Proceedings of a Meeting, May 16–17, 1991," *NIDA Res Monogr* 144 (1994): 1–286.

8. G. DeLeon, *The Therapeutic Community: Theory, Model, and Method* (New York: Springer Publishing Company, 2000).

9. M. S. Ainsworth and J. Bowlby, "An Ethological Approach to Personality Development," *American Psychologist* 46, no. 4 (1991): 333–41.

10. P. J. Flores, *Addiction as an Attachment Disorder* (Oxford: Jason Aronson, Inc., 2004.)

11. H. F. Harlow and S. J. Suomi, "Social Recovery by Isolation-Reared Monkeys," *Proceedings of the National Academy of Sciences* 68, no. 7 (1971): 1534–38.

12. D. J. Siegel, *The Developing Mind: How Relationships and the Brain Interact to Shape Who We Are*, Second ed. (New York: Guilford Press, 2012), 91.

13. M. D. Ainsworth, M. Blehar, E. Waters, and S. Wall, *Patterns of Attachment: A Psychological Study of the Strange Situation*, (Hillsdale, NJ: Lawrence Erlbaum, 1978).

14. M. Main and J. Soloman, "Procedures for Identifying Infants as Disorganized/ Disoriented During the Ainsworth Strage Situation," in *Attachement in the Preschool Years*, eds. M.T. Greenburg, D. Chcichetti, E. M. Cummings (Chicago: University of Chicago Press, 1990), 121–57.

15. See above, n. 12, p. 111.

16. See above, n. 12, p.144.

17. B. James, *Handbook for Treatment of Attachment-Trauma Problems in Children*, (New York: Lexington Books, 1994).

18. See above, n. 10.

19. L. A. Kaskutas, M. S. Subbaraman, J. Witbrodt, and S. E. Zemore, "Effectiveness of Making Alcoholics Anonymous Easier: A Group Format 12-Step Facilitation Approach," *J Subst Abuse Treat* 37, no. 3 (2009): 228–39.

20. J. Nowinski, S. Baker, and K. Carroll, *Twelve Step Facilitation Therapy Manual*, (Rockville, MD: U.S. Department of Health and Human Services, 1995).

21. L. R. Kaiser, "Spirituality and the Physician Executive: Reconciling the Inner Self with the Business of Health Care," *The Physician Executive* 26 (2000).

22. A. B. Astrow, C. M. Puchalski, and D. P. Sulmasy, "Religion, Spirituality, and Health Care: Social, Ethical, and Practical Considerations," *Am J Med* 110, no. 4 (2001): 283–87.

23. J. Bown and A. Williams, "Spirituality and Nursing: A Review of the Literature," *Journal of Advances in Health and Nursing Care* 2, no. 4 (1993): 41–66.

24. M. A. Persinger, "Religious and Mystical Experiences as Artifacts of Temporal Lobe Function," *Percept Mot Skills* 57, no. 3f (1983): 1255–62.

25. J. L. Saver, J. Rabin, and S. Salloway, "The Neural Substrates of Religious Experience," in *The Neuropsychiatry of Limbic and Subcortical Disorders*, 195–207 (Washington DC: APA Publishing, 1997).

26. A. B. Newberg, and S. K. Newberg, "Hardwired for God: A Neuropsychological Model for Developmental Spirituality," in *Authoritative Communities*, (New York: Springer, 2008), 165–86.

27. A. B. Newberg, "The Neuroscientific Study of Spiritual Practices," *Front Psychol* 5 (2014): 215.

28. B. P. "Jung's Insights Formed Basis of A. A." The New York Times, http://www.nytimes.com/1993/12/03/opinion/l-jung-s-insights-formed-basis-of-a-a-101693.html.

29. D. Berenson, "Alcoholics Anonymous: From Surrender to Transformation," *Family Therapy Networker* (1987).

30. M. Galanter, "Research on Spirituality and Alcoholics Anonymous," *Alcohol Clin Exp Res* 23, no. 4 (1999): 716–19.

31. M. Galanter, "Spirituality and Addiction: A Research and Clinical Perspective," *The American Journal on Addictions* 15, no. 4 (2006): 286–92.

32. M. Galanter, "Spirituality, Evidence-Based Medicine, and Alcoholics Anonymous," *Am J Psychiatry* 165, no. 12 (2008): 1514–17.

33. M. Galanter, H. Dermatis, G. Bunt, C. Williams, M. Trujillo, and P. Steinke, "Assessment of Spirituality and Its Relevance to Addiction Treatment," *J Subst Abuse Treat* 33, no. 3 (2007): 257–64.

34. M. Galanter, H. Dermatis, S. Post, and C. Sampson, "Spirituality-Based Recovery from Drug Addiction in the Twelve-Step Fellowship of Narcotics Anonymous," *J Addict Med* 7, no. 3 (2013): 189–95.

35. M. Galanter and L. A. Kaskutas, *Research on Alcoholics Anonymous and Spirituality in Addiction Recovery: The Twelve-Step Program Model, Spiritually Oriented Recovery, Twelve-Step Membership, Effectiveness and Outcome Research*, Springer, 2008.

36. L. A. Kaskutas, L. A. Kaskutas, J. Bond, and C. Weisner, "The Role of Religion, Spirituality and Alcoholics Anonymous in Sustained Sobriety," *Alcoholism Treatment Quarterly* 21, no. 1 (2003): 1–16.

37. S. Schoenthaler, K. Blum, E. Braverman, J. Giordano, B. Thompson, M. Oscar-Berman, R. Badgaiyan, *et al.*,,"NIDA-Drug Addiction Treatment Outcome Study (DATOS) Relapse as a Function of Spirituality/Religiosity," *Journal of Reward Deficiency Syndrome* 1, no. 1 (2015): 36–45.

38. K. Laubmeier, S. Zakowski, and J. Bair "The Role of Spirituality in the Psychological Adjustment to Cancer: A Test of the Transactional Model of Stress and Coping," *Int J Behav Med* 11, no. 1 (2004): 48–55.

39.   AA World Services, *Twelve Steps and Twelve Traditions* (New York: AA World Services, Inc., 2002.

40.   See above, n. 35.

41.   Narcotics Anonymous, *Narcotics Anonymous Basic Text*, Sixth ed. (Van Nuys, CA: Narcotics Anonymous World Services, Inc., 2008).

42.   P. Carnes, *A Gentle Path through the Twelve Steps: The Classic Guide for All People in the Process of Recovery*, Third ed. (Center City, MN: Hazelden, 2012).

43.   B. Biber, "Spiritual but Not Religious: A Humanist Perspective," American Humanist Association, http://americanhumanist.org/HNN/details/2012-11-spiritual-but-not-religious-a-humanist-perspective.

44.   Alcoholics Anonymous, *Alcoholics Anonymous*, Fourth ed. (New York: A.A. World Services, Inc., 1976).

45.   A. M. Wood, J. J. Froh, and A. W. Geraghty, "Gratitude and Well-Being: A Review and Theoretical Integration," *Clin Psychol Rev* 30, no. 7 (2010): 890–905.

CHAPTER FOURTEEN

Domain F: Relapse Prevention

Domain F focuses on pragmatic skills that prevent relapse. In Domain F, cognitive-behavioral techniques are combined with an understanding of AddictBrain. Using addictive substances over many years alters neuronal circuits dramatically. It is foolish to expect several weeks of training and therapy can unwind years of brain entrainment by powerfully addicting substances. Therefore, patients must learn how to continue the work started in their initial dose of treatment. RMT believes continued training is needed for six months to a year after a patient completes his or her initial treatment dose. This continues work on identified Recovery Skills and teaches important relapse prevention skills in Domain F. All this is contingent upon continued containment of addictive behaviors (Domain A). If the illness is not contained, any work on relapse prevention is a sham.

Throughout the first five RMT domains, many of the Recovery Skills help prevent relapse. If you step back a bit, treatment can be seen as one giant relapse prevention exercise. In fact, relapse prevention is the *raison d'être* of addiction treatment. For more granularity, RecoveryMind Training divides treatment into three distinct components:

1. Interrupting addiction behaviors.
2. Shifting the brain from AddictBrain processing to RecoveryMind thinking and acting.
3. Training the mind to prevent a relapse into addiction.

Relapse prevention can be seen as coming from static factors (illness severity, relationship status, psychiatric comorbidity, and genetics) and dynamic factors (craving, stress, and exposure to conditioned cues). This chapter covers the dynamic factors in relapse prevention—learning and practicing Recovery Skills that retrain and rewire the brain to prevent relapse. Depending on the structure of a patient's course in treatment, Domain F work should at least be touched upon during the initial, and often most intense, parts of his or her care. A patient must have accepted he or she has a chronic disease and is in the action stage of change before beginning work in Domain F.

Moderate level treatment programs (i.e., Day Hospitalization, ASAM Level 2.5 programs, or Intensive Outpatient, ASAM Level 2.1 programs) have limited time to devote to Domain F Recovery Skills. In such levels, patients acquire Domains A and B Recovery Skills and then shift their focus to relapse prevention skills after stepping down to lower levels of care (e.g., ASAM Level 2.1 or 1). In contrast, patients who are at risk for relapse require a higher level of containment; they should begin relapse prevention work while in higher levels of care to ensure the best possible prognosis. In either case, relapse prevention skills should be readdressed for many months to ensure a good outcome.

Definitions

RecoveryMind Training has specific definitions and conventions of use for relapse prevention. All staff members should become familiar with these definitions and use them in a consistent fashion. Remember, exacting definitions and terms help patients develop a more lucid and deeper understanding of their disease. The following paragraphs highlight the three most important terms and their RMT definitions.

Triggers are external or internal events that instigate thoughts or emotions related to substance procurement, use, or consequences. Triggers often introduce cravings but do not necessarily do so. Another term for "trigger" is "cue." RMT uses these terms interchangeably. The goal of trigger management is to catalog the environmental cues, stress events, emotions, and interpersonal situations that increase the propensity for relapse. The patient should develop and practice behavioral techniques to prevent a trigger from escalating into a craving. Triggers are generated by six sources:

- Environmental cues
- Visceral sensations
- Stress
- Emotional events
- Memories
- Interpersonal interactions

The first Recovery Skill in Domain F is developing a list of a patient's specific triggers. The process of delineating triggers and an appropriate response improves his or her competence in managing them when they inevitably occur in the future.

Craving is defined in the Merriam-Webster dictionary as "an intense, urgent, or abnormal desire or longing."[1] RecoveryMind Training divides cravings into two categories: overt or covert. Overt cravings are recognized as such by their victim. Covert cravings are *automatic behaviors* that set one directly on the path to relapse without conscious recognition. Overt cravings have qualities of urgency, intensity, persistence, and recurrence. The most destructive cravings also have the quality of *inevitability*—they feel as if they will continue mercilessly until the addicted individual relapses. In Domain F, a patient learns how to experience cravings without reacting to them. A second cravings management skill is transforming covert cravings into overt cravings where they can be more easily managed. Recent brain imaging studies have identified the neural correlates of craving, providing exciting new avenues for improving cravings management.[2, 3]

Relapse is defined—again using the Merriam-Webster dictionary—as "a recurrence of symptoms of a disease after a period of improvement."[4] It may seem obvious what a relapse is, but clarity is important here. One subtlety arises from the phrase "after a period of improvement." RecoveryMind Training does not consider the initial phases of treatment when calculating the period of improvement. With this in mind, if a patient leaves a short course of treatment and walks directly into a bar to get drunk, he has *not* relapsed. Such an individual has not experienced a period of improvement (or recovery, per se). During initial treatment a patient's illness is held in abeyance; recovery has not yet taken hold. Such an incident is best described as a treatment failure rather than a relapse. The approach to such a situation would be different from a true relapse (i.e., when a patient walks into a bar to drink after months of recovery).

RecoveryMind Training recognizes that many addiction symptoms persist long into recovery. Craving is the most obvious form of persistence; many people have nagging and persistent cravings that dog them for years in recovery. Although cravings are biological symptoms of addiction, their persistence or severity is not directly predictive of relapse. Further, severity and persistence of craving is not a sign of an inadequate recovery program.

To better delineate relapse, consider someone addicted to cocaine with six months of abstinence/recovery in low-dose ongoing care. One day, he gets in his car and drives to his dealer's house with the intention of buying cocaine. His dealer is not home. He leaves agitated and frustrated but does not end up using cocaine. Soon, he calms down and processes the event with his Cocaine Anonymous (CA) sponsor. Despite deliberate drug seeking behavior—a significant symptom of addiction[5]— this would also not be considered a relapse using our nomenclature. Such an individual is indeed at high risk for future relapse, and his recovery remains fragile. However, it is not defined as a relapse according to RMT.

Cues or triggers have the potential for inducing craving. Craving, in turn, prompts relapse. Patients may state, "I did not have anything trigger me; I just had a craving." Such statements are worth examining. In such a case, the relapse prevention therapist should instruct the patient to review the craving episode carefully, looking for potential trigger suspects. The therapist also has learned that this patient needs additional work in relapse prevention, searching for triggers, regardless of subtlety, that induced craving. Individuals who struggle with trigger identification often have broader difficulties in self-insight.

In Domain F, the therapist works through a patient's relapse vulnerability in its natural sequence. Start by exploring triggers, then identify high-risk situations, and then move onto practicing cravings management skills. This may be sufficient Domain F instruction for some patients. If a patient has failed to maintain recovery with this level of relapse prevention work, experienced multiple failed treatments, had a longer course of addiction or more severe physical, social, or psychological consequences, then he should explore the process model of relapse prevention pioneered by Alan Marlatt, PhD, and his colleagues. A slightly modified version of Dr. Marlatt's original relapse schema is described later in this chapter.

Identifying and Managing Triggers

Cues or triggers come from any of the human senses—sound, touch, sight, smell, and taste—as well as internal body sensations (interoceptive cues), stress, emotions, thoughts, and memories. Each recovering individual has his or her own particular set of cues and reactivity to these cues. How powerful these cues are in stimulating drug seeking and drug use is call "cue reactivity."[6] The combination of individualized cues with individualized cue reactivity creates thousands of combinations that should be explored to maximize a patient's resiliency against relapse.

At times, cues induce brain activity and never enter the patient's conscious perception.[7] In fact, early research suggests that medications (e.g., baclofen[8]) may decrease the limbic activation created by these subliminal, or unrecognized, drug cues. We all have heard stories from addicted individuals who are surprised to learn they have relapsed—after the fact. As a patient explores the vast array of his cues, he moves them from the unconscious to the conscious mind. Once they are conscious, he can develop specific skills to manage each of them. When an unconscious cue is moved into conscious awareness, it being noticed provides opportunity for successful management. If a specific relapse prevention response has been learned and practiced, the cue can be managed and the probability of relapse decreases.

Over the course of his illness, an individual may be sensitized to hundreds or even thousands of addiction-related cues or triggers. In Domain F, a therapist explores these triggers, hoping to identify and develop management plans for the most difficult of them. Triggers are divided into five categories:

1. Environmental cues (e.g., seeing a drug, smelling tobacco smoke, hearing addiction-related music).
2. Visceral events (stress level, body sensations, taste, or smell).
3. Emotional events (a feeling that the addicted individual "used to drink over").
4. Stress-related cues.
5. Memory tapes (scenes that play in the mind, especially those with strong visual "tapes").

Repeated cues that result in substance use are "conditioned." Cues are not unique to those who suffer from addiction. Everyone is conditioned by food. Those who do not have addiction may also be conditioned by alcohol use. For example, certain alcoholic beverages are paired with certain foods; when dining in a French restaurant, one might be unconsciously drawn to a particular wine based upon several past experiences there—restaurants have learned to encourage this to improve profitability. Those with substance use disorders have similar but much deeper and more complex associations with substances of abuse. When we talk of environmental cues, the most common description is "external conditioned cues." Cues are said to be **external** when they occur outside the individual. They are **conditioned**, meaning the brain is entrained to expect a using event following the external stimulus. This process is a type of operant conditioning.[9]

Added to easily identifiable external cues are four internal processes. They are visceral (i.e., in the body) events, emotional experiences, stress, and complex memory tapes regarding past use events.[10] When developing Recovery Skills in Domain F, patients should develop a list for each of the four triggers and practice their management.

Identifying and Managing Cravings

Cravings are a natural response the body develops to addiction. Raymond Anton, MD, has studied craving for decades and has likened craving to a form of obsessive-compulsive disorder.[11-15] In the motivated recovering individual, such cravings are ritualistic in nature but are certainly unwanted and ego-dystonic. At the same time, cravings are natural in and appropriate to recovery.[16] Patients will have many different responses to the experience of craving.[17, 18, 19] Some will be afraid of them. Others will minimize them and try to push through them silently when they occur. Some will act out in various ways (substitute addictive behaviors with food, relationships, or sex) without consciously acknowledging that a craving occurred in the first place while others simply feel emotionally overwhelmed. Each person has a different relationship with the craving experience. Many recovering individuals judge themselves for having cravings; I hear patients all the time say, "I must not be working a strong enough program because I am having a lot of cravings." This is simply untrue. Each person's craving experience is different, and there is no right or wrong. Despite the natural tendency to consider cravings as an indication of a faulty recovery, patients should be instructed that this is simply not the case. Cravings only indicate that the disease of addiction is still present in the brain.

RecoveryMind Training differentiates cravings as overt or covert. Overt cravings, when they occur, are recognized as such. The patient says, "I woke up this morning thinking about drinking, and after a bit, I noticed the taste of whisky in my mouth." Covert cravings are bodily hungers that beget agitation, anger, emotional overwhelm, acting-out behaviors, or relapse without registering in one's consciousness. The overt/covert distinction helps the recovering patient begin the self-discovery required for effective relapse prevention training. Often, a sponsor, family members, and/or peers in treatment identify covert cravings. Staff members should encourage everyone to examine a report or event that may be a covert craving. For example, a staff member may say, "John, your feelings seem very strong this afternoon. Could this be a covert craving related to your discussing your drug use in group this morning?"

Every person with alcohol or drug use disorder is bombarded by thousands of triggering events in the early years of recovery, and almost everybody dislikes admitting his or her vulnerabilities. This leads to one of the central paradoxes of addiction recovery; that is, the more you admit to and talk about cravings, the lower the probability of relapse. In some ways, this paradox flies in the face of common logic. Patients will assert (with a touch of bravado), "I'm doing great. I haven't had a craving for weeks." In fact, craving repression leaves the door wide open for relapse. Instead, patients are encouraged to accept idle thoughts or urges as cravings. Patients are taught to recognize cravings early on in order for them to be effectively managed before they become unbearable.

Toward these ends, whenever a patient notes a craving, he or she should be taught to use the RecoveryMind craving rating scale, which follows.

Level 1. A fleeting thought of engaging in addiction that lasts less than a minute and disappears without any response on the person's part.

Level 2. A brief thought accompanied by an urge or addiction hunger lasting any period that disappears

when the patient consciously focuses on another
subject or physically changes his or her activity.

Level 3. A craving similar to that in Level 2, but one that
lasts for multiple minutes and requires repeated
adjustment of thinking and/or physical relocation
or external support to abort the thoughts and urges.

Level 4. Any craving where the individual contemplates using
and/or considers the presumptive benefits of using
for more than ten seconds. Level 4 cravings may last
for an extended period and begin to have a quality of
inevitability—meaning they distort thinking to the
point that the patient begins to believe the only way
the cravings will go away is to use.

Level 5. Any craving that results in drug seeking or
procurement in any manner.

If we ask our patients to pay closer attention to their cravings, we
are, by inference, obligated to teach them an effective management
paradigm. RecoveryMind Training outlines a simple series of steps a
recovering individual should take to manage each craving and improve
his or her subsequent reactivity to them. The following diagram outlines
the craving management process.

When an event is recognized as a craving, several steps need to be
taken to manage that craving effectively and to prevent it from resulting
in relapse. First, the patient needs to recognize a craving has occurred.
If a specific trigger can be quickly identified, one should do so. If it is not
immediately apparent, such research is best put off until later. Second,
the individual should rate the craving using the RMT rating scale. Early
in recovery, cravings at Levels 2 and 3 can prove to be pesky at best and
risky at worst. Third, patients should determine whether they possess
sufficient skills to manage the craving with self-skills or they need
external support. This is often a tricky decision and one that, made
incorrectly, can have devastating effects.

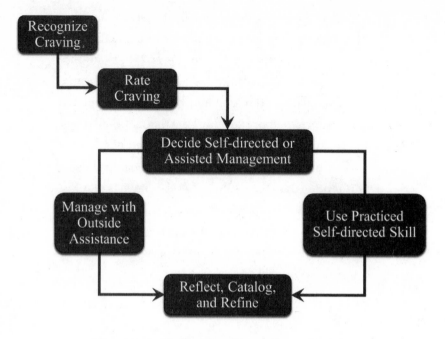

Figure 14.1 - The Craving Management Process

Lower intensity cravings may be managed by simple self-directed skills. More intense cravings may require external help and support. In treatment, patients should practice asking for help with their cravings, even if they believe the intensity of the craving is not severe. Practice prepares the patient, teaching him or her how to manage future episodes. The disclosure should sidestep embellishment, addressing the craving episode as an irritant and annoyance. This helps the craving pass quickly. Practicing self-directed craving management and asking for assistance in handling a craving are independent and mutually beneficial skills.

Individual Management

Once the patient has recognized a craving, judged its severity, and determined that outside help is not needed, self-directed craving management skills come into play. Because most individuals with addiction disorders have frequent and unpredictable cravings, it is often impractical to pull in reinforcements every time they occur. Assuming a patient has assessed that a craving can be managed without external help, he or she should immediately begin self-directed management. These simple skills include the following:

- **Thought Blocking:** Stating with an internal voice (or, better yet, say aloud), "I am not going to think about that."
- **Thought Switching:** The addicted person states (to themselves or better, aloud), "I will not think about that now, instead I will think about _____." Thought switching can often be to a current task, a past, pleasant, healthy memory, a book or movie, or a past conversation. The more the individual focuses on minute details of the replacement thought, the more effective the response. This skill is commonly combined with Thought Blocking.
- **Physical Movement:** The brain is a contextual, place-sensitive organ. Changing sensory input by movement and changing location, even a small amount, will reduce craving.
- **Labeling the Craving as Just a Craving:** Here the individual states to himself using dialog (internal or external), "Ah ha! That is a craving! Nothing more!" The proper use of language is important here. The most effective way to label a craving is to use a neutral label ("That is a craving") rather than acknowledging its pull ("I am having a terrible craving").
- **Recalling the Inaccurate Feelings That Accompany Cravings:** After labeling a craving, it may also help to run through the feeling distortions that ride alongside each craving, which are summarized in Table 14.1.

Table 14.1 - Feeling Distortions Induced by Cravings

Quality	Natural but Incorrect Interpretation	What Really Happens
Urgency	"I have to do something about this!"	If you do nothing, it will go away.
Intensity	"This craving is too intense. It will keep getting stronger!"	Cravings wax and wane over brief time spans. They become tolerable when the individual learns they naturally decrease if left alone.
Persistence	"This craving will last forever! In fact, it has already lasted forever!"	If you let a craving play out, it will eventually go away. Most cravings last five minutes or so. Sometimes they go on for thirty minutes, but they eventually go away.
Recurrence	"This craving will keep on happening until I use alcohol or other drugs (or the addiction behavior)."	Cravings do return but often do not. When they come back, they frequently change form.
Inevitability	"This craving will eventually result in relapse."	Cravings come and go and will remit spontaneously if the patient does not use.

More advanced skills for self-directed management include the following:

- **Surfing the Urge:** This skill has been described for managing difficult emotions in Chapter Eleven. Urge surfing is best taught in a group setting. In the group, patients learn that cravings come and go. Before arriving in treatment, most people with alcohol and drug use disorders have a distorted perception that urges, especially strong ones, will persist and even continue to escalate unless the person responds by using substances. After practicing urge surfing, patients realize the sense of inevitability is simply a distortion produced by the craving. It is not real or accurate. When a craving occurs, the patient recalls their experience in group therapy, and the urge de-escalates.

- **Thinking the Craving to Its Complete Conclusion:** This response is a "what if" process. The patient uses a narrative similar to the following:

  "I am having a craving to use heroin. If I react to this craving by using, I will try to smoke a little heroin just to get that fuzzy, warm blanket feeling. That will be followed by a hunger to use again. Over several days, I will fall into a continuous rut of using until I become hopelessly dependent. My girlfriend will know I relapsed, and this time she will kick me out for good. I will have nowhere to go. My life will fall apart. I will most likely continue to use until I overdose and die."

An individual with alcohol use disorder might think in the following manner:

"I want to drink. The last time I drank, I was very cruel to my wife and children. This is what alcohol is doing to me. If I drink, I will continue to hurt my family, which is the last thing I want to do. My wife will leave with our children. If I act on this craving, it will lead to an inevitable, painful loss. I know my pattern. I know where this winds up. What else could I do right now instead of ruining my life by drinking?"

Such a narrative makes sure the addicted individual follows the real sequence of events to its logical conclusion. AddictBrain always stops thoughts about using prematurely, ending at the fantasy of the short-term positive effect. We can counteract this by putting the caboose on that train of thought.

Gathering External Support

If a craving is judged as intense or unpredictable or if assistance is readily available, the recovering person is better served by asking for help. Many patients feel silly or weak when they ask for help. This alone can dissuade them from being effective at cravings management. Therefore, one of the first skills to learn in relapse prevention is openly admitting a problem exists and humbly asking for the assistance of others. This skill was addressed in Domain E, but I revisit it here. The following list outlines interpersonal craving management skills.

- **Labeling and Acknowledging**: The simplest skill comes from disclosing a craving aloud to another person. Cravings are diminished when the brain event moves from an internal thought to spoken words. Support personnel should be trained to respond by saying, "What can I do to help?" Such a question allows the recovering individual time to reevaluate severity and forces him or her to consider options. The support person should avoid moving immediately into fix-it mode. Quite often, the recovering person will notice the craving diminished dramatically the minute it was externalized.

- **Using Individual Skills with a Coach**: The support person can also assist the individual with a craving by walking him or her through one or more of the individual craving management skills described previously.

- **Changing Activity or Focus**: When the addicted person is alone, changing focus may be difficult. When alone, it is best to move and change one's physical location. Changing the current activity may also help. If a patient is with others, changing the focus of the conversation, such as switching to discussions about recovery or gratitude, is quite effective at mitigating craving. Sometimes a line of conversation inadvertently trips up an urge, or a particular place, song, or smell triggers a craving. When labeled and externalized, the patient and his or her support person eliminate the stimulus together, increasing confidence and decreasing the probability of future relapse. If this skill is practiced with friends or family, one additional benefit occurs: the recovering individual experiences deeper interpersonal connections.

- **Gradual Cue Exposure without Using**: Certain cues are unavoidable and therefore troublesome. A trained clinician or perceptive sponsor can help the patient catalog such cues and determine when it is safe to explore those cravings without responding to them. This process is called Cue Exposure and Response Prevention. Limited studies have shown that exposure to a cue while simultaneously preventing a drug or alcohol use event may decrease subsequent cravings.[20] However, the effectiveness of this paradigm is unclear.[21] Clinically, patients develop a cognitive appreciation that triggers can be managed, which increases self-efficacy in appropriate situations. Craving situations that are the most unavoidable should only be addressed when patients are stable in recovery. For example, an individual with alcohol use disorder in early recovery should avoid spending more than a few moments in a bar, if this is at all possible. However, he or she does need to learn how to be in a restaurant where alcohol is served at some point along his or her recovery journey. A gradual exposure to this environment alternated with discussion of the experience builds comfort with such unavoidable life events.

Identifying and Managing High-Risk Situations

The term "high-risk situation" is immediately identifiable to most patients. However, when identifying high-risk situations, patients often cite the most egregious of examples: "I was with my old using friend who was high on oxycodone and put out a big line on the table for me to snort." This is the proverbial three-alarm fire, not a high-risk situation as defined by RMT. When working with patients to compile a list of high-risk situations, it is most important to help them identify situations that may not, upon initial evaluation, be deemed high risk. For example, someone who is divorced and has alcohol use disorder may need to consider "having a drawn-out argument with my ex-wife about my daughter" as a high-risk situation.

When developing a relapse prevention plan, patients must write down a near exhaustive list of possible, future, high-risk situations. The list is often presented to others in group therapy; treatment peers suggest additional, potential items for the expanding list. Some patients quietly recognize their own situations while listening to the presenter's list. Once presented, the individual goes back through the list and assigns each situation to one of the following categories:

- **Address Now:** These high-risk situations are part of everyday life. The recovering person must acquire skills to manage such situations immediately. One might place the high-risk situation "Seeing beer commercials on television during sports events" in this category. One simple management would be to get up and walk away from the television during certain beer commercials.

- **Delay Exposure:** Certain high-risk situations should initially be avoided until the patient learns specific skills to manage the given situation. These high-risk situations are often those that should eventually be addressed to avoid an overly constrictive life in recovery. One example might be "Driving past a bar where I used to drink," especially when this bar is directly on the route between home and work. Early in recovery, a circuitous route avoids such a stimulus. Eventually, it would be best to drive past the bar with a sponsor on the way to an AA meeting, followed by discussion of the experience with others.

- **Avoid Forever:** Circumstances labeled "avoid forever" are extremely dangerous for recovery. Such situations commonly offer no value to the recovering individual. Many of these situations are simply a relapse waiting to happen. Recovering individuals often expose themselves to this type of high-risk situation out of false confidence or a foolish need to "prove they are strong in recovery." An example might be the addicted person who asserts he can go back to his old using friends and "be an example of how they can recover too."

Table 14.2 provides examples of high-risk situations, placing each into one of the three categories.

Table 14.2 - Examples of High-Risk Situations

High-Risk Situation	Type	Comments
Sitting in a bar for any reason and any length of time	Delay Exposure	In the first several years of recovery, this should be completely avoided. Later on, one should only proceed with extreme caution and only when there is a reason he or she has to be there (e.g., waiting for a dinner table).
Meeting up with acquaintances you used with in the past	Delay Exposure	This varies according to who the individuals are in the patient's life. Patients will commonly underestimate how dangerous using friends are to their recovery.
Getting in an argument with your spouse	Address Now	Interpersonal conflict is unavoidable. Instead of avoiding conflict, patients should be taught interpersonal effectiveness.
Sitting in front of a pile of cocaine	Avoid Forever	Some people in recovery think continuing to expose themselves to alcohol and other drugs is a sign of bravery and bravado. This is just foolhardy.
Driving past a favorite bar	Delay Exposure	One should find a different route to avoid driving past the bar. Later, desensitize the experience with one's sponsor.
Having excess money in a pocket or purse	Delay Exposure	This is especially true for individuals who have purchased drugs with cash.
Dealing with painful feelings related to addiction	Address Now	Recovery is filled with painful emotions. In treatment, such issues should be addressed head on in Domain C.
Watching movies with explicit drug or alcohol use or drug dealing	Delay Exposure	The exact process of desensitization regarding explicit movies varies from individual to individual. Movies that glorify alcohol or other drug use are the most problematic; however, even negative portrayals trigger cravings.

High-Risk Situation	Type	Comments
Placing work or social obligations over recovery	Avoid Forever	Depending on the severity of addiction, individuals must learn how much emphasis needs to be placed on recovery over work, home, and social obligations. This changes over time. Early in recovery, work and social obligations need to take a back seat.
Attending a party where the primary goal is drug or alcohol intoxication	Avoid Forever	Patients should be taught how to assess which social situations are safe and which are problematic. Social situations where intoxication is the primary goal are always unsafe. Once in recovery, most people are surprised to find such parties quite boring.
Attend a work event where alcohol will be served	Delay Exposure	The social use of alcohol is prevalent in many work environments. An individual who works around or entertains with alcohol needs specific alcohol-refusal training.
Airplane travel or boat cruise where alcohol is freely served and encouraged	Delay Exposure	Individuals whose work includes frequent airline travel have heavy alcohol exposure. Families who vacation on boat cruises are exposed to alcohol almost continuously. Both groups need specific relapse prevention plans for these activities.
Overcoming social anxiety in order to attend therapy or support groups	Address Now	Social support is a large part of the recovery process. Individuals who have social anxieties need specific training to help them obtain the benefits of the many treatment offerings that occur in a group format.
Going to a concert where drugs or alcohol are used	Delay Exposure	Concerts of all genres are associated with alcohol or other drug use. Recovering individuals should group together, controlling their immediate environment.
Attending a family function where alcohol is served	Delay Exposure	Family functions with alcohol are a double whammy, providing easy access to substances of abuse combined with the potential for strong emotional response to family dynamics and conflict.

High-Risk Situation	Type	Comments
Staying alone in a hotel or motel with a minibar	Delay Exposure	Many hotels with minibars have keys. When checking in, the recovering individual can refuse the key or ask for a room without this unneeded temptation.
Volunteering in a shelter that houses actively using people	Delay Exposure	Working in a volunteer capacity helps recovering people gain self-esteem, increase their gratitude, and feel part of humankind. However, depending on their personality structure, such jobs can create additional risks. It is best for the individual to review these decisions with a sponsor or therapist.
Spending long periods alone and away from recovery support	Delay Exposure	Recovery is a daily process that erodes when it is not maintained. Recovering individuals should have nearly constant contact with the recovering community early in their journey. Prolonged periods away from recovery support should be carefully considered.
Traveling to locations where support group meetings are unavailable	Delay Exposure	As with the previous situation, individuals who have to travel away from their support network should find alternative means of buttressing their recovery.

After developing his or her list and categorizing each situation, the patient goes back through the list a second time, entering a recovery response to each item. If time permits, staff members might review the list and have the patient role-play one or more of the more complex high-risk situations in skills group. A patient has developed Recovery Skills in relapse prevention when he or she has completed his or her high-risk list and developed proficiency when role-playing several of the most important situations.

Process Oriented Relapse Prevention

In the first half of this chapter, relapse was looked upon as a singular event. Relapse prevention in the first section uses trained skills to prevent that event. Almost every patient can comprehend relapse prevention when relapse is viewed as a single event. Many patients are well on their way to a sustained recovery after they acquire Domain F Recovery Skills that manage cues, cravings, and high-risk situations.

Other patients who have a more prolonged or severe illness, those with addictive behaviors early in life, those who suffer from the sequelae of past trauma, or those with personality types that unconsciously reinforce addiction may require more extensive relapse prevention training. Some patients in this second group describe relapses as "just happening to them." When asked about his relapse, one of my past patients said, "I just found myself in a bar with a drink in my hand!" Such a patient is begging to be led through the relapse process, looking at the antecedents to arriving at the bar and the thought patterns that preceded heading to that bar; such events set him on a direct path to inevitable relapse.

RMT's relapse prevention system is a slightly modified version of the evidence-based relapse prevention research of Marlatt and his colleagues at the University of Washington.[22-24] Using cognitive-behavioral strategies, Dr. Marlatt developed a lucid and practical relapse model almost thirty years ago. This model has undergone extensive revision since that time,[25] and one notable expansion is joining the model to mindfulness training.[26, 27] Although this model was developed three decades ago, it continues to be an extremely powerful relapse prevention paradigm, especially when combined with RecoveryMind Training. Both the original[28] and the later text[29] from the University of Washington should be studied by addiction therapists and kept on the shelf for handy reference. The following schematic shows Marlatt's earlier model adapted to RecoveryMind Training.

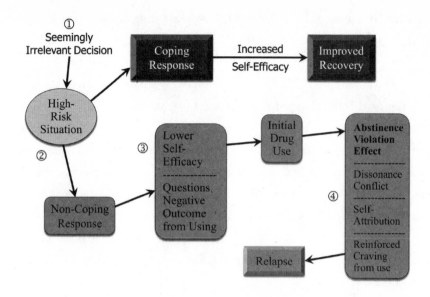

Figure 14.2 - Marlatt's Model of Relapse Prevention
(modified from the original[30])

Let us briefly review the modified Marlatt diagram. Beginning in the upper left-hand corner (①) are the words **Seemingly Irrelevant Decision** (SID). Although this concept is critical to the model, it may be difficult for patients to understand a seemingly irrelevant decision and how it places them in a high-risk situation. RecoveryMind Training helps with this confusion. A SID is a minor thought or decision that produces a cascade of troublesome events. For example, one day while on the way to work, a recovering person may impulsively decide to drive a different route. She turns left at a traffic light, thinking she is taking a more scenic route to work. Soon after, she realizes she is driving past the house of a using friend or a bar where she used to drink. This triggers intense craving and memories of her using past. What looks like a seemingly irrelevant, almost random decision, it has placed her in a high-risk situation.

Using the language of RecoveryMind Training, AddictBrain covertly injected a thought or behavior that, at first glance, seems innocuous. AddictBrain operates subtly, gently nudging the recovering person in the direction of relapse. SIDs are easy to understand in the abstract. If a patient is well along the way of internalizing the concepts of RecoveryMind Training, such an analysis might be intuitively recognizable. Note that SIDs are always easier to identify retrospectively. Asking individuals to identify a SID proactively can be a challenge.

The next inflection point (②) along the path to relapse is the **High-Risk Situation**. As previously noted, a high-risk situation is a social, geographical, emotional, or interpersonal circumstance where the recovering individual is at increased risk of relapse. Relapse prevention training teaches the individual to notice and act as soon as possible to mitigate such situations. Once trained, the recovering individual goes on alert in such circumstances, recognizing danger and the possibility of relapse. High-risk situations happen nearly every day when one is early in recovery.

Figure 14.2 illustrates how the recovering person is at a crossroads in each high-risk situation. A coping response occurs when she makes the right choice regarding such a dangerous circumstance. A coping response always involves action. Once taken, such a patient develops an increased sense of self-efficacy, and she has taken a step to reinforce her recovery. The principle of self-efficacy is difficult for a few therapists who work with twelve-step principles. Self-efficacy is different from "taking back control." The concept of self-efficacy, parsed by Albert Bandura, PhD, in the 1970s,[31, 32] contains components of increased self-esteem, the ability to make healthy choices, and a decrease in perceived helplessness.

Using RecoveryMind Training, the recovering person who responds to a high-risk situation with a coping response is using multiple resources to subvert the agenda of AddictBrain. These resources include previous relapse prevention training, the advice of one's sponsor, and often a higher power. However, self-efficacy has its limits in addiction. Danger creeps back in when the recovering individual asserts, "I outwitted that danger, and this makes me stronger. Next time, I will be able to go to my friend's house and not use methamphetamine."

The outcome of each coping response is an improvement in one's recovery program. The improvement comes from the effort taken and the sense that abstinence and recovery are attainable goals. When AddictBrain has been thwarted once or twice, some individuals confuse these short-term successes with hardened armor against future relapse. During relapse prevention training, it is important to congratulate each coping response while at the same time prevent the recovering individual from falling into the fantasy of impenetrable protection from relapse.

Let's follow Figure 14.2 down the other branch off of a high-risk situation. When an individual with alcohol use disorder fails to make a coping response, she begins a cascade of events that accumulate and build on each other, potentially leading to relapse. After failing to make a coping response, Marlatt described a series of internal states that ensue. The individual's self-esteem decreases and helplessness increases. AddictBrain whispers, "You know you're going to use." The recovering individual contemplates the possibility of a good outcome from drug or alcohol use, despite overwhelming evidence to the contrary.

At the very first moment of chemical or behavioral use, a cascade of events befalls the recovering individual. Marlatt labeled this cascade the **Abstinence Violation Effect** (AVE). I have modified his original AVE slightly in Figure 14.2. The first element in this cascade is dissonance conflict, first described and studied by Festinger.[33] Dissonance conflict arises when a particular belief or self-concept is contradicted by current actions or behaviors.[34] The conflict produces significant emotional distress. Distress often fuels relapse rather than interrupting it. The second component of AVE is self-attribution. In this model, the likelihood of the relapse process continuing is increased by how strongly the individual attributes the breach to fixed personal and global difficulties ("I have no willpower") rather than controllable causes ("I should have used better coping skills in this situation").[35, 36] Self-attribution leads to a further sense of hopelessness and defectiveness— prominent characteristics in the victims of addiction disorders.[37]

To Marlatt's original model, I added an important biological component of relapse. Once addiction's reinforcing neural pathways are entrained, reward and reinforcement from initial use drives continued use. The reward and reinforcement of addicting substances is added to the first two psychological components of the abstinence violation effect. The combination of dissonance conflict, self-attribution, and reinforced craving unleash a mighty storm of relapse. Further addiction behaviors seem inevitable, and full-blown relapse ensues.

Interventions to Prevent Relapse

Referring back to Figure 14.2, pay attention to the labels ① through ④ in the diagram. Each of these refers to specific points along the relapse prevention model where interventions prove effective. I will discuss these in turn.

Point ① Seemingly Irrelevant Decisions

The first point of intervention is noted to occur during the process of seemingly irrelevant decisions. Despite the fact that this is the first point of intervention, it is the most difficult for patients to grasp effectively, especially in early recovery. Seemingly irrelevant decisions are by their very nature *seemingly irrelevant*. Recognizing what appears to be a benign and inconsequential choice as a dangerous path to relapse requires subtlety and skill. Some patients may never be able to grasp this concept.

The single most important skill one needs to facilitate SID recognition is curiosity combined with gentle self-doubt. The recovering individual weighs each decision to determine whether it is in the service of AddictBrain or RecoveryMind. Patients should be taught to question their decisions frequently, setting aside distracting and unhelpful judgments about "right" or "wrong." Individuals who have learned to recognize their own SIDs have noted that most often these destructive decisions seem to "pop up" out of nowhere. When they arrive early in recovery, they are often accompanied by a sense of urgency. This is where self-examination and curiosity helps. Further examination establishes SIDs as promoting relapse rather than sustaining recovery.

Patients will have an easy time listing past high-risk situations, especially those that led to relapse. The therapist first acknowledges this recognition as valuable and then asks the most important question, "What were the ideas, emotions, external pressures, and decisions that got you there?" Such work leads to the exploration of seemingly irrelevant decisions and a deeper understanding of the complexity of relapse prevention strategies.

Point ② High-Risk Situations

High-risk situations were discussed earlier in this chapter. When working on the process model of relapse, it may be helpful to have patients review their list of high-risk situations. When they do so, they should consider potential SIDs that AddictBrain might use to promote each high-risk situation. This exercise is best done in group therapy with a light, almost playful air. The therapist says, "Frank, go over your list of high-risk situations. What might AddictBrain do to entice you to go there?" If Frank is stymied, group members can throw out ideas. The therapist may encourage Frank to enroll the voice of AddictBrain and listen to possible ways it could lure him into such circumstances. The more a patient explores the interplay between SIDs and high-risk situations, the more he defends himself from falling into such traps.

Point ③ Subsequent to a Non-Coping Response

Interrupting the process of relapse becomes increasingly more difficult as one proceeds down the relapse path. This does not mean, however, that relapse is inevitable. Aborting the relapse process at point ③ is best accomplished by recognizing the signs and symptoms of being there. Curiosity, when combined with knowledge of this stage in the relapse prevention model, is the most potent tool in interrupting relapse. Individuals with alcohol and drug use disorders should be taught to recognize when they feel a drop in their self-efficacy, questioning, "Why am I feeling so vulnerable at this very moment?" Similarly, RecoveryMind Training teaches the recovering individual to ring an alarm bell when certain dangerous ideas erupt. At the top of this list is the intermittent and dangerous notion that using alcohol or other drugs "Might be a good idea— just this one time." RecoveryMind Training emphasizes that certain thought patterns are extremely dangerous to the recovering individual. A subversive thought that commonly occurs at this point in the relapse process is the notion that alcohol or other drug use might not be accompanied by the negative consequences that inevitably occurred in the past.

When a recovering individual unwittingly exposes himself to a high-risk situation, he finds himself at point ③ in this relapse model. Immediate action is mandatory. RecoveryMind Training states that the individual should physically move away from the high-risk situation: "Put your wallet back in your pocket and step away from the bar. Then, don't walk but run out the door." Next, the individual should call in his support troops. This proves easiest when the individual has a previously established relationship with a sponsor or friends in recovery. He calls his sponsor and acts on immediate instructions that provide an escape from the high-risk situation. Such action reinforces future coping responses and improves recovery.

Point ④ Abstinence Violation Effect

Moving along the process of relapse, we come to the abstinence violation effect. Patients who have been traumatized by previous relapse understand the pain that occurs immediately after the first sip of alcohol or other drug use. A whole cascade of events occurs and, more often than not, they experience the full fury of the abstinence violation effect. Relapse follows. Nonetheless, some individuals can abort relapse here, surviving the maelstrom of the AVE.

The techniques for aborting full relapse at point ④ are similar to those for point ③. In relapse prevention training, patients are taught the components of the AVE so they may recognize them if they should occur. Simple understanding of each of these components provides a modicum of intellectual distance from the crisis at hand. This distance can occasionally interrupt a full-blown relapse in its embryonic state.

Putting It All Together

Let's walk through this relapse prevention model using an example. Joe is a forty-five-year-old married man who has just completed four weeks in a residential program (ASAM Level 3.5) and has just started a relapse prevention program (ASAM Level 1). His childhood friend Frank calls him up one Saturday morning and asks him to go with him to a major-league baseball game in their hometown. Frank is a boyhood friend and has no addiction issues himself. During the conversation, Frank says, "I haven't seen you for quite some time Joe, are you okay?" Joe, embarrassed about his addiction, simply states, "I've been busy for the past several months. I'll tell you about it later." Joe was given a golden opportunity to let Frank know about his recent treatment and decision for sobriety. He made a seemingly irrelevant decision (①) to put off informing Frank about his treatment, telling himself that they would have time to talk about this later in the day. Joe is excited about attending a baseball game with Frank and thinks it will be relatively safe because he knows Frank has no substance use issues.

They obtain last-minute tickets and arrive at the ballpark just as the game starts. Sitting out in the bleachers, the day is a hot but an otherwise perfect day for a ballgame. Halfway through the third inning, Frank snares a local vendor selling beer. He buys a beer for himself and offers one to Joe. Once again, Joe has an opportunity to explain his situation but now feels a bit foolish. He simply replies, "I'm not thirsty." As the day proceeds, the rising heat increases Joe's thirst. He recognizes he is in a high-risk situation (②) and chides himself for the seemingly irrelevant decision of not telling Frank earlier. Joe knows that if he had told his lifelong friend, Frank would have not purchased a beer, and the high-risk situation could have been avoided completely.

Being in a high-risk situation means Joe is at an inflection point. He must take action to avoid relapse. Let us assume he turns to Frank and says something like, "You know the oddest thing Frank, you mentioned to me on the phone that you wondered where I had been. Well, I've been in treatment for the past several months for an alcohol problem." Frank, being a good friend and having no issues with alcohol himself would likely turn to Joe and say, "Wow, that's big news. I always worried about your drinking." Frank looks down at his paper cup filled with beer and asks, "I bet my drinking this beer in front of you is not a good thing right now, is it?" Joe acknowledges this fact, and Frank quietly disposes the remainder of the beer. Joe offers to buy them both a soft drink. They discuss his treatment and reconnect in the way that old friends do. Joe recognizes that he made a seemingly irrelevant decision that placed him into a high-risk situation. However, he also happily acknowledges his coping response that resulted in increased self-efficacy. He has improved his Recovery Skills. Joe will be more comfortable discussing his addiction disorder with others when the need arises.

Next, we will next follow what occurs if Joe has a non-coping response. In this case, he sits next to Frank who casually sips his beer as the game goes on. He feels foolish for not taking better care of his recovery. A small voice in his head chastises him saying, "How could you let yourself get into this situation? When you were in treatment you thought you were so committed to recovery and now look at this fine mess!" The day gets hotter, and Joe's thirst increases. He feels more troubled. Joe feels trapped by his earlier decision and elects to say nothing about his recent treatment. Eventually, he arrives at the worst conclusion: "One sip won't hurt." He is at point ③ in the relapse prevention process. If he recognizes the signs and symptoms of this stage, he could stand up, walk away, call his sponsor, and extricate himself from what seems inevitable. This would abort relapse at point ③. In my example, however, this does not occur. Instead, he turns to Frank and asks for the sip of his beer. His good friend Frank obliges.

Immediately upon the first taste of alcohol, Joe falls into the abstinence violation effect. He decides to buy his own beer. Sitting in the bleacher, the glass of beer in his hand, Joe experiences dissonance conflict. At the beginning of this day, he was an individual committed to recovery and excited about his new life. Instead, he finds himself sitting in the stands at a ballgame with a beer in his hand. The battle between his commitment to recovery and his current situation creates dissonance conflict. The conflict is disturbing, difficult to resolve, and produces further indecision. Thoughts swirl around in his head, saying things to him, such as "I guess I wasn't as committed to recovery as I thought"; "I guess my best laid plans really don't work"; and "What's wrong with me spending all that money on treatment and getting nothing out of it?"

Joe suffers further loss of control through self-attribution. He blames himself for this setback, pronouncing himself a failure. All these thoughts and feelings combine with the initial effect of alcohol. He is at point ④ in the relapse process. The alcohol dulls the pain and allows him to push away the pain of his situation; it encourages him to continue drinking. With significant and dramatic effort, he can prevent a full-blown relapse. This would entail opening up to Frank, calling his sponsor, leaving the game, pulling other recovering people to him as protection, going directly to a twelve-step meeting, increasing psychotherapy, and ensuring everyone in his circle knows about the immediate crisis. Otherwise, he will simply continue into complete relapse.

I have labeled the four points of intervention to prevent relapse in the above story. As this story progresses, it becomes more and more difficult to abort relapse. Patients who return to treatment after relapse should be strongly encouraged to use this model to deconstruct their recent relapse. This assignment is called a "relapse autopsy." Patients who are in treatment for the first time may also benefit from this analysis if they have made a concerted effort in the past to stop using.

Dr. Marlatt's relapse prevention model helps patients understand that relapse occurs after a series of maladaptive responses—(i.e., AddictBrain thinking). It puts a systematic structure around substance use, deepening a patient's appreciation that relapse is not a single event. Relapse does not just fall out of the sky. The process model is complex and may be overkill for some patients. However, I have found that patients who have been unable to sustain recovery despite repeated attempts will benefit from a thorough examination of this model.

Recovery Skills for Domain F

The Recovery Skills in Domain F cover basic (event-based) and process-based relapse prevention. Staff members should consider disease severity, past failed treatment, and available time in treatment when making assignments in this domain. In general, the Recovery Skills should be assigned in the order shown in this section.

As in all previous domains, patients and staff routinely complete a progress assessment form that tracks and validates progress. The progress assessment form lists a domain's Recovery Skills with a three-point status rating (**B**egun, **I**ntermediate, and **C**ompleted). The patient completes the form first. This is followed by staff evaluation of the same form. Once complete, the patient and staff meet to reconcile discrepancies between the two evaluations. In this manner, the patient and his or her caregivers have a clear understanding of progress in treatment.

A Recovery Skill in this domain is complete when the following tasks occur:

1. The patient can accurately verbalize an understanding of the following terms: trigger, craving, high-risk situation, and relapse.
2. The patient can describe the interaction and difference between a trigger, craving, high-risk situation, and a relapse.
3. The patient has created and reviewed a list of triggers or cues and has identified at least one cue in each of the five cue categories (environmental, visceral, stress-related, emotional, and memory tapes).
4. The patient has kept a list of cravings over a period of several weeks or more. He or she has reviewed the list in group therapy and graded each craving's severity.
5. The patient has identified four or more of these cravings as especially troublesome and has committed to memory an automatic response to each.
6. The patient understands and has demonstrated competency in three or more of the six individual craving management skills.

7. The patient understands and has practiced each interpersonal craving management technique. He or she has identified one technique as a favorite.

8. The patient has participated in training on "surfing the urge."

9. The patient has an extensive list of high-risk situations and a plan to manage each one.

10. The patient has a complete description of each of the emotional states that create the highest risk for relapse and has a memorized response plan when each one occurs.

11. The patient knows the high-risk situations that fit in the Avoid Forever category and has shared this list with his or her family and sponsor and agrees to avoid these high-risk situations for the first five years of recovery.

12. The patient has participated in training on the process model of relapse and has described how it fits with his or her personal recovery.

13. The patient has recognized and reviewed several past and at least one current seemingly irrelevant decision.

14. If a past relapse has occurred, the patient has assessed this relapse using Marlatt's model and discussed future alternatives to relapse.

Chapter Fourteen Notes

1. As defined by the online version of the Merriam-Webster Dictionary. http://www. merriam-webster.com/dictionary/craving, accessed Jan 18, 2015.

2. D. Seo, C. M. Lacadie, K. Tuit, K. Hong, R. Constable, and R. Sinha, "Disrupted Ventromedial Prefrontal Function, Alcohol Craving, and Subsequent Relapse Risk," *JAMA Psychiatry* 70, no. 7 (2013): 727–39.

3. N. D. Volkow and R. D. Baler, "Brain Imaging Biomarkers to Predict Relapse in Alcohol Addiction," *JAMA Psychiatry* 70, no. 7 (2013): 661–3.

4. As defined by the online version of the Merriam-Webster Dictionary, http://www. merriam-webster.com/dictionary/relapse, accessed Jan 18, 2015.

5. ASAM, "The Definition of Addiction," ASAM, http://www.asam.org/docs/publicy-policy-statements/1definition_of_addiction_long_4-11.pdf?sfvrsn=2.

6. A. J. Jasinska, E. A. Stein, J. Kaiser, M. J. Naumer, and Y. Yalachkov, "Factors Modulating Neural Reactivity to Drug Cues in Addiction: A Survey of Human Neuroimaging Studies," *Neuroscience & Biobehavioral Reviews* 38 (2014): 1–16.

7. A. R. Childress, R. N. Ehrman, Z. Wang, Y. Li, N. Sciortino, J. Hakun, W. Jens, *et al.*, "Prelude to Passion: Limbic Activation by 'Unseen' Drug and Sexual Cues," *PLoS One* 3, no. 1 (2008): e1506.

8. K. A. Young, T. R. Franklin, D. C. Roberts, K. Jagannathan, J. J. Suh, R. R. Wetherill, Z. Wang, *et al.*, "Nipping Cue Reactivity in the Bud: Baclofen Prevents Limbic Activation Elicited by Subliminal Drug Cues," *J Neurosci* 34, no. 14 (2014): 5038–43.

9. B. F. Skinner, *Science and Human Behavior* (New York: Macmillan, 1953).

10. RecoveryMind Training calls these "Addiction Memory" events. They are postulated to be similar and stored in the brain in a manner similar to post traumatic stress disorder (PTSD).

11. R. F. Anton, "What Is Craving? Models and Implications for Treatment," *Alcohol Res Health* 23, no. 3 (1999): 165–73.

12. "Alcohol Craving: A Renaissance," *Alcohol Clin Exp Res* 23, no. 8 (1999): 1287–8.

13. "Obsessive-Compulsive Aspects of Craving: Development of the Obsessive Compulsive Drinking Scale," *Addiction* 95, Suppl 2 (2000): S211–17.

14. R. F. Anton, D. H. Moak, and P. Latham, "The Obsessive Compulsive Drinking Scale: A Self-Rated Instrument for the Quantification of Thoughts About Alcohol and Drinking Behavior," *Alcohol Clin Exp Res* 19, no. 1 (1995): 92–99.

15. R. F. Anton, D. H. Moak, and P. K. Latham, "The Obsessive Compulsive Drinking Scale: A New Method of Assessing Outcome in Alcoholism Treatment Studies," *Arch Gen Psychiatry* 53, no. 3 (1996): 225–31.

16. See above, n. 11.

17. See above, n. 12.

18. B. A. Flannery, A. J. Roberts, N. Cooney, R. M. Swift, R. F. Anton, and D. J. Rohsenow, "The Role of Craving in Alcohol Use, Dependence, and Treatment," *Alcohol Clin Exp Res* 25, no. 2 (2001): 299–308.

19. B. A. Flannery, J. R. Volpicelli, and H. M. Pettinati, "Psychometric Properties of the Penn Alcohol Craving Scale," *Alcohol Clin Exp Res* 23, no. 8 (1999): 1289–95.

20. H. Rankin, R. Hodgson, and T. Stockwell, "Cue Exposure and Response Prevention with Alcoholics: A Controlled Trial," *Behav Res Ther* 21, no. 4 (1983): 435–46.

21. R. C. Havermans and A. T. M. Jansen, "Increasing the Efficacy of Cue Exposure Treatment in Preventing Relapse of Addictive Behavior," *Addict Behav* 28, no. 5 (2003): 989–94.

22. S. Bowen, N. Chawla, and G. Marlatt, *Mindfulness-Based Relapse Prevention for Addictive Behaviors: A Clinician's Guide* (New York: Guilford Press, 2010).

23. M. E. Larimer, R. S. Palmer, and G. A. Marlatt, "Relapse Prevention. An Overview of Marlatt's Cognitive-Behavioral Model," *Alcohol Res Health* 23, no. 2 (1999): 151–60.

24. A. Marlatt and D. Donovan, *Relapse Prevention, Maintenance Strategies in the Treatment of Addictive Behaviors*, Second ed. (New York: Guilford Press, 2007).

25. See above, n. 23.

26. K. Witkiewitz, G. A. Marlatt, and D. Walker, "Mindfulness-Based Relapse Prevention for Alcohol and Substance Use Disorders," *Journal of Cognitive Psychotherapy* 19, no. 3 (2005): 211–28.

27. S. Bowen, K. Witkiewitz, S. L. Clifasefi, J. Grow, N. Chawla, S. H. Hsu, H. A. Carroll, *et al.*, "Relative Efficacy of Mindfulness-Based Relapse Prevention, Standard Relapse Prevention, and Treatment as Usual for Substance Use Disorders: A Randomized Clinical Trial," *JAMA Psychiatry* (2014).

28. See above, n. 24.

29. See above, n. 22.

30. See above, n. 24.

31. A. Bandura, "Self-Efficacy Mechanism in Human Agency," *American Psychologist* 37, no. 2 (1982): 122.

32. A. Bandura, "Self-Efficacy: Toward a Unifying Theory of Behavioral Change," *Psychol Rev* 84, no. 2 (1977): 191.

33. L. Festinger, *A Theory of Cognitive Dissonance* (Stanford, CA: Stanford University Press, 1957).

34. L. Festinger, "Cognitive Dissonance," *Scientific American* 207, no. 4 (1962): 93–107.

35. R. A. Cormier, "Predicting Treatment Outcome in Chemically Dependent Women: A Test of Marlatt and Gordon's Relapse Model," University of Windsor, 2000.

36. M. A. Walton, F. G. Castro, and E. H. Barrington, "The Role of Attributions in Abstinence, Lapse, and Relapse Following Substance Abuse Treatment," *Addict Behav* 19, no. 3 (1994): 319–31.

37. Ibid.

Examples of Worksheets and Forms

In Section Two of this text, I frequently referred to the structural elements of RecoveryMind Training that ensure patients learn specific Recovery Skills through treatment. Some Recovery Skills are taught and internalized using role-play. Others are taught though worksheets and reinforced by discussion in Assignment Group. I also described how a patient performs a routine self-assessment, which then goes to his or her therapist or treatment team. Staff members use the same evaluation form that is then reviewed by the patient and his or her caregivers. Each domain has a unique progress assessment form that tracks specific Recovery Skills.

This appendix contains examples from a companion volume *RecoveryMind Training: An Implementation Guide.* The guide covers each Recovery Skill in every domain, describes the purpose of each worksheet, and provides an overview of the different types of therapy groups. The guide also contains all the worksheets and progress assessment forms for the six domains. The examples in this appendix (two worksheets and one progress assessment form) come from the implementation guide.

As you read Section Two of this text, you should glance at these forms from time to time. This will help you visualize the RecoveryMind Training care model. You will discover that RecoveryMind Training is not simply a conceptual model. It is a pragmatic, integrated system that builds full spectrum addiction care, whether it occurs in a single therapist's office or a treatment center staffed by individuals from many healthcare disciplines.

Recovery Reflection

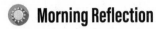 **Morning Reflection**

Name: _____ Date: _____ Time in Recovery: _____

Recovery Schedule

My first goal is to remain sober and to continue to grow in recovery. Today I will:

1. Attend a twelve-step meeting at this time _____ and this location _____ .

2. Focus my attention on this step _____ in this manner (read, write, discuss a particular feeling or thought) _____

_____ .

3. Spend time on the phone, in electronic communication, or in person with _____ .
    I will ask him or her for help with _____

_____

I have this specific issue I want to discuss with others in recovery today: _____

_____ .

4. This particular emotion is especially important for me to experience / avoid / explore / feel / talk about _____

_____ .

5. I have made a commitment to myself or others to accomplish these additional tasks:

    a. _____

    b. _____

    c. _____

    d. _____

Mindfulness Meditation

The next task in your reflection is mindfulness meditation. You should receive specific meditation training before implementing this part of your reflection. Skip this section if you have not yet been trained.

This is a brief review of the steps used in meditation. Find a quiet place and sit upright in a chair; rest your hands softly on your thighs. You may choose to place your hands in positions that you have learned in meditation skills training. Allow your eyes to close gently. Relax your face with just a hint of a smile. Focus on your breath as it moves in and out of your nose or mouth. When a thought, urge, or feeling comes to you, watch it drift away like a leaf going down a stream. When you become distracted, gently return to your breath.

When first learning, practice this for several minutes. Extend meditation time as you become more comfortable. When your meditation period is complete, slowly open your eyes and sit for a moment, reacquainting yourself with your surroundings. If you are unable to meditate, you may use one of the audio files that help with mindfulness. Ask for help with any part of your meditation practice that you are confused about or find difficult.

Emotional Awareness

Since your last Recovery Reflection, you may have experienced strong or surprising feelings or emotions. This is normal. Record these feelings in the list provided. Place an asterisk after any feeling that was especially uncomfortable or one you wanted to suppress or avoid.

Since my last Recovery Reflection, I noticed the following feelings or emotions:

_____ related to _____

_____ related to _____

_____ related to _____

_____ related to _____

Deception Detection

Every individual with an addiction disorder displays some level of dishonesty to themselves or others. Write about any deceptions or dishonesties you have thought or uttered to another person since your last reflection. Do not ignore seemingly small dishonesties or "white lies." Dig deep for dishonesties from long ago as well. Place an asterisk next to any of these you want to discuss in group therapy—even if you are not ready yet to do so. Describe the deception or dishonesty in full. Then check *each* box (☑) that applies.

Deception or Dishonesty: _____

_____

This occurred in: ☐ The past several days ☐ The recent past
                        ☐ My past   ☐ Is it Ongoing?

This deception is: ☐ Shading the truth   ☐ Self-deception
                     ☐ Lying to others   ☐ Related to my addiction

Deception or Dishonesty: _____

_____

This occurred in: ☐ The past several days ☐ The recent past
                        ☐ My past   ☐ Is it Ongoing?

This deception is: ☐ Shading the truth   ☐ Self-deception
                     ☐ Lying to others   ☐ Related to my addiction

Deception or Dishonesty: _____

_____

This occurred in: ☐ The past several days ☐ The recent past
                        ☐ My past   ☐ Is it Ongoing?

This deception is: ☐ Shading the truth   ☐ Self-deception
                     ☐ Lying to others   ☐ Related to my addiction

Craving Recognition

Describe and rate craving events you have experienced since your last Recovery Reflection. If you have not been trained in using the RecoveryMind craving scale, skip the check boxes. If you have been trained, place a check in the applicable boxes.

Craving Description: _____

_____

Intensity rating: ❏ One ❏ Two ❏ Three ❏ Four ❏ Five

The craving: ❏ Is a conditioned cue from this trigger

                  _____

                  ❏ Is emotions-based from the feeling

                  _____

                  ❏ Is related to this stress

                  _____

                  ❏ Is memory-induced from the memory of

                  _____

Craving Description: _____

_____

Intensity rating: ❏ One ❏ Two ❏ Three ❏ Four ❏ Five

The craving: ❏ Is a conditioned cue from this trigger

                  _____

                  ❏ Is emotions-based from the feeling

                  _____

                  ❏ Is related to this stress

                  _____

                  ❏ Is memory-induced from the memory of

                  _____

☾ Evening Reflection

Name: _____ Date _____

Mindfulness Meditation

If you have completed meditation training, spend five to fifteen minutes in mindfulness meditation. Meditation slows down your thinking and allows you to contemplate your day and find peace when you experience emotional turmoil.

Emotional Awareness

In the time since your last Recovery Reflection, you may have experienced strong or surprising feelings or emotions. This is normal. Record these feelings in the list provided. Place an asterisk after any feeling that was especially uncomfortable or one you wanted to suppress or avoid.

Since my last Recovery Reflection, I noticed the following feelings or emotions:

_____ related to _____

_____ related to _____

_____ related to _____

_____ related to _____

Deception Detection

Every individual with an addiction disorder displays some level of dishonesty to themselves or others. Write about any deceptions or dishonesties you have thought or uttered to another person since your last reflection. Do not ignore seemingly small dishonesties or "white lies." Dig deep for dishonesties from long ago as well. Place an asterisk next to any of these you want to discuss in group therapy—even if you are not ready yet to do so. Describe the deception or dishonesty in full. Then check *each* box (☑) that applies.

Deception or Dishonesty: _____

_____

This occurred in: ❑ The past several days   ❑ The recent past
                   ❑ My past   ❑ Is it Ongoing?

This deception is: ❑ Shading the truth   ❑ Self-deception
                    ❑ Lying to others   ❑ Related to my Addiction

Deception or Dishonesty: _____

_____

This occurred in: ❑ The past several days   ❑ The recent past
                   ❑ My past   ❑ Is it Ongoing?

This deception is: ❑ Shading the truth   ❑ Self-deception
                    ❑ Lying to others   ❑ Related to my Addiction

Craving Recognition

Describe and rate craving events you have experienced since your last Recovery Reflection. If you have not been trained in using the RecoveryMind craving scale, skip the check boxes. If you have been trained, place a check in the applicable boxes.

Craving Description: _____

_____

Intensity rating: ❑ One   ❑ Two   ❑ Three   ❑ Four   ❑ Five

The craving: ❑ Is a conditioned cue from this trigger

                  _____

                  ❑ Is emotions-based from the feeling

                  _____

❏ Is related to this stress

_____

❏ Is memory-induced from the memory of

_____

Craving Description: _____

_____

Intensity rating: ❏ One ❏ Two ❏ Three ❏ Four ❏ Five

The craving: ❏ Is a conditioned cue from this trigger

_____

❏ Is emotions-based from the feeling

_____

❏ Is related to this stress

_____

❏ Is memory-induced from the memory of

_____

Healthy Attachment

Human beings need each other to survive. Our natural temperament and our past experiences form the basis of how we connect or attach to other people in our life and whether the attachment is healthy or unhealthy. AddictBrain exaggerates unhealthy attachment and suppresses healthy connections. In treatment and early recovery, we have to reevaluate our modes of interacting with those around us. Make a note of at least one episode today where you experienced a connection to another person. Describe what was important about the connection. Describe how you felt and the elements of the connection that were healthy and unhealthy. Briefly note ways you plan to make it better in the days ahead.

Describe the connection experience. _____

_____

What feelings did you experience? What was significant about this experience? _____

_____

_____

What was healthy about the interaction? (Examples: I expressed my feelings clearly; I expressed gratitude for the time with them; I was angry without attacking.) _____

_____

_____

What was unhealthy about the interaction? (Examples: I was verbally hurtful; I made fun of them; I was so interested in them that I lost sight of myself.) _____

_____

_____

Step Review

When we "work the steps," we seek understanding of what a step means, notice our reaction to it, and consider how it applies to us. We discuss our reactions to twelve-step concepts with others. We must also write about our work with each step. When we write down our thoughts, we clarify them, and they become more real to us. In the last section of Recovery Reflection, review your thoughts and reactions to the particular step you have been working on today. Consider both the positive and the negative. Do not write what you think others want to hear. At the same time, remain open to change.

The step I committed to work on today was Step _____.

What I learned about this step today was: _____

_____

_____

I resist or struggle with the parts of this step in this way: _____

_____

_____

I find relief or acceptance in this step in this way: _____

_____

_____

I have noticed a change in my attitude or acceptance about this step, in that: _____

_____

_____

AddictBrain's Emotional Games

AddictBrain is constantly plotting inside your head, hoping to keep you using or goad you into relapse. It does this by changing your perspective, rearranging priorities, creating cravings, and modifying your emotions. This worksheet helps you look at how your feelings and emotional states helped drive your substance use in the past and increase your relapse risk in the future.

Question 1: If you have completed Worksheet C1, review it now for emotions you discovered were especially difficult for you to experience or seemed to trigger substance use. If you have not been assigned this worksheet, take a moment and write down painful emotions, ones you have suppressed, or ones that seem to trigger substance use.

Enter the most important of these emotions in column ①. Spend some time thinking about each of the emotions you listed. To the best of your ability, consider why each specific emotion is hard for you. It may be that an emotion is difficult because it seems to never go away, or it reminds you of an especially difficult time in your life. Note these characteristics of each emotion in column ②. Now, return to consider your addiction disease. Think like a spy who is trying to defeat his or her enemy. How could that spy use each of these emotions to defeat his foe? If AddictBrain was the spy, how would he or she sabotage your recovery by playing on each of these difficult emotions? Enter this information in column ③.

The first row of this worksheet contains an example of how to complete this worksheet.

①	②	③
An especially difficult emotion for me	What makes this emotion difficult	In the past or in the future, AddictBrain may use this emotion against me in the following way
Grief	*I have difficulty with grief and would avoid it. It seems like it is always there right under the surface.*	*AddictBrain keeps my grief about my son's death alive. It knows I hate to feel this way. My son would want me to feel better. AddictBrain wants me to hurt so I continue to drink.*

Question 2: With the help of your peers and staff members, come up with a list of ways you can uncouple these emotions from AddictBrain. List several ideas in the space provided.

_____

_____

_____

_____

_____

_____

_____

_____

_____

_____

_____

_____

_____

_____

_____

_____

Domain A Progress Assessment Form

Containment Review: RecoveryMind Training

Domain A Recovery Skills	Date:						Date:						Date:					
	Patient			Staff			Patient			Staff			Patient			Staff		
	B	I	C	B	I	C	B	I	C	B	I	C	B	I	C	B	I	C
Understands the concepts and types of containment.																		
Intellectually accepts that AddictBrain needs to be contained.																		
Recognizes and has experienced how AddictBrain has altered past thoughts and behaviors.																		
Has identified and practiced current and potential future ways AddictBrain can sabotage recovery.																		
Has a workable plan for addiction containment at the current level of care.																		
Recognizes how past experiences, emotions, and personality issues may affect containment.																		
Is effectively using containment tools to prevent past experiences, emotions, and personality from sabotaging recovery.																		
Has a workable plan for addiction containment after moving on from this level of care.																		

This evaluation is completed at regular intervals while working on Domain A assignments, first by the patient (self-assessment) and then by the staff. The patient begins by entering the current date at the top of the column. He or she then places a check mark in each row corresponding to the Recovery Skills he or she is working on. If work on a given skill has not begun, no entry is made. Otherwise, the patient places a check mark in the **B** column if the he or she has begun work on the respective skill. The **I** column should be checked if the patient is in an intermediate or midway through his or her work on this item, and the **C** column should be checked if the patient has completed the respective recovery skill.

The free spaces at the bottom of this form can be used to list patient-specific Domain A Recovery Skills.